Deep Learning in Internet of Things for Next Generation Healthcare

This book presents the latest developments in deep learning-enabled healthcare tools and technologies and offers practical ideas for using the IoT with deep learning (motion-based object data) to deal with human dynamics and challenges including critical application domains, technologies, medical imaging, drug discovery, insurance fraud detection, and solutions to handle relevant challenges. This book covers real-time healthcare applications, novel solutions, current open challenges, and the future of deep learning for next-generation healthcare. It includes detailed analysis of the utilization of the IoT with deep learning and its underlying technologies in critical application areas of emergency departments such as drug discovery, medical imaging, fraud detection, Alzheimer's disease, and genomes.

- Presents practical approaches of using the IoT with deep learning vision and how it deals with human dynamics
- Offers novel solutions for medical imaging, including skin lesion detection, cancer detection, enhancement techniques for MRI images, automated disease prediction, fraud detection, genomes, and many more
- Includes the latest technological advances in the IoT and deep learning with their implementations in healthcare
- Combines deep learning and analysis in the unified framework to understand both IoT and deep learning applications
- Covers the challenging issues related to data collection by sensors, detection and tracking of moving objects, and solutions to handle relevant challenges

Postgraduate students and researchers in the departments of computer science working in the areas of the IoT, deep learning, machine learning, image processing, big data, cloud computing, and remote sensing will find this book useful.

Deep Learning in Internet of Things for Next Generation Healthcare

Edited by

Lavanya Sharma and Pradeep Kumar Garg

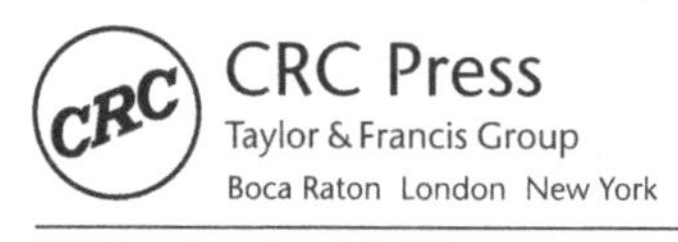

CRC Press is an imprint of the
Taylor & Francis Group, an **informa** business
A CHAPMAN & HALL BOOK

Designed cover image: ShutterStock

First edition published 2024
by CRC Press
2385 NW Executive Center Drive, Suite 320, Boca Raton FL 33431

and by CRC Press
4 Park Square, Milton Park, Abingdon, Oxon, OX14 4RN

CRC Press is an imprint of Taylor & Francis Group, LLC

ISBN: 9781032586106 (hbk)
ISBN: 9781032588674 (pbk)
ISBN: 9781003451846 (ebk)

DOI: 10.1201/9781003451846

Typeset in Times
by Apex CoVantage, LLC

Dedicated to my Dada Ji (Late. Shri Ram Krishan Choudhary Ji)
– Dr. Lavanya Sharma

Dedicated to my Parents (Late Shri Ramgopal Garg and Late Smt Urmila Garg)
– Prof. Pradeep Kumar Garg

Contents

Preface

This book explores the utilization of the Internet of Things (IoT) and deep learning for next-generation healthcare. Using a series of current tools of data collection and applications, such as drug discovery, human detection and tracking, e-health departments, geospatial data, healthcare assistive devices, medical imaging, and many more, this publication will help readers to get a deeper knowledge and implement deep learning with IoT-based approaches.

This book consists of four parts and provides an overview of basic concepts from the rise of communication devices to the IoT with deep learning, critical application domains, tools, technologies, and solutions to handle the relevant challenges in healthcare. The book provides a detailed description to readers with practical ideas on using deep learning in the IoT with visual surveillance (motion-based object data) to deal with human dynamics, challenges involved in surpassing diversified architecture, communications, big data, integrity, and security and privacy aspects. The use of deep learning in the IoT has proved most advantageous for healthcare companies to efficiently monitor and control their day-to-day processes, such as security, drug discovery, robotics, implementation, distribution of their products, and medical imaging.

Overall this publication, *Deep Learning in Internet of Things for Next Generation Healthcare*, will help readers to understand the use of deep learning approaches in the IoT with value to clinicians as well as organizations.

Editor Biographies

Brief Biography of Dr. Lavanya Sharma

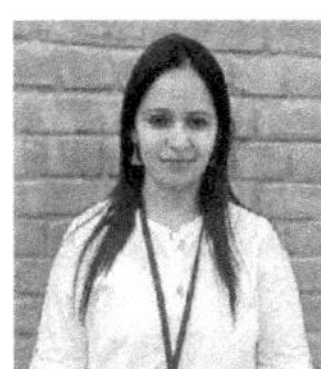

Dr. Lavanya Sharma is an assistant professor, Amity Institute of Information Technology at Amity University UP, Noida, India. She did her M.Tech. (computer science and engineering) in 2013 at Manav Rachna College of Engineering, affiliated with Maharshi Dayanand University, Haryana, India. She did her Ph.D. at Uttarakhand Technical University, India, as a full time Ph.D. scholar in the field of digital image processing and computer vision in April 2018 and received a TEQIP scholarship for the same. Her research work is on motion-based object detection using a background subtraction technique for smart video surveillance. She has been a recipient of several prestigious awards during her academic career. She has more than 40+ research papers to her credit, including Elsevier (SCI indexed), Inderscience, IGI Global, IEEE Explore, and many more. She has authored six books, and five with Taylor & Francis, CRC Press. She has done various certified courses from IIRS (ISRO Dehradun Unit) and also guided 90+. She also contributed as an organizing committee member to Springer's Springer and IEEE conferences. She is an editorial member/reviewer of various journals of repute and active program committee member of various IEEE and Springer conferences. Her primary research interests are digital image processing and computer vision, artificial intelligence, mobile ad-hoc networks, and the Internet of Things. Her vision is to promote teaching and research, providing a highly competitive and productive environment in academic and research areas with tremendous growing opportunities for society and her country.

Brief Biography of Professor P.K. Garg

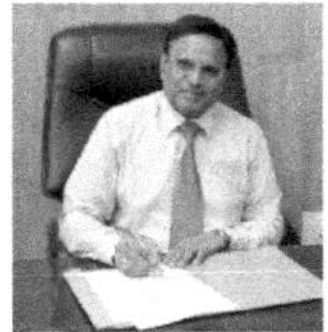

Professor P.K. Garg worked as a vice chancellor, Uttarakhand Technical University, Dehradun. Presently he is working in the department of Civil Engineering, IIT Roorkee, as a professor. He completed a B.Tech. (civil engineering) in 1980 and M.Tech. (civil engineering) in 1982, both from the University of Roorkee (now IIT Roorkee). He is a recipient of the Gold Medal at IIT Roorkee to stand first during the M.Tech. program, Commonwealth Scholarship Award for doing his Ph.D. at the University of Bristol (UK), and Commonwealth Fellowship Award to carry out post-doctoral research work at the University of Reading (UK). He joined the Department of Civil Engineering at IIT Roorkee in 1982, and, gradually advancing, his career rose to the position of Head of the department in 2015.

Professor Garg has published more than 300 technical papers in national and international conferences and journals. He has undertaken 26 research projects and provided technical services to 83 consultancy projects on various aspects of civil engineering, generating funds for the Institute. He has authored three textbooks on remote sensing, theory and principles of geoinformatics, and introduction to unmanned aerial vehicles and produced two technical films on the story of mapping. He has developed several new courses and practical exercises in geomatics engineering. Besides supervising a large number of undergraduate projects, he has guided about 72 M.Tech. and 27 Ph.D. thesis students. He is instrumental in prestigious MHRD-funded projects on e-learning and the development of virtual labs, pedagogy, and courses under NPTEL. He has served as an expert on various national committees, including the Ministry of Environment & Forest; EAEC Committee; NBA (AICTE); and Project Evaluation Committee, DST, New Delhi.

Professor Garg has reviewed a large number of papers for national and international journals. Considering the need to train human resources in the country, he has successfully organized 42 programs in advanced areas of surveying, photogrammetry, remote sensing, GIS, and GPS, as well as ten conferences and workshops. He is a life member of 24 professional societies, out of which he is a fellow of eight societies. For academic work, Professor Garg has traveled widely, nationally and internationally.

Editor Biographies

Contributors

Himanshu Kumar Agrawal
I-Hub for Robotics and Autonomous Systems Innovation Foundation (ARTPARK)
Indian Institute of Science
Bengaluru, India

Naman Kumar Agrawal
Science & Technology
NITI Ayoog
New Delhi, India

Sonal Agrawal
Krishi Neer
New Delhi, India

Surendiran Balasubramanian
Department of Computer Science and Engineering
National Institute of Technology Puducherry
Karaikal, India

Pallavi S. Bangare
Department of E&TC, Sinhgad Academy of Engineering
Savitribai Phule Pune University
India

Mukesh Carpenter
Department of Surgery
Alshifa Multispecialty Hospital
Okhla, New Delhi, India

Mrinalika Durairaju
Department of Computer Science and Engineering
Shiv Nadar University
Chennai, India

Mrinalini Durairaju
Department of Computer Science and Engineering
Shiv Nadar University
Chennai, India

Pradeep Kumar Garg
Civil Engineering Department
Indian Institute of Technology
Roorkee, India

Sanjay Ghosh
Civil Engineering Department
Indian Institute of Technology Roorkee
Uttarakhand, India

Yaman Hooda
Department of Civil Engineering, School of Engineering and Technology
Manav Rachna International Institute of Research and Studies
Faridabad, Haryana, India

V. Jokanović
Institute of Nuclear Science "Vinča"
Beograd, Serbia
and
ALBOS doo
Beograd, Serbia

Rashmi Kandwal
HealthcareMN
Minneapolis, MN, USA

Vallidevi Krishnamurthy
Vellore Institute of Technology
Chennai, India

Rajeev Kumar
Atal Innovation Mission
NITI Ayoog
New Delhi, India

Jimmy Mehta
Department of Mechanical Engineering, School of Engineering and Technology
Manav Rachna International Institute of Research and Studies
Faridabad, Haryana, India

Sahil Mehta
Electrical and Instrumentation Engineering Department
Thapar Institute of Engineering and Technology
Patiala, Punjab, India

Tanvi Misra
Atal Innovation Mission
NITI Ayoog
New Delhi, India

Kishor P. Patil
Department of E&TC, Sinhgad Academy of Engineering
Savitribai Phule Pune University
Pune, India

Prithvi Sai Penumadu
Atal Innovation Mission
NITI Ayoog
New Delhi, India

Nisheeth Saxena
Department of Computer Science and Engineering
Birla Institute of Technology
Mesra, Ranchi, India

Sudhriti Sengupta
Amity Institute of Information Technology
Amity University
Noida, India

Lavanya Sharma
AIIT, Amity University
Noida, India

Vipasha Sharma
Civil Engineering Department
Indian Institute of Technology Roorkee
Uttarakhand, India

Haobam Derit Singh
Department of Civil Engineering, Faculty of Engineering and Technology
Manav Rachna International Institute of Research and Studies
Faridabad, Haryana, India

Nishi Srivastava
Department of Physics
Birla Institute of Technology
Mesra, Ranchi, India

Naba Suroor
Science & Technology
NITI Ayoog
New Delhi, India

Sakthivel V
Vellore Institute of Technology
Chennai Campus, India
and
Konkuk Aerospace Design-Airworthiness Research Institute
Konkuk University
Seoul, South Korea

1 Rise of Communication Devices in IoT

Yaman Hooda, Haobam Derit Singh, Jimmy Mehta, and Sahil Mehta

1.1 INTRODUCTION

The term Internet of Things (IoT) was coined by Auto-ID Centre in the late 1900s. The Internet of Things is considered a technological advancement to internet due to its characteristics of enhancing pervasive connection between the digital world and physical world. With the application of radio frequency identification (RFID) tags, which are composed of low-cost and tiny microchips and antennas, a unique contactless system was developed for the benefit of society. Interaction with individuals over the world through a system of networks provides an efficient networking system of querying and tracking objects in a shorter span of time. To date, the network of IoT is expanding gradually in its applications and incorporation with heterogeneous technological advancements, applications, objects and communication protocols for allowing the provision of different facilities available in cloud services or cloud servers.

IoT-based devices, which are generally devised and produced for specified related applications, include water sensors, smart cameras, smart plugs, motion sensors, smart bulbs and smart watches. Also, such devices are inherently resource constrained in their limited energy, memory and processing power. In contrast, non-IoT devices such as computer systems, laptops, smart phones, and tablets serve different purposes, as they can be equipped with huge datasets. IoT devices, which are specific function oriented, are fabricated with major characteristics such as data exchange, connectivity systems and sensing ability [1]. Such devices successfully incorporate a speedy rate into different domains of everyday life. This is made possible due to the evolution and multi-disciplinary technological advancements in different aspects of the IoT, leading to the formation of various types of IoT architectural networks. For setting up an IoT network, the basis on which its architecture is chosen depends upon the properties of the demand based on the intended applications. The process of finalising the network is a three-layered architectural framework [2, 8–20].

The various challenges developed due to technological advancements in the domain of fresh IoT networking ecosystems are illustrated in Figure 1.1.

Studies conducted in the past decade reveal that the proliferating growth rate of diverse IoT devices and services with individual functionalities are now facing trouble in one of the following categories:

- Privacy and security challenges
- Device management
- Enforcement of security rules
- Attack detection
- Tracking of locations
- Anomaly detection
- Authentication
- Identification of faulty devices

DOI: 10.1201/9781003451846-1

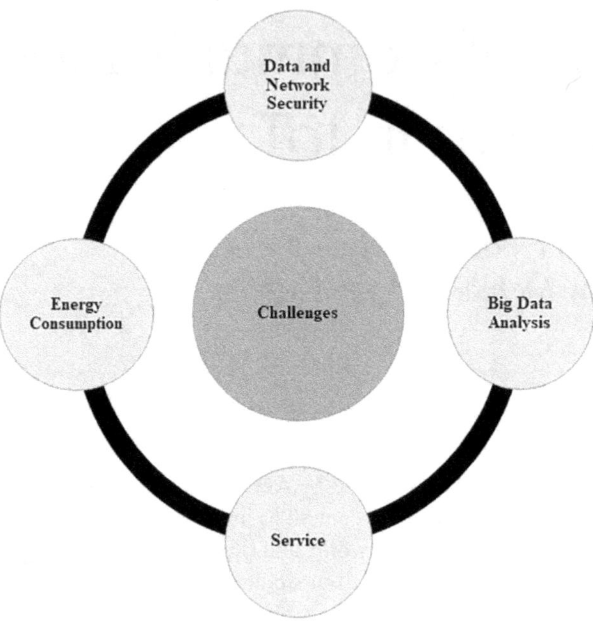

FIGURE 1.1 Challenges due to emerging IoT advancements.

The possible reason behind this is because of the resource-constrained behaviour of the IoT, which leads to forcing the devices connected in an IoT network to have a connection to the internet with naïve security arrangements. Such vulnerable situations allow opponents to take advantage of performing different types of spoofing and malicious attacks [3, 4]. For mitigation purposes, studies have been conducted and various approaches have been proposed on the basis of signal processing and trace analysis of network traffic, such as in Figure 1.2.

The same can be achieved by implementing algorithms of either deep learning (DL) or machine learning (ML). Algorithms of both DL and ML find application in various processes, including decision-making and device classification, on the basis of observations made on the input/source of the data.

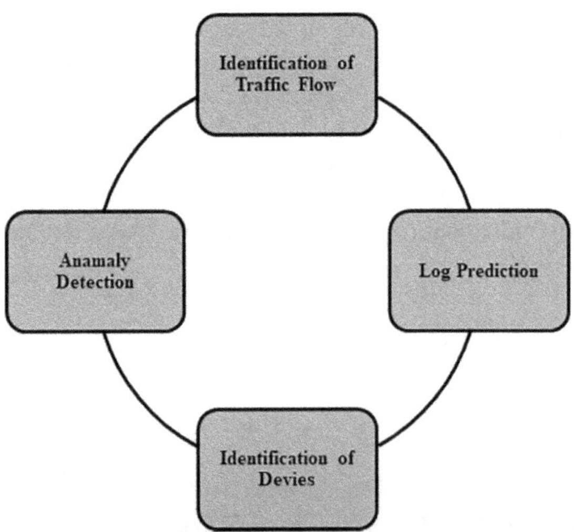

FIGURE 1.2 Emerging approaches in mitigation studies for DL and IoT.

1.2 INTERNET OF THINGS

The Internet of Things refers to the network of physical objects, devices, vehicles, buildings and other items that are embedded with sensors, software and other technologies to collect and exchange data over the internet [5, 21–30]. This enables these objects to connect, communicate and interact with each other and with humans, leading to various applications and benefits across different industries.

The key components of the Internet of Things include:

1. *Devices and Sensors:*
   These are the physical objects that are equipped with sensors, actuators and other hardware to collect data from their surroundings. Examples include smart thermostats, wearable fitness trackers, industrial machines and more.
2. *Connectivity:*
   IoT devices communicate through various connectivity options such as Wi-Fi, Bluetooth, cellular networks, Zigbee, LoRaWAN and more. These technologies enable seamless data transfer and remote control.
3. *Data Processing:*
   Collected data is sent to cloud servers or edge devices for processing, storage and analysis. Advanced analytics and machine learning algorithms can extract meaningful insights from this data.
4. *Cloud Computing:*
   Cloud platforms provide the infrastructure and resources needed to store and process the massive amounts of data generated by IoT devices. This allows for scalable and cost-effective data management.
5. *Data Analytics and Insights:*
   Once the data is collected, it can be analysed to extract valuable insights. This can lead to improved decision-making, predictive maintenance, optimisation of operations and more.
6. *Automation and Control:*
   IoT enables automation and remote control of devices and processes. For example, smart homes allow users to control lights, thermostats and security systems from their smartphones.
7. *Security and Privacy*:
   The interconnected nature of IoT raises concerns about security and privacy. As more devices are connected to the internet, protecting data and ensuring secure communication become crucial.

The IoT finds applications not only in the domain of computer sciences but also in inter-disciplinary applications in industries focusing on agriculture, healthcare systems, manufacturing and production, smart cities and smart infrastructure, intelligent transportation systems, sustainable energy and solid waste management systems and many more [6, 7]. Despite the enormous application areas, it also faces some challenges. Some of the major challenges faced by the IoT include:

- Data security
- Interoperability
- Standardisation
- Ethical implications in the collection of data
- Ethical implications in utilising personal information

The IoT has the potential to transfigure businesses by providing understanding, mechanisation and connectivity that were not possible before.

The IoT is a network made up of physical elements or "things" which are rooted with various software, sensor and emerging technologies for the only purpose of connecting with each other, exchanging information in the form of data amongst various devices or systems by using the power of the internet. The basic technologies which form the background of "things" consist of the junction of various phases of different technologies such as machine learning, commodity sensors, real-time analytics and embedded systems. Conventional areas of networking of wireless sensors, embedded systems and building automation contribute to the formation of the Internet of Things in the real world.

In September 1985, the term and concept of the Internet of Things first made their appearance in a speech given by Peter Lewis at the 15th Annual Congressional Black Caucus Foundation in Washington, D.C. Lewis stated that, "The Internet of Things, or IoT, is the integration of people, processes and technology with connectable devices and sensors to enable remote monitoring, status, manipulation and evaluation of trends of such devices." But the actual revolution in the field of the IoT was in 2010, when it was reported that the things-to-people ratio grew to 1.85 from 0.08 in 2003, as estimated by CISCO Systems by considering their concept of the IoT as the point in time when there were more things than people connected to the internet. Sometimes the background of the IoT also refers to installing short-range sensors (such as mobile transceivers) in various gadgets for the formation of modes of communication between things and people while performing the work of daily necessities.

One of the main characteristics of IoT devices is that they can upgrade their software without involvement or with negligible involvement by the user. Also, for communication between devices, the process of the setup of new devices with existing devices is simple and doesn't consume much time. With the advancement in the technology and the development of interoperable communication, the IoT enables devices to connect to each other with the same or different architectures. The functional block of IoT systems offers different skills of identification, sensing, inclination, process of communication or transfer of data and data management. The various parts of this functional block are shown in Figure 1.3.

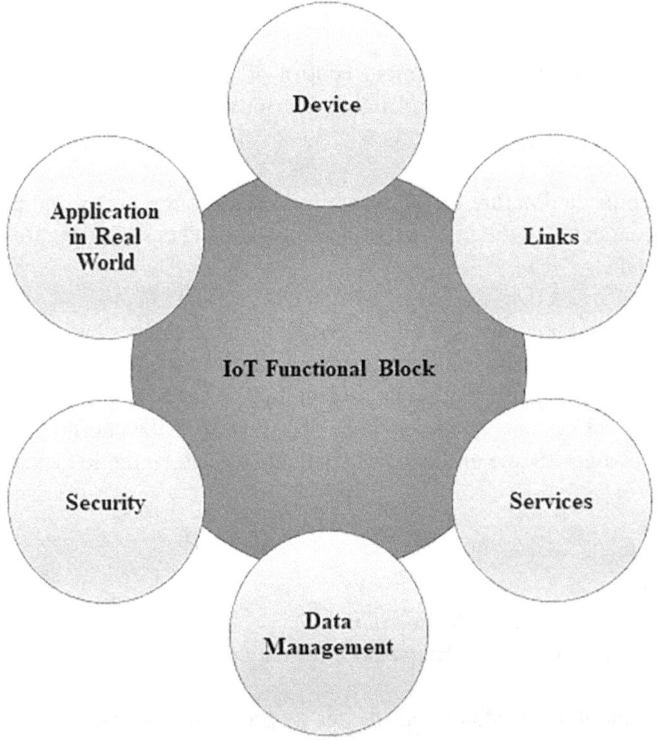

FIGURE 1.3 IoT functional block components.

Currently, IoT finds applications in nearly all phases of life. Data management becomes more effective and efficient with the formation of IoT-enabled data centres. With the help of IoT in automation, devices in residential and commercial buildings can easily be managed. Also, the concept of smart cities has come into existence because of the application of the IoT in factories, transportation industries and construction companies.

1.3 EXISTING SCENARIO OF COMMUNICATION DEVICES IN IoT SYSTEMS

The networking system of the IoT involves numerous devices. In the past few decades, there is an increasing rate of development and application of communication devices in IoT networking. Communication devices play a vital role in the ecosystem of the IoT, as they enable communicating devices to transfer information and data flawlessly. The information shared by IoT networking includes a setup of connection of various physical objects, actuators, sensors and devices to the internet, making them collect and share information for a wide range of applications. Following are communication devices that have been implemented in present applications of the IoT in different domains:

1. *Cellular Modules:*
   IoT devices can use cellular networks (3G, 4G and now 5G) to connect to the internet. Cellular IoT is ideal for remote areas and mobile applications.
2. *Bluetooth Modules:*
   Bluetooth enables short-range wireless communication between devices, often used for connecting devices like smartphones, wearables and home automation devices.
3. *Wi-Fi Modules:*
   These modules allow devices to connect to existing Wi-Fi networks, enabling data exchange over a local area network (LAN) or the internet.
4. *Zigbee Modules:*
   Zigbee is a low-power, low-data-rate wireless communication protocol designed for small-scale applications like home automation, industrial control and healthcare monitoring.
5. *Long Range (LoRa) Modules:*
   LoRa technology enables long-range, low-power communication between IoT devices and gateways, making it suitable for applications like smart agriculture and smart cities.
6. *6LoWPAN Modules:*
   6LoWPAN (IPv6 over low-power wireless personal area networks) is designed for low-power, low-data-rate communication in IoT applications.
7. *Near Field Communication (NFC) Modules:*
   NFC allows short-range communication between devices when they are brought close together, commonly used for contactless payments and access control.
8. *RFID Modules:*
   RFID devices enable the identification and tracking of objects using radio waves. They are used in supply chain management, inventory tracking and access control.
9. *Ethernet Interfaces:*
   In scenarios where devices have a wired connection, Ethernet interfaces are used to establish a connection to the internet or local network.
10. *Remote Sensing and Geoinformatics:*
    For IoT applications in remote or isolated areas, satellite communication modules can provide connectivity where traditional networks are unavailable.
11. *Thread Modules:*
    A thread is a communication protocol built on IPv6 that allows secure and scalable connectivity in smart homes and buildings.
12. *MQTT and CoAP Protocols:*
    These are lightweight communication protocols designed for IoT applications with low bandwidth and low power requirements.

1.4 EMERGING COMMUNICATION DEVICES IN IoT SYSTEMS

With the advancements in the technological domain worldwide, it has been observed that fresh communication devices/networking systems are developed and have started to be used in some parts of the world for the benefit of society. Such technological advancements in the domain of the IoT are going to stay on the market and will boom in the future with more applications in different domains. Some of the emerging communication devices/systems in IoT systems are as follows:

1. *5G Technology:*

   5G is a term refers to the fifth generation of mobile or cellular networking systems. The main objective of this revolutionary cellular network is that it provides very high data speed in GB per second with very low latency. It has an excellent support and dependability for users around the world, with a consistent experience. With the tremendous speed, the exchange of data and information is possible with a faster communication media, simultaneously necessitating fresh devices or modification in existing devices to have the proper coordination to accomplish the assigned tasks. Also, with a low latency rate for the existing technology and devices, 5G provides information to IoT devices in delicate situations such as information needed while performing medical surgery. With a high bandwidth, 5G provides IoT devices a platform to connect to servers in high numbers without compromising quality.

   With all the advantages, there are some disadvantages too. To blend the upcoming technology of 5G with existing IoT devices and networking systems, there are some challenges to be taken into consideration:

   - Since almost all the components of 5G are virtual, there are high chances of leaking information, leading to greater security risks. Moreover, with the increasing rate of users, there will be a necessity for strong security measures.
   - The towers for 5G communication need to be placed closer as they use shortwave for sharing information. Hence, the challenge lies in providing a greater number of communication towers without hampering the environment or society.
   - There will be an immense implementation cost for the installation of new network devices, which consists of more advanced equipment with a high-frequency operation of bandwidth.

   The application of the IoT has a vast domain. Some prominent applications of the 5G-induced IoT are shown in Figure 1.4.

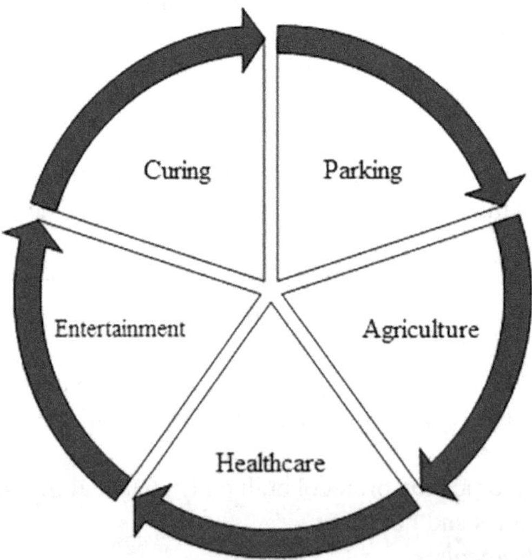

FIGURE 1.4 Application domains of the geospatial technologies in private healthcare systems.

- With the advancement in parking facilities through 5G networking, one can park their vehicle at a desired parking slot without going to it instead. Moreover, one can summon it directly.
- In the agricultural sector, 5G–IoT networking is playing an essential role for farmers in monitoring crops and livestock. Also, control of various equipment desired on agricultural land also becomes easier with the innovation of 5G technology in the IoT.
- The blending of 5G communication in IoT-related devices has proved beneficial in the healthcare sector when surgeries have to be performed with low-latency equipment.
- The characteristic of the low latency of the 5G communication system is beneficial in providing entertainment to all generations. From fast streaming to fast downloading and playing high-end American Automobile Association (AAA) games, 5G communication is increasing the efficiency of IoT networking and devices for transmission of data and information.
- With a networking system for transmission of data at high frequency and bandwidth, one can maintain and monitor their house when they are not physically present at the home. Also, one can track the devices connected to the internet at home with the help of 5G communication more effectively and efficiently.

2. *IoT Edge Computing:*

The concept of edge computing in the IoT can prove a game changer, as it increases the storing capacity, processing capacity and analysis rate of IoT devices, thus making them more independent. The main advantage of this technology includes improved effectiveness of prevailing IoT devices, development of new devices and deployment of possible topologies.

A conventional IoT system has a working principle of gathering, transmitting and analysing data in a feedback loop process. The algorithms of artificial intelligence (AI)–ML learning aid the analytical process in real-time scenarios for help in deriving insights from a huge data set. The phenomenon of edge computing involves the movement of computing, storage and functions—networking near or at the physical designated point of the data sources or users. By moving computing services near the desired designated point, the user benefits from a much more reliable, faster, enhanced experience, thereby enabling organisations/institutions to deploy various types of applications that are latency sensitive.

When combined with the IoT, edge computing enables organisations/institutions to flexibly deploy workloads on IoT hardware, resulting in improved performance with high throughput data and low latency, which is missing in traditional networking systems of the IoT. The applications of the IoT are more often employed as a monitoring system, which has the basic function of collection and analysis of data for triggering informed actions. The applications of the IoT may have a process rate on an hourly or daily basis or in response to external triggers. Edge computing is benefitting IoT networking systems by locating devices near the computing processes, thereby reducing network traffic. Moreover, in contrast to IoT devices sending small data packets for analysis to central management systems, edge computing–enabled IoT systems optimise frequency and bandwidth and thus are responsible for sending all the relevant data in big chunks of datasets. Not with the data transfer and data storage, edge computing in IoT systems will also restrict the security issues in better ways. Data security can be managed efficiently, as the new concept focuses on the localised approach rather than automatically providing all datasets on cloud-based systems. For implementing edge computing with the IoT, there is a need of a fresh architecture, which consists of either of the following (Figure 1.5).

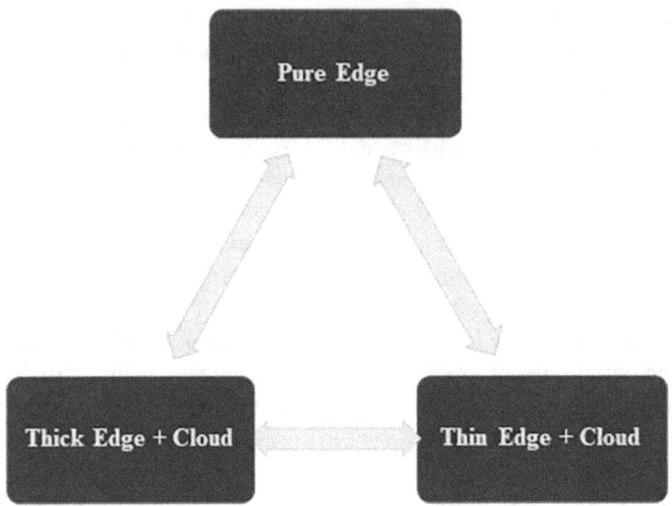

FIGURE 1.5 Edge computing architectures.

- *Pure Edge:*

  The architecture of pure edge refers to a system that deploys every resource on the premises. Such an architecture is most suitable for security-related organisations/institutions or where the requirements of compliance do not allow transmission of data to a cloud system. This kind of architecture requires a large initial investment.
- *Thick Edge + Cloud:*

  Thick edge + cloud architecture consists of three basic components of cloud-based resources, on-premises data centres and devices. This type of architectural framework allows an existing leverage investment system based on the premises' data stations but also enables cloud systems for the purpose of analysis, aggregation and storage of the data.
- *Thin Edge + Cloud:*

  The thin edge + cloud approach connects edge resources to the cloud service available to the users directly, without any on-premise data stations, as observed in the thick edge + cloud approach. This architectural system has several advantages:
  - Flexible in nature.
  - Lightweight
  - Lowest upfront cost

  Moreover, this system may raise security issues, as it provides less control over the operating environment.

3. *Satellite IoT Connectivity:*

   The application of satellite-based IoT solutions is being employed in different domains from agriculture to engineering and management to national security. With technological advancements, this pre-existing domain also has the potential to develop more and can prove beneficial for society with desired modifications. In the past decade, due to a tremendous growth in the IoT market and observation of limited coverage of the area for terrestrial networking, it has been noted that researchers and industrialists are gearing their interest towards satellite-based IoT networking connections.

   One of the major breakthroughs is the rise of low orbit earth (LEO)-based satellite IoT networking systems. Per the report shared by IoT Analytics for 2022–2026, it has been reported there has been a gradual increase in satellite IoT connection systems based on LEO constellations. The two reasons for adopting this technology are summarised as follows:

- *Low-Power Communication System:*

  LEO satellite networking systems can deploy at a distance lower than 200 km. The short distance range to the earth implies lower losses in signal propagation, which means a reduction in the power requirements of the user's equipment. Thereby, such a system is ideal with low-powered IoT equipment for communication purposes.
- *Fast Design and Easy Deployment:*

  This technology enables different organisations/institutions for mass production of the components and thus propose for off-the-shelf parts commercially. It shows a drastic reduction in the time and cost of designing and developing satellites. This technological advancement follows a quicker, cost-effective path in building and deployment of a satellite networking constellation system for the IoT. With all these advantages for better design and easy and economical installation and maintenance, it has been a favourite option for operators of incumbent satellite communication systems.

Satellite and terrestrial networking operations have shown an increasing partnership with offering hybrid connectivity solutions. These solutions include IoT devices to apply terrestrial connectivity as the first option and switch to satellites for areas where there is no coverage of the terrestrial network. Such a solution requires different chipsets that are embedded into the satellite terminal or end-user devices. Furthermore, there has been an advancement in the technological background of chipsets where a single communication chipset is only required for satellite or terrestrial connectivity. The same can also be achieved by providing some modifications to the prevailing IoT devices with the help of a firmware upgrade with minimal or no requirements in the change of hardware, which allows vendors leverage the prevailing ecosystems, devices and certifications. Also, the combination of satellite networking and IoT can present a concrete option for users with applications covering both domains of low bandwidth and high bandwidth.

4. *Blockchain for IoT Security*

One of the main concerns with IoT technology which has been hindering its deployment for the large-scale market is data security. It has been observed that existing IoT devices were suffering security vulnerabilities, making them a good target for distributed denial of service (DdoS) attacks. DdoS attacks refer to a situation where "multiple compromised computer systems bombard a target such as a central server with a huge volume of simultaneous data requests, thereby causing a denial of service for users of the targeted system." The outcomes of such DdoS attacks are commotion in the working of organisations, and they sometimes have a direct impact on the lives of individuals. Therefore, IoT devices that are unsecured in nature become a simple target for cyber criminals for exploiting the protection of weak security networking systems and thus hacking them by introducing DdoS attacks.

One of the breakthrough technologies that has the ability to help address IoT security as well as scalability challenges is blockchain or distributed ledger technology (DLT). It is considered a "game changer" because of its special characteristics and benefits. A blockchain system consists of a distributed ledger in digital format which exists on the internet. This ledger is shared amongst all the participants in the system, and moreover, all the events and transactions are recorded and validated in the ledger, and the information cannot be removed or amended subsequently, hence providing a better way of sharing and recording information for different communities of users. Within this community, some specific members have their own copy of the ledger and have a specific task of validation of any fresh collective transactions by undergoing a consensus procedure prior to getting accepted by the ledger.

There are different ways in which blockchain can be useful in alleviating concerns regarding security and scalability associated with the IoT, as follows (Figure 1.6):

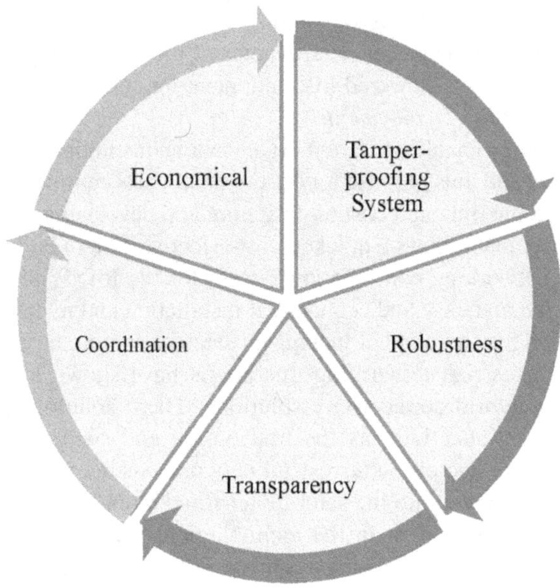

FIGURE 1.6 Ways of blockchain aiding IoT concerns of security and scalability.

- *Tamper-Proof System:*
  One of the biggest advantages is that the distributed ledger is tamper-proof in a blockchain system, which inherently removes the necessity of trust amongst the parties involved. The tremendous amount of data produced by IoT devices cannot be controlled by a single organisation. With this application, a number of organisations can team up without fearing loss of data and information, with a transparent working environment.
- *Robustness:*
  With the application of blockchain in storing IoT data, the former multiplies different security layers and subsequently does not allow hackers to bypass the arrangement for getting access to the networking system. Blockchain in IoT devices enables a higher level of robustness in data encryption, which makes it impossible to overwrite the existing data and information virtually.
- *Transparency:*
  Blockchain in IoT devices provides transparency by enabling everyone to access the network to track transactions that occurred in the past. This transparent system is accessed by those who have already been authorised to access the data as well as the networking system. A transparent system provides a dependent way of identification of a specific source of malfunctioning of data (such as data leakages) and taking quicker remedial action.
- *Coordination:*
  Blockchain and IoT networking systems provide better coordination between all the connected devices around the world, resulting in a faster rate of processing of transactions of data and information. With an increasing rate of interconnected devices, distributed ledger technology enables a feasible solution in supporting the processing of a greater amount of data transactions.

- *Economical:*

  Blockchain allows IoT-based organisations reduction of their costs with the elimination of the processing overheads observed in IoT gateways. This cost reduction can only be possible because of the trust between the different parties in a networking system. Also, the overhead costs that can be minimised with the employment of blockchain in IoT include traditional communication, protocol and hardware overhead costs.

5. *Integration of AI and ML in IoT:*

   In every form, artificial intelligence is the technological advancement that has impacted nearly all the major domains of the industries worldwide. Advancements in the application of AI lie in advancements in the process of data collection, data analysis and data processing. The vital contributor behind all of these advancements is a robust IoT networking system.

   IoT applications based on AI and ML services may consist of the following components.

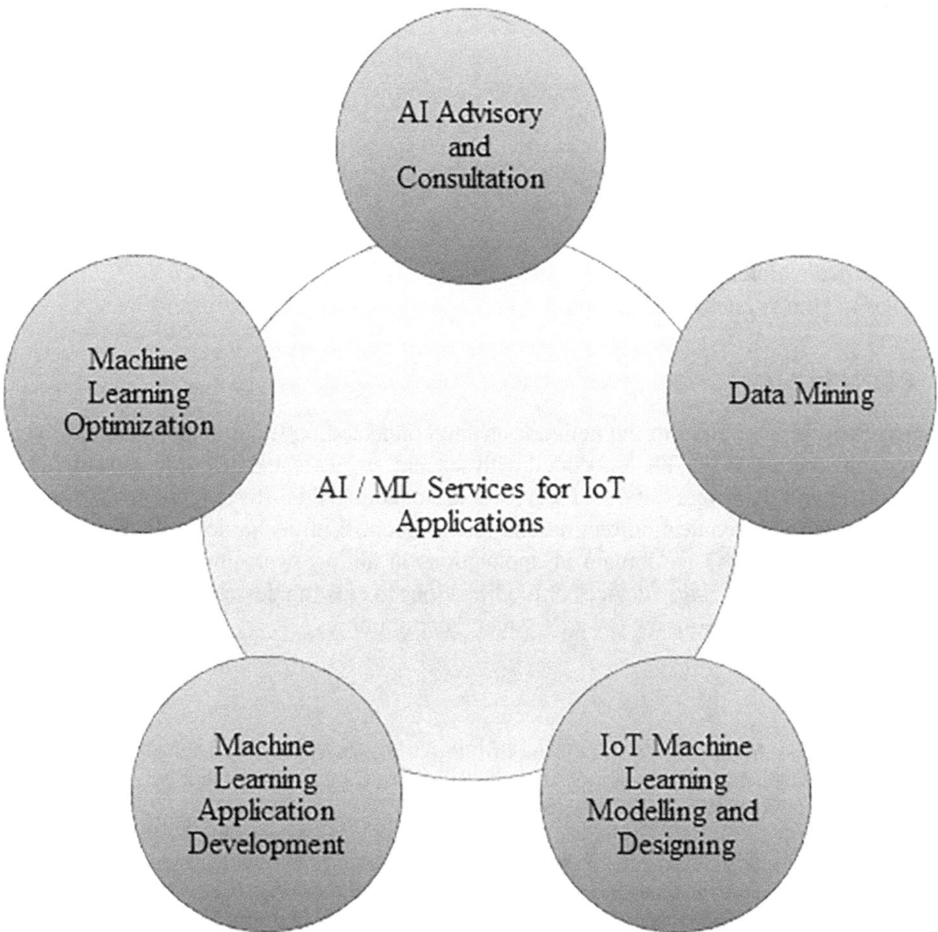

FIGURE 1.7 AI/ML services for IoT applications.

To develop a model based on the services of machine learning to IoT applications, several factors must be taken into consideration. The procedure involved in developing such a model is summarised in Figure 1.8.

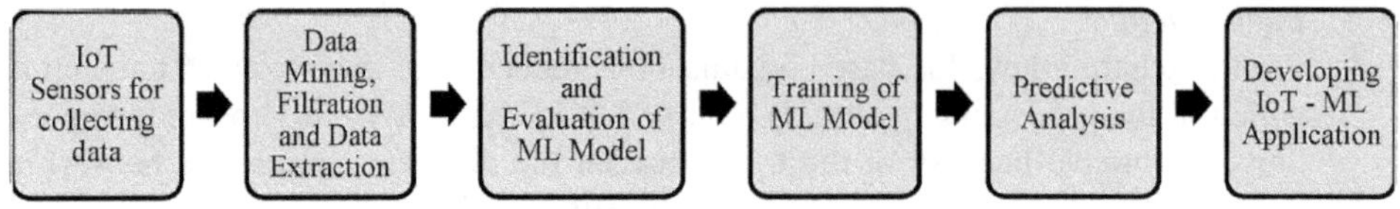

FIGURE 1.8 Procedure in developing ML–IoT applications.

Some of the application areas that will majorly depend upon the networking of AI/ML–IoT technologies are listed as follows:

- Navigation
- Automotive entertainment
- Driving modes—control
- Intelligent mobile apps
- Road condition assessment
- Heath monitoring devices
- Smart location tracking
- Control of cabin conditions
- Connectivity with mobile devices
- Parking assistance
- Driver behaviour monitoring
- Sports applications/wearables
- Predictive maintenance for battery monitoring
- Solar tracking systems in Industry 4.0

1.5 CONCLUSION

The Internet of Things refers to the network of interconnected physical objects, devices, vehicles, buildings and other items that are embedded with sensors, software and network connectivity. These objects collect and exchange data over the internet, enabling them to communicate, interact and perform tasks without requiring direct human intervention. With technological advancements, the IoT will grow and expand its domain of applications in almost every industry. To deal with this expansion, new communication devices or modifications to existing devices are requires so that they can be adopted by users and grow towards "smart" communities.

REFERENCES

1. Yongwan Chun, Mei-Po Kwan, Daniel A. Griffith (2019), Uncertainty and Context in GIScience and Geography: Challenges in the Era of Geospatial Big Data. Int. J. Geogr. Inf. Sci. 33 (6), 1131–1134. https://doi.org/10.1080/13658816.2019.1566552.
2. Alan T. Murray, Tony H. Grubesic, Ran Wei, Elizabeth A. Mack (2015), A Hybrid Geocoding Methodology for Spatio-Temporal Data. https://doi.org/10.1111/j.1467-9671.2011.01289.x.
3. Yaman Hooda, Haobam Derit Singh (2023), Digital Reforms in Public Services and Infrastructure Development & Management. In Technological Prospects and Social Applications of Society 5.0, 219–237, Chapman and Hall/CRC.
4. Haobam Derit Singh, Yaman Hooda (2023), Resilience of Digital Society to Natural Disasters. In Technological Prospects and Social Applications of Society 5.0, 185–199, Chapman and Hall/CRC.
5. Y. Hooda, P. Kuhar, K. Sharma, N. K. Verma (2021), Emerging Applications of Artificial Intelligence in Structural Engineering and Construction Industry. J. Phys. Conf. Ser. 1950 (1), 012062. https://doi.org/10.1088/1742-6596/1950/1/012062.

6. P. Kuhar, K. Sharma, Y. Hooda, N. Verma (2021), Internet of Things (IoT) based Smart Helmet for Construction. J. Phys. Conf. Ser. 1950, 012075.
7. Y. Hooda (2022), IoT and Remote Sensing. In Computer Vision and Internet of Things, 111–140, Chapman and Hall/CRC.
8. G. Jha, L. Sharma, S. Gupta (2021a), E-health in Internet of Things (IoT) in Real-Time Scenario. In P. K. Singh, S. T. Wierzchoń, S. Tanwar, M. Ganzha, J. J. P. C. Rodrigues (eds) Proceedings of Second International Conference on Computing, Communications, and Cyber-Security. Lecture Notes in Networks and Systems, vol. 203, Springer. https://doi.org/10.1007/978-981-16-0733-2_48
9. G. Jha, L. Sharma, S. Gupta (2021b), Future of Augmented Reality in Healthcare Department. In P. K. Singh, S. T. Wierzchoń, S. Tanwar, M. Ganzha, J. J. P. C. Rodrigues (eds) Proceedings of Second International Conference on Computing, Communications, and Cyber-Security. Lecture Notes in Networks and Systems, vol 203, Springer. https://doi.org/10.1007/978-981-16-0733-2_47).
10. Lavanya Sharma (2019), The Rise of the Visual Surveillance to Internet of Things. In From Visual Surveillance to Internet of Things, Taylor & Francis, CRC Press.
11. Lavanya Sharma (2020a), Human Detection and Tracking Using Background Subtraction in Visual Surveillance. In Towards Smart World: Homes to Cities using Internet of Things, 317–329, Taylor & Francis, CRC Press.
12. Lavanya Sharma (2020b), The Future of Smart Cities. In Towards Smart World: Homes to Cities using Internet of Things, 1–19, Taylor & Francis, CRC Press.
13. Lavanya Sharma (2020c), The Rise of Internet of Things and Smart Cities. In Towards Smart World: Homes to Cities Using Internet of Things, 1–19, Taylor & Francis, CRC Press.
14. Lavanya Sharma (2022a), Analysis of Machine Learning Techniques for Airfare Prediction. In Computer Vision and Internet of Things: Technologies and Applications, 211–231, Taylor & Francis, CRC Press.
15. Lavanya Sharma (2022b), Computer Vision in Surgical Operating Theatre and Medical Imaging. In Computer Vision and Internet of Things: Technologies and Applications, 75–96, Taylor & Francis, CRC Press.
16. Lavanya Sharma (2022c), Innovation and Emerging Computer Vision and Artificial Intelligence Technologies in Coronavirus Control. In Computer Vision and Internet of Things: Technologies and Applications, 177–192, Taylor & Francis, CRC Press.
17. Lavanya Sharma (2022d), Preventing Security Breach in Social Media: Threats and Prevention Techniques. In Computer Vision and Internet of Things: Technologies and Applications, 53–62, Taylor & Francis, CRC Press.
18. Lavanya Sharma (2022e), Self-Driving Cars: Tools and Technologies. In Computer Vision and Internet of Things: Technologies and Applications, 99–110, Taylor & Francis, CRC Press.
19. Lavanya Sharma (2022f), Computer-Aided Lung Cancer Detection and Classification of CT Images Using Convolutional Neural Network. In Computer Vision and Internet of Things: Technologies and Applications, 247–262, Taylor & Francis, CRC Press.
20. Lavanya Sharma (2022g), Rise of Computer Vision and Internet of Things. In Computer Vision and Internet of Things: Technologies and Applications, 5–17, Taylor & Francis, CRC Press.
21. Lavanya Sharma et al. (2022), An Overview of Security Issues of Internet of Things. In Computer Vision and Internet of Things: Technologies and Applications, 29–40, Taylor & Francis, CRC Press.
22. L. Sharma, M. Carpenter (Eds.). (2022a), Computer Vision and Internet of Things: Technologies and Applications (1st ed.), Chapman and Hall/CRC. https://doi.org/10.1201/9781003244165
23. Lavanya Sharma, Mukesh Carpenter (2022b), Use of Robotics in Real-Time Applications. In Computer Vision and Internet of Things: Technologies and Applications, 41–50, Taylor & Francis, CRC Press.
24. Lavanya Sharma, Nirvikar Lohan (2019), Internet of Things with Object Detection. In Handbook of Research on Big Data and the IoT, 89–100, IGI Global. doi:10.4018/978-1-5225-7432-3.ch006.
25. Lavanya Sharma, P. K. Garg (2019a), Block based Adaptive Learning Rate for Moving Person Detection in Video Surveillance. In From Visual Surveillance to Internet of Things, Taylor & Francis, CRC Press.
26. Lavanya Sharma, P. K. Garg (2019b), Future of Internet of Things. In From Visual Surveillance to Internet of Things, Taylor & Francis, CRC Press.
27. Lavanya Sharma, P. K. Garg (2019c), IoT and Its Applications. In From Visual Surveillance to Internet of Things, Taylor & Francis, CRC Press.
28. Lavanya Sharma, P. K. Garg (2019d), Smart E-healthcare with Internet of Things: Current Trends Challenges, Solutions and Technologies. In From Visual Surveillance to Internet of Things, Taylor & Francis, CRC Press.

29. Lavanya Sharma, P. K. Garg, Naman Agarwal (2019), A Foresight on e-Healthcare Trailblazers. In From Visual Surveillance to Internet of Things, Taylor & Francis, CRC Press.
30. S. Sharma, S. Verma, M. Kumar, L. Sharma (2019), Use of Motion Capture in 3D Animation: Motion Capture Systems, Challenges, and Recent Trends. In 2019 International Conference on Machine Learning, Big Data, Cloud and Parallel Computing (COMITCon), 289–294. doi:10.1109/COMITCon.2019.8862448

2 Architecture Framework for Deep Learning Systems and IoT

An Overview

Sahil Mehta, Jimmy Mehta, Yaman Hooda, and Haobam Derit Singh

2.1 INTRODUCTION

In today's data-driven world, big data is ubiquitous, generated by virtually everything around us. However, this data's sheer complexity and scale often render traditional methods and databases ineffective in processing and analysis. Figure 2.1 provides a schematic definition of big data, portraying it as a multifaceted phenomenon at the intersection of technology, culture, and academia [1, 2].

As depicted in Figure 2.1, the essence of big data revolves around three key pillars:

- Technology: It hinges on the maximization of computing power and the precision of algorithms, enabling the accumulation, analysis, linkage, and comparison of vast datasets.
- Analyses: Big data's significance lies in its capacity to unveil patterns that underpin social, economic, technological, and legal phenomena, empowering data-driven insights and assertions.
- Mythology: There exists a pervasive belief in the transformative power of big data, wherein it promises a higher form of knowledge and intelligence, capable of unlocking previously unattainable insights with an aura of objectivity, accuracy, and truth [3, 4].

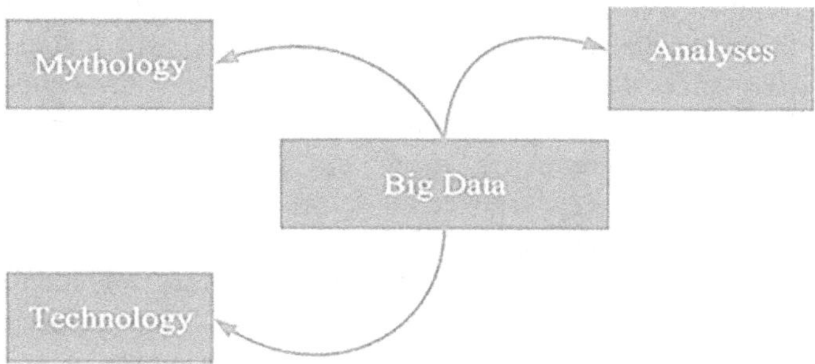

FIGURE 2.1 Pillars of big data.

The conventional landscape of machine learning (ML) and statistical algorithms, often referred to as "shallow learning," faced insurmountable challenges in harnessing big data's potential due to its inherent characteristics, collectively referred to as the "Vs": volume, velocity, variety, and veracity [2]. These characteristics pose significant limitations for traditional ML algorithms, making them unsuitable for the demands of modern data analysis. Shallow learning methods struggled to deliver

DOI: 10.1201/9781003451846-2

high-quality outcomes; could not decipher online communities and political movements; and relied on complex, intricate features. Deep learning (DL) emerged as a powerful paradigm shift in data analysis [5]. It solved the problem of big data by addressing the limitations of shallow learning methods. Before 2006, training deep architectures to discern complex patterns remained an elusive goal. Traditional neural networks were constrained by their inability to effectively balance the layers of the network, leading to issues like vanishing gradients and overfitting. This hindrance compelled the exponential growth of neuron layers to mitigate these problems, ultimately hampering their performance. However, DL introduced a novel feature extraction and selection approach, effectively alleviating these challenges [6–8]. By training networks layer by layer through a process known as greedy layer-wise unsupervised pre-training, DL models autonomously identify and harness relevant features from data, making them adept at handling vast and intricate datasets.

Consequently, DL has become a pivotal tool in diverse domains, ranging from computer vision, speech recognition, and text processing to medical diagnostics, finance, digital advertising, fraud detection, and agriculture. Its natural structure, rooted in artificial neural networks, forms the basis of its effectiveness in classification tasks. In essence, deep learning represents a seismic shift in our ability to harness the potential of big data, enabling computers to learn autonomously and uncover previously inaccessible insights across various industries. As we delve deeper into this era of data-driven decision-making, the relationship between big data and deep learning continues to be one of mutual empowerment, ushering in a new era of knowledge discovery and innovation [7, 8].

In addition to this, another major technological development is the Internet of Things (IoT). As we proceed into the 22nd century, we find ourselves on the cusp of a remarkable technological transformation. Our lives are becoming increasingly intertwined with the very objects and devices that make our daily routines more convenient. This phenomenon is being propelled by a new wave of wearable technology, which is, in turn, driving the rapid expansion of the Internet of Things. In recent years, the IoT has transcended its status as a buzzword, evolving into a tangible reality with profound implications. It's no longer a concept confined to science fiction; it has permeated our world. Consider the devices you encounter daily: the smartwatch on your wrist that monitors your health, the fitness tracker bands that help you stay active, the smart cities that optimize urban living, and the industrial enterprises that enhance productivity. These connected "things" aren't just passive tools; they actively work to improve our lives [9, 10].

The promise of IoT lies in its ability to catalyze innovation. It achieves this by enabling data collection, analysis, exploitation, and management through a robust, forward-looking, scalable, and secure architecture. While IoT architectures can take on diverse forms tailored to different industries, they share a common goal: to establish an ecosystem that is not only cost effective but also highly functional, flexible, scalable to meet evolving needs, and easily maintainable. In essence, the emergence of IoT signifies a paradigm shift in how we interact with technology and the world around us. It heralds an era where connectivity and intelligence are embedded in the fabric of our lives, fostering unprecedented opportunities for progress, efficiency, and convenience. As we journey further into this connected future, the boundaries of what's possible expand, paving the way for many transformative innovations yet to come [11–13, 18–40].

Thus, in today's world, deep learning and the Internet of Things are revolutionizing industries and enhancing our daily lives. DL's data analysis capabilities and IoT's interconnected devices reshape our lives and work. The future holds boundless opportunities for innovation and progress as these technologies continue to shape our world. Therefore, this work focuses on the architecture framework of these two trending technologies in Sections 2.2 and 2.3, their practical applications in Section 2.4, and their future scope in Section 2.5.

2.2 ARCHITECTURE FRAMEWORK FOR IoT

The IT landscape is currently abuzz with emerging concepts like data science, analytics, artificial intelligence, and the Internet of Things. But what do these terms truly encompass? The Internet of

Things signifies the extensive interlinking of a myriad of devices—from wearables, watches, tablets, remote controls, and sensors to household appliances—within the purview of human interaction. In essence, this technological solution aggregates data from many devices, which is subsequently transmitted to data centers and servers for in-depth analysis, culminating in the facilitation of automation and subsequent actions. Yet the journey from your command to task accomplishment traverses an intricate and predominantly invisible architectural framework, hinging on an array of elements and their interactions. IoT architecture encapsulates this intricate web of components, including sensors, actuators, cloud services, protocols, and various layers constituting the IoT network systems. Generally, this architecture is structured into layers, offering administrators the means to assess, supervise, and sustain system integrity [41–55]. The IoT architecture essentially follows a four-step process: data originates from connected devices equipped with sensors; traverses a network; and culminates in the cloud for processing, analysis, and storage. As IoT continues to evolve, it promises to expand further, ushering in novel and enhanced user experiences.

Regarding the different layers of IoT architecture, it is essential to note that IoT technology has witnessed a surge in popularity, resulting in diverse applications designed to align with distinct use cases. Consequently, there is no universally defined standard architecture; instead, the complexity and quantity of architectural layers vary based on the specific business objectives at hand [51–60]. A four-layer architecture model prevails as the conventional and widely embraced format. Figure 2.2 elucidates these layers: the perception layer, network layer, processing layer, and application layer [14–16].

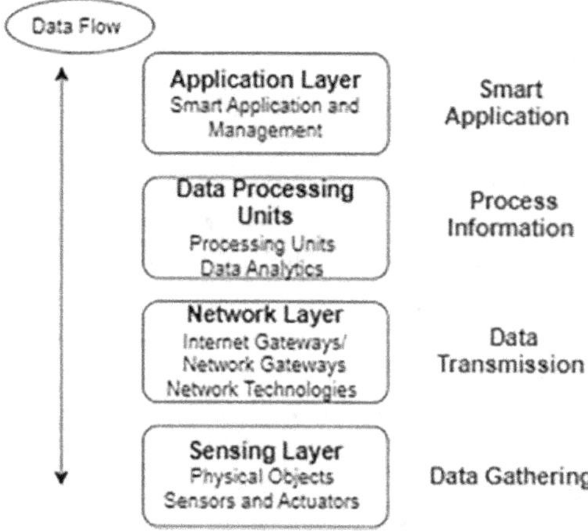

FIGURE 2.2 Four-stage IoT architecture.

Particularly, the layers are explained as:

- Perception/Sensing Layer—The initial tier within an IoT system encompasses the realm of "things" or endpoint devices, bridging the divide between the physical and digital realms. This layer, known as perception, encompasses the physical domain, housing sensors and actuators proficient in gathering, receiving, and processing data across the network. These sensors and actuators can establish connections either wirelessly or through wired interfaces. The architecture remains agnostic regarding the components' scope and their geographical distribution.
- Network Layer—The network layer provides a comprehensive framework for data movement within the IoT application. One finds data acquiring systems (DASs) and internet/network gateways within this stratum. DAS undertakes data aggregation and

conversion functions, involving tasks like collecting data from sensors and transforming analog data into digital formats. It is pivotal in transmitting and processing data amassed by sensor devices. On the other hand, the network layer facilitates the seamless connection and communication of these devices with servers, intelligent devices, and network components. Furthermore, it manages all data transmissions on behalf of these devices.

- Processing Layer—Serving as the cognitive center of the IoT ecosystem, the processing layer is where data is typically analyzed, pre-processed, and stored before its dispatch to the data center. Subsequently, the data becomes accessible to software applications responsible for monitoring, managing, and orchestrating further actions. This is where the concept of edge IT or edge analytics comes into play, enabling real-time decision-making at the network's periphery.
- Application Layer—The application layer is the interface where user interaction unfolds, furnishing user-specific services. For instance, it might encompass applications like a smart home system, allowing users to activate a coffee maker with a mere tap on a mobile app or providing a dashboard that offers insights into the status of various devices within a system. The Internet of Things finds versatile deployment across domains such as smart cities, smart residences, and healthcare, each tailored to its unique applications and requirements [14–16].

Phases of IoT Solutions Architecture—After delving into the intricacies of IoT layers and their potential advantages for businesses, the question arises: how can enterprises harness these layers to derive maximum value from the IoT? While the term "Internet of Things" may encompass interconnected devices and communication protocols, the data generated by these devices often remains confined within silos, fragmented and isolated. Consequently, these fragmented insights in isolation seldom offer sufficient grounds to justify a substantial resource investment in an IoT strategy. To unlock the full potential of IoT, organizations must facilitate unhindered device interactions and strive for optimal synergy among devices and systems. Ensuring that the existing infrastructure aligns with the IoT architecture is imperative. Figure 2.3 presents the various stages of IoT architecture implementation within enterprises:

- Connected Devices/Objects: The initial step in building an IoT architecture is establishing the physical layer within the environment. Without "smart" or interconnected devices, the Internet of Things would not exist. Typically, these devices are wireless sensors or actuators situated in the perception layer. Sensors are responsible for gathering and evaluating data from the environment, making it ready for further analysis, while actuators measure changes detected by the sensors. These sensors and actuators can be interconnected either wirelessly or through wired connections, enabling them to perform sensing and actuation tasks. Local area networks (LANs) and personal area networks (PANs) serve as the means for connecting these sensors and actuators.

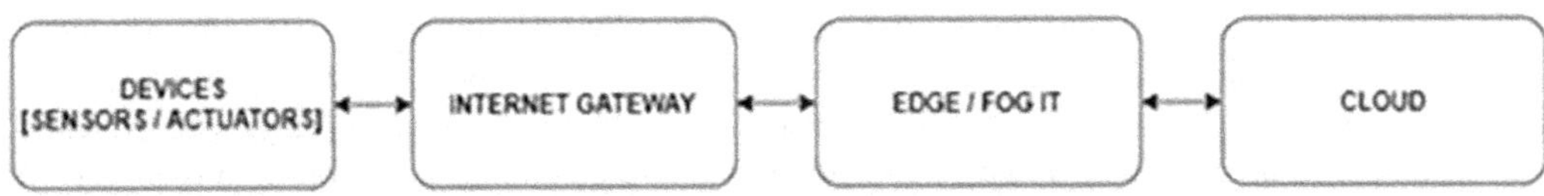

FIGURE 2.3 Stages of IoT solutions architecture.

- Internet Gateway: Once the first step is effectively executed, the subsequent phase involves the setup of an internet gateway. Since sensors and actuators collect data in analog format, a mechanism is required to convert this analog data into digital data for processing purposes. The internet gateway fulfills this crucial role. During this stage, raw data is received from the devices and undergoes pre-processing before transmission to the cloud. Data acquisition systems are employed to transform analog data into digital formats. These systems connect with sensors and actuators, aggregating and converting the data into digital form for transmission over the network via the internet gateway. Additional functionalities, such as analytics and security enhancements, can be integrated to boost performance and efficiency.
- Edge IT Systems: The third stage in an IoT architecture encompasses pre-processing and advanced data analytics. Given IoT systems' substantial volume of data and the resulting bandwidth demands, edge IT systems are pivotal in alleviating strain on the core IT infrastructure. These systems employ machine learning and visualization techniques to derive insights from the collected data. Machine learning algorithms extract valuable insights from the data, while visualization techniques understandably present the information. Directly transmitting data to the server or data center can impede system speed and LAN or router bandwidth. Analog data is generated rapidly and consumes significant storage space, underscoring the importance of data conversion to digital form. Typically, not all data collected by sensors and actuators holds equal value to the organization, so only pertinent data undergoes processing and transmission to data centers and servers.
- Data Centers and Cloud Storage: Following proper pre-processing, analysis, and thorough scrutiny, the data is relayed to data centers and servers for ultimate analysis and reporting. Data centers and cloud services fall within the management services category and are typically responsible for data processing through analytics, device management, and security protocols. Moreover, the cloud facilitates data transfer to end-user applications across various domains such as healthcare, retail, environment, emergency, and energy. After analysis, the data may be directed to cloud-based servers or data centers for final processing. Utilizing cloud platforms can reduce hardware expenditures, although data security remains a concern. Conversely, physical servers or data centers offer heightened security but entail higher costs.

2.3 ARCHITECTURE FRAMEWORK FOR DEEP LEARNING SYSTEMS

A multitude of architectures and algorithms are employed within the realm of deep learning, showcasing diversity and breadth. This section delves into six distinct deep learning architectures that have evolved over the past two decades. Remarkably, long short-term memory (LSTM) and convolutional neural networks (CNNs) emerge as prominent figures in this compilation, standing as both of the earliest methods and among the most extensively applied in various application domains. This section categorizes deep learning architectures into supervised and unsupervised learning paradigms, unveiling a roster of prominent deep learning models. These include convolutional neural networks, recurrent neural networks (RNNs), long short-term memory networks, gated recurrent unit (GRU) networks, self-organizing maps (SOMs), autoencoders (AEs), and restricted Boltzmann machines (RBMs). Additionally, it provides insights into deep belief networks (DBNs) and deep stacking networks (DSNs), as shown in Figure 2.4 [17–40].

- Supervised Deep Learning—In supervised learning, we delve into a problem space where the target variable to be predicted is explicitly labeled within the training data. This section provides an overview of two widely acclaimed supervised deep learning architectures: convolutional neural networks and recurrent neural networks, along with some of their variations.

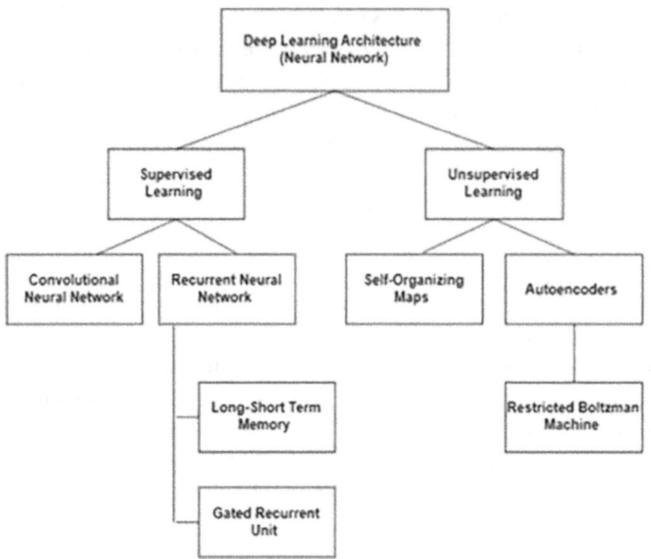

FIGURE 2.4 Deep learning architecture.

- Convolutional Neural Networks (CNNs)—CNNs draw inspiration from the biological visual cortex, making them particularly suited for image processing tasks. The inception of CNNs can be attributed to Yann LeCun, with an initial focus on applications like handwritten character recognition, such as postal code interpretation. As a deep network, CNNs consist of layers that progressively identify features, beginning with low-level attributes like edges and culminating in higher-level characteristics of the input. The LeNet CNN architecture comprises several layers responsible for feature extraction and subsequent classification (as shown in Figure 2.5). The input image is divided into receptive fields, feeding into a convolutional layer that extracts features. Following this, a pooling step reduces the dimensionality of the extracted features, typically via max pooling, while preserving critical information. This process repeats with additional convolution and pooling layers, eventually connecting to a fully connected multilayer perceptron. The network's final output layer consists of nodes that recognize distinct image features, such as one node for each identified number. Training the network involves utilizing the backpropagation algorithm. Incorporating deep processing layers, convolution operations, pooling techniques, and a fully connected classification layer has paved the way for diverse applications of deep learning neural networks. Beyond image processing, CNNs have demonstrated their effectiveness in video recognition and numerous tasks within the realm of natural language processing. Applications include—Image recognition, video analysis, and natural language processing.

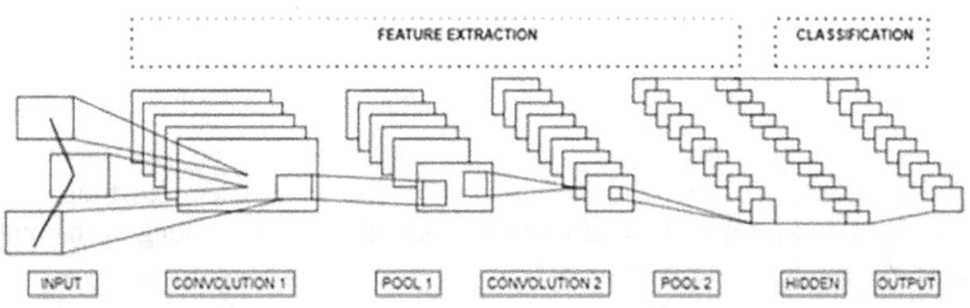

FIGURE 2.5 CNN architecture.

- Recurrent neural networks form the foundational architecture upon which various other deep learning models are constructed. Unlike typical multilayer networks with purely feed-forward connections, RNNs incorporate feedback connections that loop back into previous layers or even the same layer, as shown in Figure 2.6. This feedback mechanism empowers RNNs to retain a memory of past inputs and effectively model temporal dependencies. RNNs encompass a diverse array of architectures, and in the following section, we'll delve into one of the widely recognized topologies known as long short-term memory. The critical distinction lies in internal feedback connections within the network, which can originate from hidden layers, the output layer, or a combination thereof. RNNs can be "unfolded" over time and trained using the conventional backpropagation algorithm or a modified version known as backpropagation through time (BPTT). Example applications include speech recognition and handwritten text recognition.

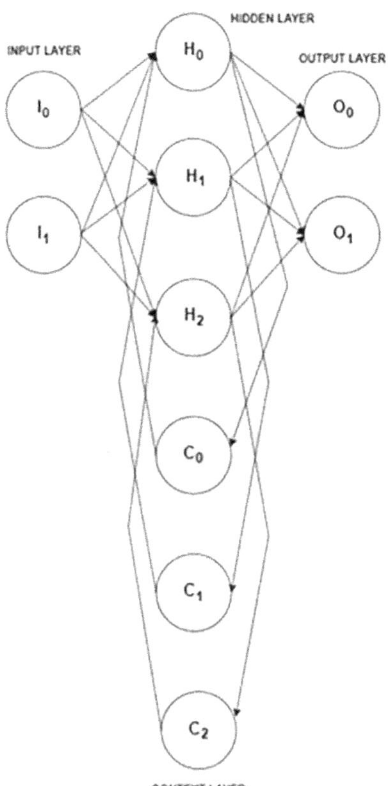

FIGURE 2.6 RNN architecture.

- LSTM networks, introduced by Hochreiter and Schmidhuber in 1997, have gained popularity in recent years for various applications, including smartphones and conversational speech recognition. Unlike traditional neural networks, LSTMs introduce memory cells that can store information for short or long durations based on input, allowing them to focus on relevant data. These memory cells include input, forget, and output gates controlled by weights optimized through methods like BPTT. Recent applications combine CNNs and LSTMs to create image and video captioning systems, where CNNs process visual data, and LSTMs generate natural language captions. LSTM architecture is shown in Figure 2.7.

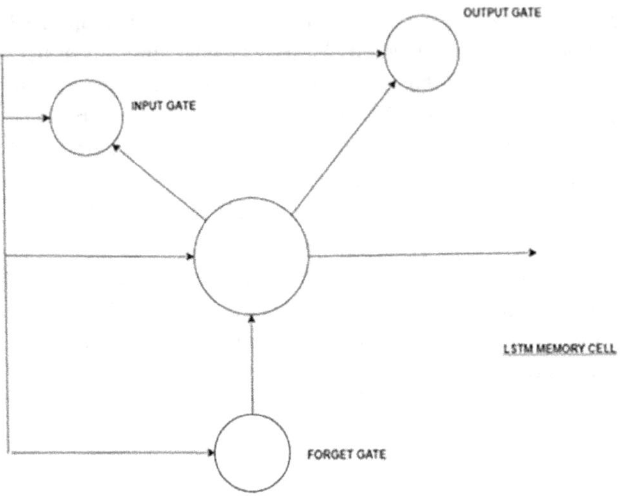

FIGURE 2.7 LSTM architecture.

- In 2014 a more streamlined version of the LSTM, known as the gated recurrent unit, was introduced. The GRU model features two gates, omitting the output gate found in LSTM as shown in Figure 2.8. These gates are the update gate, which determines the retention of previous cell contents, and the reset gate, which governs the integration of new input with the existing cell contents. By configuring the reset gate to 1 and the update gate to 0, a GRU can emulate a standard RNN. GRUs offer simplicity, faster training, and enhanced execution efficiency compared to LSTMs. However, LSTMs may exhibit greater expressiveness and improved performance with larger datasets. Example applications include, Natural language text compression, handwriting recognition, speech recognition, gesture recognition, and image captioning.

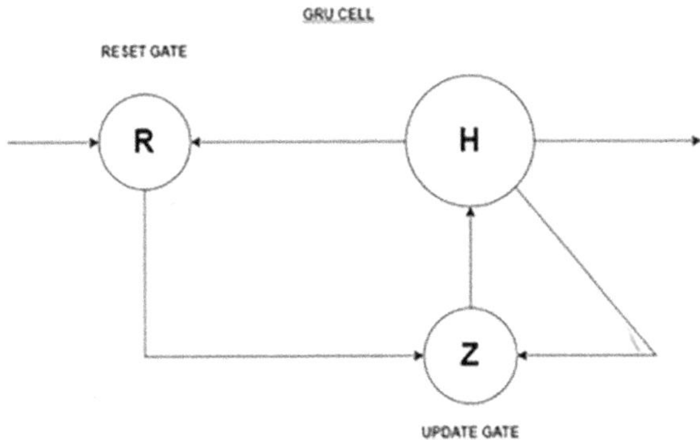

FIGURE 2.8 GRU architecture.

- Unsupervised Deep Learning—Unsupervised learning pertains to scenarios in which the training data lacks target labels. This section delves into three unsupervised deep learning architectures: self-organized maps, autoencoders, and restricted Boltzmann machines. We will also explore how deep belief and stacking networks are constructed upon the foundational unsupervised architecture.
- Self-organized maps, also known as Kohonen maps, are unsupervised neural networks introduced by Dr. Teuvo Kohonen in 1982. Unlike traditional artificial neural networks,

SOMs reduce input dimensionality and use node weights as characteristics as shown in Figure 2.9. They start with random weights for each input feature, calculate Euclidean distances between output nodes and inputs, and identify the best matching unit (BMU). This BMU becomes the input representation, and other units are assigned to clusters based on their proximity. SOMs do not employ activation functions or backpropagation, making them suitable for various tasks like dimensionality reduction, high-dimensional input clustering into 2D output, and cluster visualization.

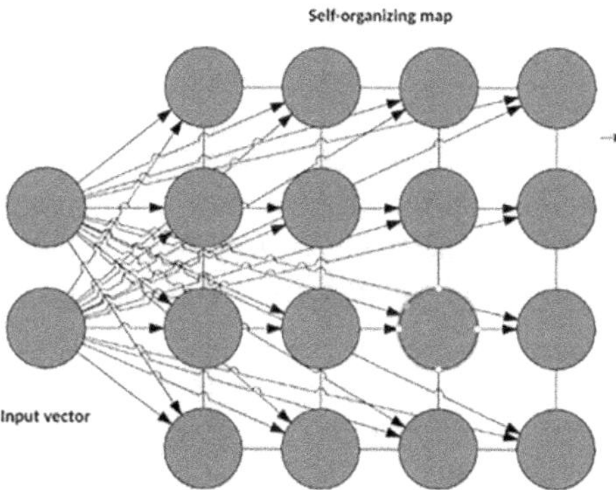

FIGURE 2.9 SOM architecture.

- Autoencoders, originating to approximately 1987, represent a distinctive variant of artificial neural networks (ANNs) structured into three fundamental layers: the input layer, the hidden layer, and the output layer, as shown in Figure 2.10. The functionality of autoencoders is founded on a two-step process. The input layer is initially encoded into the hidden layer by implementing a specialized encoding function. Notably, the number of nodes residing in the hidden layer is significantly less than those present in the input layer. This condensed hidden layer encapsulates a compressed representation of the original input data. Subsequently, the output layer undertakes the challenging task of reconstructing the input, employing a decoder function to achieve this objective. During the training phase of autoencoders, a critical error function is calculated by assessing the disparity between the input and output layers. This error serves as the basis for iteratively adjusting the weights to minimize the discrepancy. An interesting characteristic of autoencoders, distinguishing them from conventional unsupervised learning methods, is their adoption of backward propagation, which facilitates continuous learning. This unique feature classifies autoencoders as self-supervised algorithms. Practical applications of autoencoders encompass diverse domains, such as dimensionality reduction, data interpolation, and data compression/decompression.

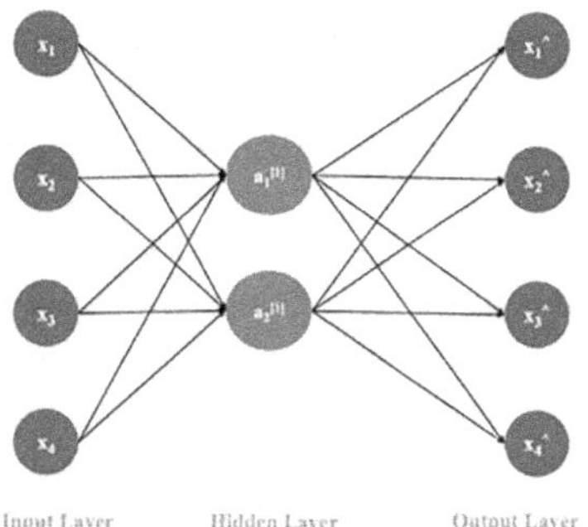

FIGURE 2.10 Autoencoders architecture.

- Restricted Boltzmann machines, initially conceptualized by Paul Smolensky in 1986 and termed harmoniums, have gained prominence in recent years. An RBM is characterized by a two-layered neural network comprising the input and hidden layers, as shown in Figure 2.11. Unlike traditional Boltzmann machines, which establish connections between nodes within the same layer, RBMs simplify the architecture due to computational complexity. In RBMs, each node in the hidden layer connects to every node in the visible layer, forming a comprehensive network structure. The training process for RBMs involves calculating the probability distribution of the training dataset through a stochastic approach. At the commencement of training, each neuron becomes activated randomly. Additionally, RBMs integrate hidden and visible bias. The hidden bias contributes to constructing the activation during the forward pass, while the visible bias aids in reconstructing the input data. One distinctive trait of RBMs is their generative nature, as they invariably produce reconstructed inputs distinct from the original ones. This inherent randomness sets them apart from deterministic models like autoencoders. Notable applications of RBMs encompass dimensionality reduction and collaborative filtering.

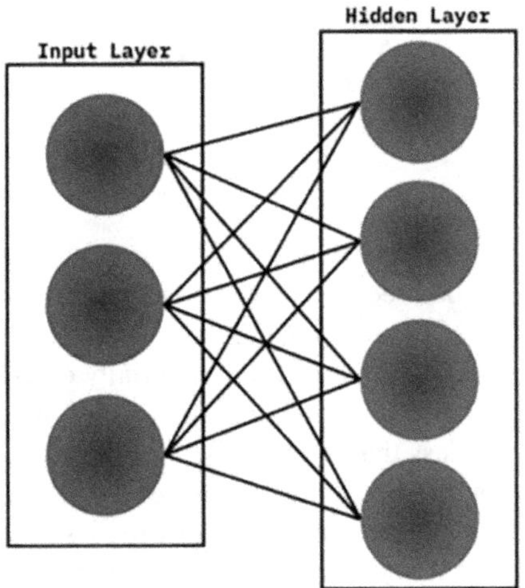

FIGURE 2.11 RBM architecture.

- Deep belief networks present a distinctive network architecture coupled with an innovative training algorithm. A DBN typically constitutes a multilayer network, often characterized by depth and an abundance of hidden layers, as shown in Figure 2.12. DBNs are included in pairs of connected layers, where each pair forms a restricted Boltzmann machine. This unique arrangement transforms a DBN into a stack of RBMs, making it a powerful construct for various tasks. In a DBN, the input layer serves as the conduit for raw sensory inputs. Each successive hidden layer progressively learns abstract representations of this input data. The output layer, treated differently from the other layers, is primarily responsible for network classification. The training process for DBNs unfolds in two phases: unsupervised pretraining and supervised fine-tuning. During unsupervised pretraining, each RBM learns to reconstruct its input layer, with subsequent RBMs leveraging the outputs of the previous hidden layer as their inputs. This iterative process continues until all layers are pretrained. Once pretraining concludes, supervised fine-tuning commences. In this phase, meaningful labels are assigned to the output nodes, imbuing them with contextual significance within the network. The full network is then trained using gradient descent learning or backpropagation to complete the training process. DBNs find applications in diverse fields such as image recognition, information retrieval, natural language understanding, and failure prediction.

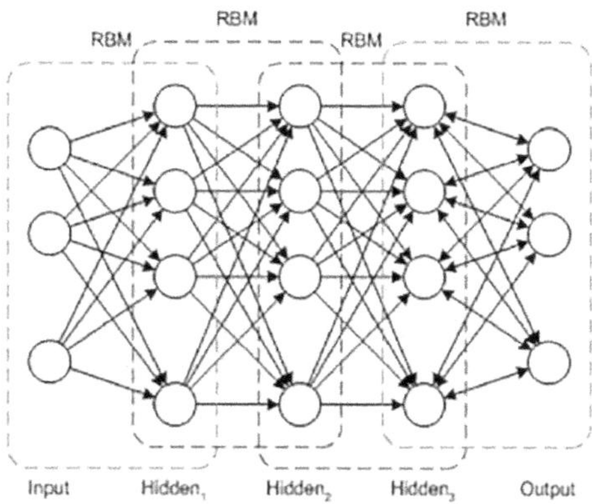

FIGURE 2.12 DBN architecture.

- Deep stacking networks, also known as deep convex networks, represent a distinct architectural approach within the realm of deep learning. Their unique perspective on training complexity sets DSNs apart from conventional deep learning frameworks. While DSNs feature a deep structure akin to other deep networks, they differentiate themselves by functioning as a collection of individual networks, each with its own set of hidden layers, as shown in Figure 2.13. This architectural choice stems from a central challenge in deep learning: the escalating training complexity associated with each additional layer. DSNs address this challenge by reframing training as a set of individuals, parallel training problems rather than a monolithic one. A DSN comprises a series of modules, with each module representing a subnetwork within the overarching DSN hierarchy. In a typical DSN configuration, multiple modules are established. Each module consists of an input layer, a single hidden layer, and an output layer. These modules are stacked hierarchically, with the inputs of each module encompassing the outputs of the previous layer, along with the original input vector. This layered arrangement enables the DSN to acquire a deeper understanding of complex classifications beyond the capacity of a single module. Importantly, DSNs offer the advantage of training individual modules in isolation, allowing for efficient parallel training. Supervised training is carried out using backpropagation for each module, rather than employing backpropagation across the entire network. DSNs outperform traditional deep belief networks in many applications, rendering them a favored and efficient network architecture. DSNs find practical utility in a variety of domains, including information retrieval and continuous speech recognition.

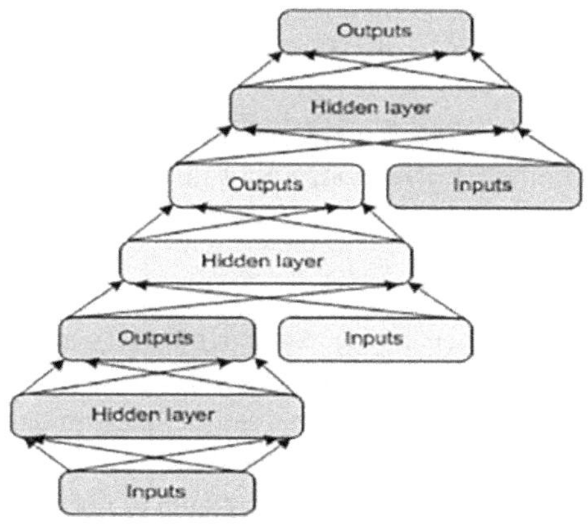

FIGURE 2.13 DSN architecture.

2.4 APPLICATIONS

2.4.1 Deep Learning Systems

- Automating the Colorization of Black-and-White Images: Traditionally, adding color to black-and-white images was a labor-intensive manual process. Deep learning now allows for automated colorization, where objects and their content are identified within the image, simulating the human eye's approach to colorizing.
- Adding Sound to Silent Movies: DL models, trained on a dataset of 1000 examples, enable the automatic addition of sounds to silent movies. These models are trained on videos capturing various drumstick sounds striking different surfaces, creating diverse audio responses. DL associates video frames with a database of pre-recorded sounds, selecting the most suitable background audio to match the movie's scenes, enhancing the overall cinematic experience.
- Object Detection and Classification in Photos: DL has revolutionized object detection in photographs, facilitating the identification of various objects and drawing bounding boxes around them. This advancement simplifies image comprehension by categorizing objects within photographs, enabling more intricate variations in tasks related to object detection.
- Automated Machine Translation: DL plays a crucial role in automating machine translation tasks, allowing for the translation of words, sentences, or phrases from one language to another. This process, applicable to both text and image translation, is performed seamlessly with DL algorithms, eliminating the need for extensive pre-processing.
- Generating Handwriting Automatically: DL is instrumental in automatically generating handwriting for words or phrases. DL models establish a relationship between movement and pen strokes by utilizing coordinate data from human-written text, collected using a pen. This learning process enables the generation of new handwriting examples based on these collected samples.
- Medical Image Analysis and DL: DL has extensive medical image analysis application. For instance, it aids in predicting the survival time of glioblastoma patients based on phenotype and genotype imaging. Various DL techniques are employed for tasks like brain image segmentation and segmentation in medical image analysis, addressing a range of medical image-related challenges.
- Intelligent Transportation Systems and DL: DL has transformed intelligent transportation systems (ITSs) by enhancing traffic congestion prediction and traffic sign recognition. Its application extends to self-driving cars, where DL models detect obstacles and pedestrians, contributing to safer autonomous driving.
- DL and 3D Objects: DL has gained widespread use in handling 3D objects, enabling tasks such as robotic grasping, object recognition, and model classification. Different DL architectures are employed to classify and recognize 3D objects, simplifying complex recognition challenges.
- Natural Language Processing (NLP) and DL: DL is extensively employed in NLP, powering applications like grammar correction, author mimicry, sentiment analysis, spam classification, and social media analysis. DL models like LSTM and CNN play pivotal roles in these diverse NLP applications.
- Voice Generation and DL: DL techniques have significantly impacted voice generation and speech synthesis, effectively generating voice parameters and synthesizing high-quality speech signals. These techniques find application in various voice-related tasks.
- Health Monitoring and DL: Deep neural networks, one-dimensional CNNs, and vision-based methods, including two-dimensional CNNs, are extensively used in health monitoring and structural damage detection. They contribute to detecting damage and anomalies from vibration and image datasets in infrastructure and structural assessments.

2.4.2 IoT

- Smart Homes: The IoT enables the automation and remote control of various home devices such as thermostats, lights, security cameras, and appliances. Smart home systems allow homeowners to increase energy efficiency, enhance security, and create more convenient living spaces.
- Wearable Health Devices: The IoT plays a crucial role in wearable health technology, allowing individuals to monitor their health and fitness levels. Devices like fitness trackers and smart watches collect data on heart rate, activity levels, sleep patterns, and more, providing valuable insights for personal health management.
- Connected Vehicles: IoT technology is used in connected cars to provide real-time data on vehicle performance, navigation, and safety. It can also enable features like remote diagnostics, predictive maintenance, and autonomous driving capabilities.
- Smart Cities: The IoT is used in smart city initiatives to improve urban infrastructure and services. Applications include smart traffic management, waste management, environmental monitoring, and public safety enhancements.
- Industrial IoT (IIoT): In the industrial sector, IoT sensors and devices are used to monitor and optimize manufacturing processes, track equipment performance, and enhance supply chain management. The IIoT increases efficiency, reduces downtime, and lowers operational costs.
- Agriculture: IoT sensors are used in precision agriculture to monitor soil conditions, weather, and crop health. This data helps farmers make informed decisions about irrigation, fertilization, and pest control, ultimately increasing crop yields.
- Healthcare: IoT devices are used in healthcare for remote patient monitoring, medication adherence tracking, and asset management within healthcare facilities. These applications improve patient outcomes and streamline healthcare operations.
- Retail: IoT technology is used in retail for inventory management, supply chain optimization, and personalized shopping experiences. Smart shelves, beacons, and customer tracking systems enhance the retail industry.
- Environmental Monitoring: IoT sensors are deployed to monitor air quality, water quality, and weather conditions. This data is critical for environmental agencies and researchers to assess and respond to environmental changes and emergencies.
- Energy Management: The IoT helps optimize energy consumption in commercial buildings and industries. Smart meters, sensors, and energy management systems allow organizations to reduce energy costs and minimize their environmental impact.
- Logistics and Supply Chain: IoT-enabled tracking systems improve visibility and transparency in logistics and supply chain operations. This includes real-time tracking of shipments, monitoring of temperature-sensitive cargo, and inventory management.
- Asset Tracking: Many industries, including logistics, manufacturing, and construction, use IoT for asset tracking. This involves attaching IoT sensors to valuable assets to monitor their location and condition in real time.
- Smart Grids: The IoT is used in modernizing electrical grids to create smart grids. This technology enables utilities to monitor and manage electricity distribution more efficiently, respond to outages faster, and integrate renewable energy sources.

2.5 CONCLUSIONS AND FUTURE SCOPE

In conclusion, the convergence of deep learning and the Internet of Things (IoT) represents a transformative force in today's technology landscape. DL's ability to extract intricate patterns and insights from vast datasets has revolutionized various domains and found a natural partner in the IoT ecosystem. As we reflect on the current state of these technologies and look toward the future, several key takeaways and future directions emerge.

DL has demonstrated its prowess in tasks ranging from image recognition and natural language processing to medical image analysis and predictive modeling. It offers versatile tools like deep belief networks, convolutional neural networks, and recurrent networks, which can be tailored to specific applications. However, ongoing research should aim to create more robust and efficient DL frameworks that seamlessly handle noisy, real-world IoT data, ensuring scalability and real-time processing.

For IoT, the present landscape is marked by unprecedented connectivity, enabling devices to interact, gather data, and enhance user experiences. Yet challenges such as security, data privacy, and interoperability persist. Future IoT developments should prioritize comprehensive security measures, standardized protocols, and data governance frameworks to ensure the integrity and confidentiality of data transmitted through interconnected devices.

The future scope of DL and IoT is promising. Enhanced DL algorithms will empower IoT systems to predict and respond to events more intelligently, optimizing energy consumption, traffic management, and resource allocation. Furthermore, DL-driven predictive analytics will revolutionize healthcare, agriculture, and urban planning, fostering a more sustainable and efficient world. IoT deployments are expected to expand across diverse sectors in the coming years, from smart cities and healthcare to manufacturing and agriculture. Collaboration between DL and the IoT will pave the way for autonomous vehicles, smart infrastructure, and precision agriculture, revolutionizing industries and improving the quality of life. To fully realize this potential, researchers, policymakers, and industry leaders must work together to address the ethical, regulatory, and technical challenges ahead. As DL and the IoT continue to evolve, their integration promises a future of boundless possibilities, reshaping industries and enhancing human experiences in unprecedented ways.

REFERENCES

[1] Boyd, D., Crawford, K.: Critical questions for big data: provocations for a cultural, technological, and scholarly phenomenon. Inf. Commun. Soc. 15(5), 662–679 (2012). https://doi.org/10.1080/1369118x.2012. 678878

[2] Webb, G.I., Pazzani, M.J., Billsus, D.: Machine learning for user modeling. User Model. User-Adapted Interact. 11(1), 19–29 (2001). https://doi.org/10.1023/a:1011117102175

[3] Liu, Y., Starzyk, J.A., Zhu, Z.: Optimized approximation algorithm in neural networks without overfitting. IEEE Trans. Neural Netw. 19(6), 983–995 (2008). https://doi.org/10.1109/tnn.2007.915114

[4] Gheisari, M., Wang, G., Bhuiyan, M.Z.A.: A survey on deep learning in big data. In: IEEE International Conference on Computational Science and Engineering (CSE) and IEEE International Conference on Embedded and Ubiquitous Computing (EUC), pp. 173–180. IEEE (2017).

[5] Srivastava, N., Hinton, G., Krizhevsky, A., Sutskever, I., Salakhutdinov, R.: Dropout: a simple way to prevent neural networks from overfitting. J. Mach. Learn. Res. 15(1), 1929–1958 (2014).

[6] Hinton, G.E., Simon, O., Teh, Y.-W.: A fast learning algorithm for deep belief nets. Neural Comput. 18(7), 1527–1554 (2006). https://doi.org/10.1162/neco.2006.18.7.1527

[7] Motahari Kia, M.M., Alzubi, J.A., Gheisari, M., Zhang, X., Rahimi, M., Qin, Y.: A novel method for recognition of Persian alphabet by using fuzzy neural network. IEEE Access 6, 77265–77271 (2018).

[8] Dreiseitl, S., Ohno-Machado, L.: Logistic regression and artificial neural network classification models: a methodology review. J. Biomed. Inf. 35(5–6), 352–359 (2002). https://doi.org/10.1016/s1532-0464(03) 00034-0

[9] www.geeksforgeeks.org/architecture-of-internet-of-things-iot/, accessed on September 25, 2023.

[10] Kumar, S., Tiwari, P., Zymbler, M.: Internet of things is a revolutionary approach for future technology enhancement: a review. J. Big Data 6, 111 (2019). https://doi.org/10.1186/s40537-019-0268-2

[11] Mouha, R.: Internet of Things (IoT). J. Data Analysis Infor. Proc. 9, 77–101 (2021). https://doi.org/10.4236/jdaip.2021.92006

[12] Rahmani, A.M., Bayramov, S., Kiani Kalejahi, B.: Internet of things applications: opportunities and threats. Wireless Pers. Commun. 122, 451–476 (2022). https://doi.org/10.1007/s11277-021-08907-0

[13] Abashidze, I., Dąbrowski, M.: Internet of things in marketing: opportunities and security issues. Manag. Sys. Prod. Eng. 4(24), 217–221 (2016).

[14] www.interviewbit.com/blog/iot-architecture/, accessed on August 21, 2023.

[15] www.interviewbit.com/blog/iot-applications/, accessed on August 25, 2023.

[16] www.architectureandgovernance.com/app-tech/an-architectural-framework-for-end-to-end-iot-systems/, accessed September 10, 2023.

[17] https://developer.ibm.com/articles/cc-machine-learning-deep-learning-architectures/, accessed September 13, 2023.

[18] Jha, G., Sharma, L., Gupta, S.: E-health in Internet of Things (IoT) in real-time scenario. In: Singh P.K., Wierzchoń S.T., Tanwar S., Ganzha M., Rodrigues J.J.P.C. (eds) Proceedings of Second International Conference on Computing, Communications, and Cyber-Security. Lecture Notes in Networks and Systems, vol. 203. Springer (2021). https://doi.org/10.1007/978-981-16-0733-2_48

[19] Jha, G., Sharma, L., Gupta, S.: Future of augmented reality in healthcare department. In: Singh P.K., Wierzchoń S.T., Tanwar S., Ganzha M., Rodrigues J.J.P.C. (eds) Proceedings of Second International Conference on Computing, Communications, and Cyber-Security. Lecture Notes in Networks and Systems, vol. 203. Springer (2021). https://doi.org/10.1007/978-981-16-0733-2_47.

[20] Sharma, L.: The rise of the visual surveillance to Internet of Things. In: From Visual Surveillance to Internet of Things. Taylor & Francis, CRC Press (October 2019).

[21] Sharma, L.: Human detection and tracking using background subtraction in visual surveillance. In: Towards Smart World: Homes to Cities Using Internet of Things. Taylor & Francis, CRC Press, pp.317–329 (December 2020).

[22] Sharma, L.: Analysis of machine learning techniques for airfare prediction. In: Computer Vision and Internet of Things: Technologies and Applications. Taylor & Francis, CRC Press, pp.211–231 (May 2022a).

[23] Sharma, L.: Computer vision in surgical operating theatre and medical imaging. In: Computer Vision and Internet of Things: Technologies and Applications. Taylor & Francis, CRC Press, pp.75–96 (May 2022b).

[24] Sharma, L.: Computer-aided lung cancer detection and classification of CT images using convolutional neural network. In: Computer Vision and Internet of Things: Technologies and Applications. Taylor & Francis, CRC Press, pp.247–262 (May 2022c).

[25] Sharma, L.: Innovation and emerging computer vision and artificial intelligence technologies in coronavirus control. In: Computer Vision and Internet of Things: Technologies and Applications. Taylor & Francis, CRC Press, pp.177–192 (May 2022d).

[26] Sharma, L.: Preventing security breach in social media: Threats and prevention techniques. In: Computer Vision and Internet of Things: Technologies and Applications. Taylor & Francis, CRC Press, pp.53–62 (May 2022e).

[27] Sharma, L.: Self-driving cars: Tools and technologies. In: Computer Vision and Internet of Things: Technologies and Applications. Taylor & Francis, CRC Press, pp.99–110 (May 2022f).

[28] Sharma, L.: Rise of computer vision and Internet of Things. In: Computer Vision and Internet of Things: Technologies and Applications. Taylor & Francis, CRC Press, pp.5–17 (May 2022g).

[29] Sharma, L.: The future of smart cities. In: Towards Smart World: Homes to Cities Using Internet of Things. Taylor & Francis, CRC Press, pp.1–19 (December 2020).

[30] Sharma, L.: The rise of Internet of Things and smart cities. In: Towards Smart World: Homes to Cities Using Internet of Things. Taylor & Francis, CRC Press, pp.1–19 (December 2020).

[31] Sharma, L., Carpenter, M. (Eds.): Computer Vision and Internet of Things: Technologies and Applications (1st ed.). Chapman and Hall/CRC (2022a). https://doi.org/10.1201/9781003244165

[32] Sharma, L., Carpenter, M.: Use of robotics in real-time applications. In: Computer Vision and Internet of Things: Technologies and Applications. Taylor & Francis, CRC Press, pp.41–50 (May 2022b).

[33] Sharma, L., et al.: An overview of security issues of Internet of Things. In: Computer Vision and Internet of Things: Technologies and Applications. Taylor & Francis, CRC Press, pp.29–40 (May 2022).

[34] Sharma, L., Garg, P.K.: Block based adaptive learning rate for moving person detection in video surveillance. In: From Visual Surveillance to Internet of Things. Taylor & Francis, CRC Press (October 2019).

[35] Sharma, L., Garg, P.K.: Future of Internet of Things. In: From Visual Surveillance to Internet of Things. Taylor & Francis, CRC Press (October 2019).

[36] Sharma, L., Garg, P.K.: IoT and its applications. In: From Visual Surveillance to Internet of Things. Taylor & Francis, CRC Press (October 2019).

[37] Sharma, L., Garg, P.K.: Smart E-healthcare with Internet of Things: Current trends challenges, solutions and technologies. In: From Visual Surveillance to Internet of Things. Taylor & Francis, CRC Press (October 2019).

[38] Sharma, L., Garg, P.K., Agarwal,N.: A foresight on e-healthcare Trailblazers. In: From Visual Surveillance to Internet of Things. Taylor & Francis, CRC Press (October 2019).

[39] Sharma, L., Lohan, N.: Internet of things with object detection. In: Handbook of Research on Big Data and the IoT. IGI Global, pp.89–100 (March 2019). doi:10.4018/978-1-5225-7432-3.ch006.

[40] Sharma, S., Verma, S., Kumar M., Sharma, L.: Use of motion capture in 3D animation: Motion capture systems, challenges, and recent trends. In: 2019 International Conference on Machine Learning, Big Data, Cloud and Parallel Computing (COMITCon), pp.289–294 (2019). doi:10.1109/COMITCon.2019.8862448

3 Deep Learning and Human Vision in IoT

Jimmy Mehta, Yaman Hooda, Haobam Derit Singh, and Sahil Mehta

3.1 INTRODUCTION

Deep learning and human vision are two interrelated concepts that contribute significantly to the Internet of Things (IoT) landscape. Deep learning is a subset of machine learning that involves training multi-layered artificial neural networks (deep architectures) to learn patterns from data and make predictions or decisions [4, 6]. Human vision refers to the visual perception process in humans, including object recognition, motion detection, and depth perception. The integration of deep learning and human vision into the IoT has resulted in transformative applications that leverage visual data to improve understanding, decision making, and interaction [1, 3, 5, 8–30]. A breakdown of the technical aspects of this integration follows:

- *Image and video data in IoT:*
  IoT devices, such as cameras and sensors, collect large amounts of image and video data from the environment. This visual data can be rich in information and context, allowing applications to mimic human visual perception.
- *Deep learning for feature extraction:*
  Convolutional neural networks (CNNs), in particular, are excellent at extracting hierarchical characteristics from images using deep learning models. These models learn to recognize edges, textures, forms, and even intricate patterns inside images in the context of human vision. CNNs may automatically identify pertinent features for IoT applications from unprocessed visual data without the need for explicit feature engineering.
- *Classification and recognition:*
  The classification and recognition of objects is one of the most important uses of deep learning and human vision in IoT. Deep learning models can be taught to identify and categorize objects in frames of pictures or videos. Security (intruder detection), retail (product identification), healthcare (medical image analysis), and other fields all make use of these capabilities.
- *Motion detection and tracking:*
  Deep learning models have the capacity to examine sequential visual input in order to identify motion and track moving objects. This is essential in applications like surveillance where tracking things over time is necessary to spot anomalies or suspect activity. Long short-term memory (LSTM) networks and recurrent neural networks are two examples of designs that can deal with sequential data, such as video frames [1, 2].
- *Depth perception and 3D construction*:
  Another aspect of human vision that can be replicated in IoT with deep learning is depth perception, which is essential for comprehending spatial relationships. Neural networks are able to estimate depth information and rebuild 3D scenes by processing stereo images or utilizing depth sensors. This has uses in robots, autonomous navigation, virtual reality, and augmented reality.

DOI: 10.1201/9781003451846-3

- *Interaction that is human-centric*:
  Natural human–device interaction is made possible by IoT deep learning and human vision. IoT devices are capable of deducing emotions, movements, and even facial expressions from visual information. Applications like emotion-aware user interfaces, gesture-controlled smart home appliances, and accessibility options for those with disabilities result from this.
- *Edge computing on a real-time basis:*
  IoT devices frequently have limited resources and may be unable to send all data to the cloud for processing owing to latency issues. This is where edge computing for real-time analysis comes in. Deep learning models can be implemented at the edge, enabling on-device real-time analysis and decision-making. This is especially helpful for applications like autonomous driving or industrial automation that call for quick reactions.
- *Transfer learning and pre-trained models:*
  Deep learning models can be tailored for particular IoT applications with smaller datasets after being trained on large datasets. Utilizing pre-trained models through transfer learning speeds up training and enhances performance. This is especially helpful in situations when it is difficult to acquire huge labelled datasets.

Also, increasingly important are privacy and security as IoT devices collect visual data. By enabling on-device processing, deep learning can assist in lowering the need to transfer sensitive data. Without centralized data, methods like federated learning enable model training across remote devices. Artificial intelligence known as "deep learning" mimics how the human brain generates signals and organizes data for use in decision-making. Other names for it include deep neural learning and deep neural networks. Deep learning networks may learn from unlabeled or unstructured data without supervision. Simply speaking, deep learning is a type of algorithm that appears to be particularly effective at anticipating events. Deep learning is built on the concept of recurrent training. It teaches the computer to identify a voice or image and to comprehend a particular pattern. When the computer recognizes a word or voice, it can automatically pick it up.

Machine learning techniques employ labelled sample data to uncover patterns, while deep learning algorithms use huge volumes of data as input and analyses it to extract features from an object. Deep learning is required to maintain model performance since machine learning algorithms performance degrades as data volume rises.

3.1.1 Why Is Classical Machine Learning Less Effective Than Deep Learning?

Practically speaking, machine learning and deep learning complement one other, but not the other way around. In situations where the dataset is modest and well curated, or when the data has undergone appropriate preprocessing, machine learning can be effective. Data preparation necessitates human input. Additionally, it implies that machine learning algorithms would underfit and fail to extract information from huge, complicated datasets. Machine learning is typically referred to as shallow learning since it is so successful with tiny datasets. On the other hand, deep learning is quite effective with large datasets.

3.2 IMPORTANCE OF HUMAN VISION IN IoT SYSTEMS

The integration of human vision into Internet of Things systems holds significant importance in enhancing the overall functionality, user experience, and real-world applications of these interconnected devices. Human vision, as a sensory input, enables IoT systems to interact with and understand the physical environment, facilitating improved decision-making, automation, and human–machine collaboration [3–5, 8–30].

1. *Environmental perception and contextual awareness:*
   Human vision provides IoT systems with the ability to perceive and interpret their surroundings. Cameras and other visual sensors can capture real-time images and videos, allowing IoT devices to understand the context, detect objects, recognize faces, assess environmental conditions, and even anticipate potential risks or anomalies. This contextual awareness enables smarter and more responsive actions.
2. *Object detection and recognition:*
   Human vision is crucial for object detection and recognition in IoT applications. Cameras integrated into IoT devices can identify objects like vehicles, pedestrians, obstacles, and equipment. This capability is vital in various domains such as smart transportation, security, retail, and manufacturing, where object recognition helps in automating processes, ensuring safety, and enhancing operational efficiency.
3. *Enhanced user experience:*
   Human vision integration enhances the user experience by enabling intuitive interactions with IoT systems. Visual interfaces, augmented reality (AR), and virtual reality (VR) experiences become possible, making interactions more natural and user-friendly. For instance, smart home devices with cameras allow users to remotely monitor their homes and control various functionalities through visual interfaces.
4. *Safety and security application:*
   Human vision-enabled IoT systems play a pivotal role in safety and security applications. Surveillance cameras, coupled with advanced image analysis algorithms, enable real-time monitoring of public spaces, homes, and industrial environments. Intrusion detection, facial recognition, and anomaly detection are some of the applications that contribute to ensuring safety and preventing potential threats.
5. *Healthcare and medical applications:*
   IoT systems equipped with human vision capabilities find applications in the healthcare sector. Remote patient monitoring, telemedicine, and assisted living scenarios are facilitated by cameras that monitor patients' conditions and help healthcare providers make informed decisions. In surgical settings, IoT-assisted tools can enhance precision and enable remote collaboration.
6. *Data-driven decision making:*
   Human vision data collected by IoT devices can be processed and analyzed to generate valuable insights. Patterns, trends, and correlations in visual data can aid in optimizing processes, improving resource allocation, and predicting future trends. This data-driven approach enhances decision-making in various domains, from agriculture to urban planning.
7. *Collaboration between humans and machines:*
   By integrating human vision capabilities, IoT systems can better collaborate with humans. For instance, drones with cameras can be deployed for tasks like search and rescue operations, infrastructure inspection, and environmental monitoring. These machines can assist humans by providing visual information from hard-to-reach or hazardous areas.

In conclusion, the integration of human vision into IoT systems brings a multitude of benefits, ranging from enhanced contextual understanding to improved safety, user experience, and collaboration between humans and machines. This synergy between IoT and human vision has the potential to revolutionize various industries and domains, paving the way for smarter, more connected, and more efficient systems.

3.3 CHALLENGES AND OPPORTUNITIES IN COMBINING DEEP LEARNING AND HUMAN VISION FOR IoT

Combining deep learning and human vision within the context of IoT presents a dynamic landscape filled with both challenges and opportunities. The synergy of these two technologies holds great promise in enhancing the capabilities of IoT systems, enabling richer interactions and more intelligent decision-making [6, 7]. However, several technical hurdles must be overcome to fully harness their potential.

3.3.1 Challenges

The use of human vision data for deep learning in IoT raises significant privacy and security concerns. The collection and transmission of visual information requires strong encryption, data anonymization, and secure storage to prevent unauthorized access and potential breaches. Bandwidth and latency: IoT devices often operate in resource-constrained environments with limited bandwidth and processing power. Transferring high-resolution image data for deep learning analysis can exhaust network resources and cause latency, affecting real-time applications. Energy efficiency: Deep learning models, especially those involving complex neural architectures, require significant computational resources. Balancing the power-hungry nature of deep learning algorithms with the power limitations of IoT devices remains a significant challenge. Embedding deep learning into IoT devices requires lightweight models that can run efficiently on limited hardware. Developing and implementing such models without loss of accuracy poses a challenge due to the inherent complexity of deep neural networks. Also, IoT devices operate in diverse and dynamic environments where the lighting conditions, perspective, and appearance of objects can change dramatically. Ensuring the robustness and adaptability of deep learning models to these changing scenarios is a constant challenge.

3.3.2 Opportunities

The various opportunities are summarized in Figure 3.1.

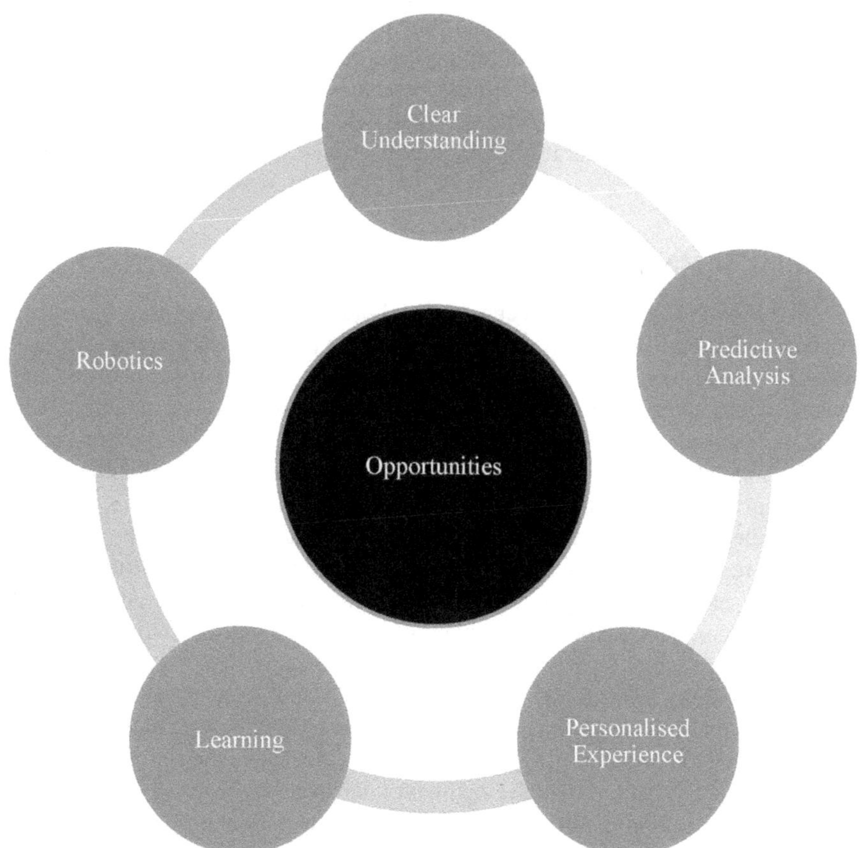

FIGURE 3.1 Opportunities after combining deep learning and human vision.

1. *Understanding context:*
   Human vision enabled by deep learning enables IoT devices to comprehend the context of their surroundings. Contextual knowledge improves situational awareness, anomaly detection, and object recognition, improving decision-making efficiency.
2. *Predictive analytics:*
   Deep learning models can find patterns and trends that humans might miss by analyzing visual data. With the use of this predictive capabilities, proactive measures can be made in response to user behaviour, environmental changes, and potential dangers.
3. *Personalized experience:*
   IoT systems can adapt user interfaces based on visual inputs by integrating deep learning with human vision. Smart homes, retail, and healthcare can all benefit from this personalization, which raises customer pleasure and engagement.
4. *Continuous learning:*
   Deep learning models can be made to learn and adapt continually as situations change, which will increase their accuracy and flexibility. The durability and efficiency of IoT systems are improved by this cycle of constant learning.
5. *Collaboration between humans and robots:*
   The combination of deep learning with human vision can result in cooperative interactions between people and technology. For instance, robots with these qualities can help people in challenging situations or dangerous settings.

Also, edge intelligence enables IoT devices to perform real-time analysis locally without constant dependency on cloud resources by combining edge computing and deep learning. This improves application responsiveness by lowering latency and bandwidth utilization. In conclusion, the integration of deep learning and human vision into IoT systems presents a range of fascinating opportunities for revolutionizing a number of different fields and sectors. Even though issues like privacy, resource shortages, and model complexity still exist, overcoming these obstacles paves the way for a time when IoT devices will be capable of sophisticated perception, cognition, and collaboration, which will ultimately change how we use and benefit from connected technologies.

3.4 MATERIAL SCIENCE AND THE IoT

The integration of the IoT into materials engineering holds the promise of transformative advancements in various fields. The convergence of these two fields allows for the creation of "smart materials" integrated with sensors and actuators, enabling real-time monitoring, analysis and adaptive response to conditions and environment changes. This synergy represents a paradigm shift in material design, manufacturing, and application, with potential benefits spanning several sectors. One of the key benefits of combining IoT with materials engineering is the improved ability to monitor the structural health of critical infrastructure. By embedding sensors into materials such as concrete, metal, or composites, engineers can continuously monitor parameters such as stress, strain, and temperature. This real-time data can aid in the early detection of potential structural weaknesses, enabling predictive maintenance strategies to optimize infrastructure life, reduce downtime, and improve safety. The combination of IoT and materials engineering also has important implications for the manufacturing sector. Smart materials can communicate their status during production, allowing for quick quality control and defect detection. Manufacturers can optimize production parameters based on real-time feedback, helping to increase productivity, reduce waste, and increase process efficiency. In addition, the ability of materials to self-regulate their properties in response to changing conditions could lead to the development of self-healing materials, minimizing the need for manual intervention and prolonging the life span and product durability. In the healthcare sector, IoT-integrated materials offer revolutionary possibilities. Implantable medical devices could become "intelligent implantable devices," providing continuous physiological data and alerting healthcare providers of abnormalities. This real-time monitoring can lead to personalized treatment and early intervention strategies. In addition, wearable sensors embedded in tissue could enable remote health monitoring, enabling proactive healthcare management and early disease detection. The fusion of the IoT and materials engineering also has the potential to revolutionize sustainability and environmental sensing efforts. Smart materials can be designed to detect pollutants, monitor air and water quality, and even harness energy from the environment. This paves the way for real-time environmental monitoring, informed policy decisions, and the development of environmentally friendly energy extraction technologies. However, this convergence also poses challenges. Material design with embedded sensors requires consideration of factors such as power source and communication protocols and compatibility with the manufacturing process. Ensuring data security and privacy is paramount in an interconnected hardware ecosystem. Furthermore, the integration of IoT technologies creates complexity in terms of system integration, data interpretation, and decision making. In conclusion, merging IoT with materials engineering heralds a new era of innovation in various industries. The ability to create smart materials that can sense, communicate, and adapt offers a range of benefits from improved infrastructure resilience and manufacturing efficiency to advanced healthcare and management. While challenges remain, the potential rewards are transformative, driving the development of smarter, more responsive materials that will shape the future of technology and society.

3.5 VISUAL PERCEPTION PROCESSES

Visual perception is a complex process by which the human brain interprets and understands visual information gathered from the environment. It involves several interconnected processes (Figure 3.2).

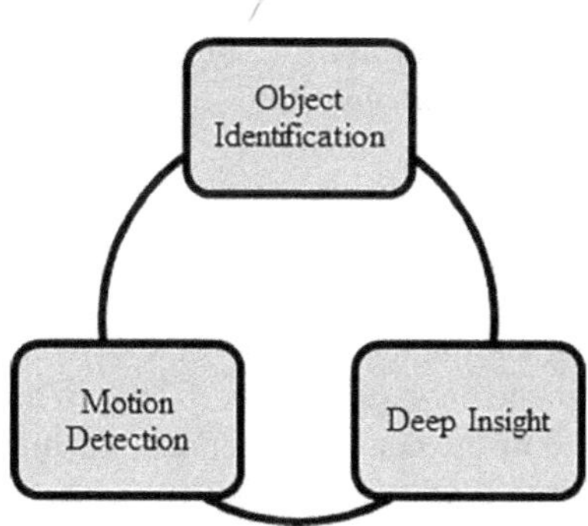

FIGURE 3.2 Distinguished segments of a typical GPS system.

1. *Object identification:*

   Object recognition is the ability to identify and classify objects present in a visual scene. The process is based on a combination of low-level functionality (such as edges, textures, and colors) and high-level functionality (such as shapes, patterns, and context). The visual cortex, especially the ventral tegmental area, plays an important role in processing these features. Neurons in this area are selectively tuned to respond to specific patterns, allowing for the recognition of familiar objects. Object recognition involves complex computational mechanisms, such as hierarchical processing. In this process, image information flows through different layers of neurons, with each layer detecting increasingly complex features. Deep neural networks, inspired by brain processing, have successfully mimicked this hierarchical feature extraction for tasks such as image classification and object detection.

2. *Motion detection:*

   Motion detection involves determining the movement of objects in the visual field. This process is essential for understanding the dynamics of the environment and detecting potential threats or changes. Motion-sensing neurons, called "motion sensors" or "optical flow sensors," are located in the visual regions of the brain, including the medial temporal region (MT) and the temporal region above (MST). Motion detection can be explained by concepts like the "aperture problem" and "matching problem". Aperture problems arise when the direction of the subject's movement is not clear based on the local area of the visual field. The brain overcomes this by integrating information from multiple directions to infer the actual motion of the object. The matching problem involves matching the features of the same object on different images to track its movement over time. Computer algorithms, such as optical flow estimation and tracking, simulate these processes and are used in applications such as video analytics and self-driving cars.
3. *Deep insight*:

   Depth perception is the ability to perceive the relative distance of objects from the viewer. The brain does this by using signals from monocular (one eye) and binocular (both eyes) vision. Monocular cues include perspective, relative size, shadows, and texture gradients. Binocular signs, like binocular disparity, occur due to slight separation between the eyes, causing each eye to receive a slightly different image of the same scene. Stereopsis is the most well-known binocular signal, which relies on the brain comparing the difference in images received by the two eyes to determine the depth of an object. The process is computationally complex, involving precise matching of features between two images to calculate disparities. Depth perception is critical for tasks such as navigation, object manipulation, and 3D scene reconstruction in computer vision.

Overall, visual perception processes such as object recognition, motion detection, and depth perception are complex and multifaceted. They involve the interaction of neural circuits, feature extraction, hierarchical processing, and computational algorithms to understand the visual world and enable us to navigate and interact efficiently.

3.5.1 Emerging Trends in Deep Learning and Human Vision in the IoT

Emerging trends in deep learning and human vision in the context of the IoT are leading to innovative applications and advancements in various fields. These trends leverage the synergy between deep learning techniques, inspired by the neural networks of the human brain and the capabilities of IoT devices. Let's explore these trends with examples:

1. *Edge computing for real-time processing:*

   IoT devices generate huge amounts of data, and sending all that data to the cloud for processing can cause latency issues. Deep learning models are increasingly efficient and can run on edge devices, allowing real-time data processing at the source. In the context of human vision, peripherals equipped with deep learning algorithms can perform tasks like object detection and facial recognition without requiring a persistent cloud connection. For example, a security camera equipped with a deep learning model can identify intruders and send an immediate alert to the owner or security officer.
2. *Human-centered surveillance*:

   IoT devices equipped with cameras and sensors can be used to monitor human health and activity. Deep learning algorithms can analyze video streams to detect gestures, emotions, and even vital signs. In the healthcare sector, wearable devices can analyze a person's gait and posture to detect abnormalities that may indicate a risk of falling. This information can be important for care or rehabilitation programs for the elderly.

3. *Improved accessibility:*

   Deep learning enables IoT devices to improve accessibility for visually impaired people. The wearable's camera can record the environment, and deep learning models can process this visual data to provide auditory or tactile feedback to the user. For example, a wearable camera can identify subjects, read text, and describe scenes to visually impaired users.
4. *Image quality control and anomaly detection:*

   Deep learning algorithms improve intuitive quality control processes in manufacturing. IoT-connected cameras can capture product images, and deep learning models can quickly analyze those images to detect errors, ensuring consistent quality. For example, in the automotive industry, IoT-enabled cameras can identify paint defects or structural irregularities on an assembly line.
5. *Retail analytics and personalized advertising:*

   IoT devices in retail environments, such as smart shelves and cameras, can collect data about customer behavior. Deep learning models can analyze this data to understand customer preferences, optimize store layouts, and personalize ads. For example, smart shelves equipped with cameras and deep learning algorithms can determine when products are out of stock and automatically place orders with suppliers. Also, IoT-enabled materials analysis is used in wearable devices and smart fabrics to improve user experience. Wearable devices may include sensors that monitor vital signs, body temperature, and movement. Smart fabrics can incorporate sensors that monitor sweat composition or skin response. This data is transmitted to a smartphone or cloud platform for analysis, allowing users to monitor health, adjust activity, or receive real-time alerts.
6. *Smart cities and traffic management:*

   IoT devices in smart city environments can monitor traffic flow and pedestrian movements. Deep learning models can process this data to optimize traffic signals and improve overall traffic management. In human vision, these models can analyze video feeds to detect traffic violations or accidents in real time, allowing for faster responses from emergency services. Also, IoT-enabled materials analysis is used in structural health monitoring of buildings, bridges, and other infrastructure. Sensors embedded in concrete, steel or other building materials can continuously monitor factors such as tension, stress, temperature, and humidity. These sensors transmit data wirelessly to a central server for analysis. This real-time data helps engineers assess the structural integrity of their infrastructure, detect potential failures, and predict maintenance needs. For example, if a bridge's concrete sensors detect increased pressure due to heavy traffic, engineers can take proactive measures to prevent possible damage or breakdown. In manufacturing, IoT-based materials analysis can improve quality control processes. Sensors can be integrated into the production line to monitor various material properties during the production process. For example, sensors can measure the temperature, viscosity, and composition of materials during the production of polymers or chemicals. Real-time data analytics can help manufacturers identify deviations from desired specifications and adjust production parameters accordingly. This ensures consistent product quality and reduces waste.
7. *Interaction of natural language with visual data:*

   IoT devices equipped with cameras and microphones can collect visual and auditory data. Deep learning models can combine these methods to enable natural language interaction with visual data. For example, users can ask questions about what they see through wearables, and deep learning models can provide well-informed answers. These emerging trends illustrate the convergence of deep learning and human vision in the IoT ecosystem.
8. *Agriculture and precision farming:*

   IoT-enabled materials analysis is used in precision agriculture to optimize crop growth. Soil sensors can measure moisture, nutrient content, and pH in soil. This data is fed to a cloud platform where analytics and machine learning algorithms help farmers make informed decisions about irrigation, fertilization, and crop rotation. By adopting farming practices tailored to specific soil conditions, farmers can achieve higher yields while conserving resources.

3.5.2 IoT Technologies for Sustainable Development

The rapid advancement of information technologies has led to the need for "energy digitalization" in a certain context. To achieve global energy transition goals in the coming decades, it will be crucial to increasingly implement renewable energy technologies and formulate effective policies, as highlighted. Building upon this idea, the exploration of alternative renewable energy sources holds significant value.

In recent years, various energy scenarios or possibilities have been examined. These scenarios involve a significant portion of renewables through hybrid energy solutions. Additionally, there's consideration for applying alternative energy sources like hydrogen technologies across different sectors, including applications in vehicles. The research primarily aims to assess the technical and economic feasibility of diverse energy concepts to establish an optimal mix of technologies that can facilitate a seamless energy transition.

IoT-enabled materials analysis contributes to environmental monitoring by analyzing air and water quality. Sensors located in urban areas can measure contaminants such as particles, volatile organic compounds, and gases. Data from these sensors is transmitted to a central database for analysis. This information helps local authorities act quickly to reduce pollution levels and improve public health. For example, if air quality sensors detect high levels of pollution near a plant, regulators can step in to enforce emissions control measures.

Energy and environmental considerations are pivotal in smart cities, often interconnected concepts.

3.5.2.1 Summary

By combining IoT device capabilities with complex deep learning algorithms, industries are poised to create transformative applications that enhance the human experience, improve efficiency, and drive innovation in many different industries. In conclusion, the IoT ecosystem holds enormous potential for developing intelligent and observant applications thanks to the merging of deep learning and human vision. IoT devices can gain valuable insights from visual data by simulating features of human visual perception and using deep learning's capabilities, which will improve interaction, automation, and decision-making across a variety of areas.

REFERENCES

[1] Chun Y., Kwan M.-P., Griffith D.A. Uncertainty and context in GIScience and geography: challenges in the era of geospatial big data. *Int. J. Geogr. Inf. Sci.* 2019;33(6):1131–1134. https://doi.org/10.1080/13658816.2019.1566552.

[2] Murray A.T., Grubesic T.H., Wei R., Mack E.A. A hybrid geocoding methodology for spatio-temporal data. 2015. https://doi.org/10.1111/j.1467-9671.2011.01289.x.

[3] Hooda Y. IoT and Remote Sensing. In *Computer Vision and Internet of Things*. Taylor & Francis Group; USA: 2022, pp. 111–140.

[4] Hooda Y., Singh H.D. Digital Reforms in Public Services and Infrastructure Development & Management. In *Technological Prospects and Social Applications of Society 5.0*. Taylor & Francis Group; USA: 2023, pp. 219–237.

[5] Singh H.D., Hooda Y. Resilience of Digital Society to Natural Disasters. In *Technological Prospects and Social Applications of Society 5.0*. Taylor & Francis Group; USA: 2023, pp. 185–199.

[6] Hooda Y., Kuhar P., Sharma K., Verma, N.K. Emerging applications of artificial intelligence in structural engineering and construction industry. *J. Phys. Conf. Ser.* 2021;1950(1):012062. https://doi.org/10.1088/1742-6596/1950/1/012062.

[7] Kuhar P., Sharma K., Hooda Y., Verma N. Internet of things (IoT) based smart helmet for construction. *J. Phys. Conf. Ser.* 2021;1950:012075.

[8] Sharma, L., & Carpenter, M. (Eds.). (2022). Computer Vision and Internet of Things: Technologies and Applications (1st ed.). Chapman and Hall/CRC. https://doi.org/10.1201/9781003244165
[9] Lavanya Sharma, "Computer-Aided Lung Cancer Detection and Classification of CT Images Using Convolutional Neural Network", Computer Vision and Internet of Things: Technologies and Applications", Taylor & Francis, CRC Press, pp. 247–262, May 2022.
[10] Lavanya Sharma, "Analysis of Machine Learning Techniques for Airfare Prediction", Computer Vision and Internet of Things: Technologies and Applications", Taylor & Francis, CRC Press, pp. 211–231, May 2022.
[11] Lavanya Sharma, "Innovation and Emerging Computer Vision and Artificial Intelligence Technologies in Coronavirus Control", Computer Vision and Internet of Things: Technologies and Applications", Taylor & Francis, CRC Press, pp. 177–192, May 2022.
[12] Lavanya Sharma, "Self-Driving Cars: Tools and Technologies", Computer Vision and Internet of Things: Technologies and Applications", Taylor & Francis, CRC Press, pp. 99–110, May 2022.
[13] Lavanya Sharma, "Computer Vision in Surgical Operating Theatre and Medical Imaging", Computer Vision and Internet of Things: Technologies and Applications", Taylor & Francis, CRC Press, pp. 75–96, May 2022.
[14] Lavanya Sharma, "Preventing Security Breach in Social Media: Threats and Prevention Techniques", Computer Vision and Internet of Things: Technologies and Applications", Taylor & Francis, CRC Press, pp. 53–62, May 2022.
[15] Lavanya Sharma, Mukesh Carpenter, "Use of Robotics in Real-Time Applications", Computer Vision and Internet of Things: Technologies and Applications", Taylor & Francis, CRC Press, pp. 41–50, May 2022.
[16] Lavanya Sharma et.al., "An Overview of Security Issues of Internet of Things", Computer Vision and Internet of Things: Technologies and Applications", Taylor & Francis, CRC Press, pp. 29–40, May 2022.
[17] Lavanya sharma, "Rise of Computer Vision and Internet of Things", Computer Vision and Internet of Things: Technologies and Applications", Taylor & Francis, CRC Press, pp. 5–17, May 2022.
[18] Lavanya sharma, "Human Detection and Tracking Using Background Subtraction in Visual Surveillance", Towards Smart World: Homes to Cities using Internet of Things", Taylor & Francis, CRC Press, pp. 317–329, December 2020.
[19] Lavanya sharma, "The Rise of Internet of Things and Smart Cities", Towards Smart World: Homes to Cities using Internet of Things", Taylor & Francis, CRC Press, pp. 1–19, December 2020.
[20] Lavanya sharma, "The Future of Smart Cities", Towards Smart World: Homes to Cities using Internet of Things", Taylor & Francis, CRC Press, pp. 1–19, December 2020.
[21] Lavanya Sharma, Nirvikar Lohan, "Internet of things with object detection", in Handbook of Research on Big Data and the IoT, IGI Global, pp. 89–100, March, 2019. (ISBN: 9781522574323, DOI: 10.4018/978-1-5225-7432-3.ch006).
[22] Lavanya Sharma, "The Rise of the Visual Surveillance to Internet of Things", From Visual Surveillance to Internet of Things", Taylor & Francis, CRC Press, October 2019.
[23] Lavanya Sharma, P K Garg "Block based Adaptive Learning Rate for Moving Person Detection in Video Surveillance", From Visual Surveillance to Internet of Things, Taylor & Francis, CRC Press, October 2019.
[24] Lavanya Sharma, P K Garg "Smart E-healthcare with Internet of Things: Current Trends Challenges, Solutions and Technologies", From Visual Surveillance to Internet of Things, Taylor & Francis, CRC Press, October 2019.
[25] Lavanya Sharma, P K Garg, Naman Agarwal "A foresight on e-healthcare Trailblazers", From Visual Surveillance to Internet of Things", Taylor & Francis, CRC Press, October 2019.
[26] Lavanya Sharma, P K Garg "IoT and its applications", From Visual Surveillance to Internet of Things, Taylor & Francis, CRC Press, October 2019.
[27] Lavanya Sharma, P K Garg "Future of Internet of Things", From Visual Surveillance to Internet of Things, Taylor & Francis, CRC Press, October 2019.
[28] Jha G., Sharma L., Gupta S. (2021) Future of Augmented Reality in Healthcare Department. In: Singh P.K., Wierzchoń S.T., Tanwar S., Ganzha M., Rodrigues J.J.P.C. (eds) Proceedings of Second International Conference on Computing, Communications, and Cyber-Security. Lecture Notes in Networks and Systems, vol 203. Springer, Singapore. https://doi.org/10.1007/978-981-16-0733-2_47).
[29] Jha G., Sharma L., Gupta S. (2021) E-health in Internet of Things (IoT) in Real-Time Scenario. In: Singh P.K., Wierzchoń S.T., Tanwar S., Ganzha M., Rodrigues J.J.P.C. (eds) Proceedings of Second International Conference on Computing, Communications, and Cyber-Security. Lecture Notes in Networks and Systems, vol 203. Springer, Singapore. https://doi.org/10.1007/978-981-16-0733-2_48
[30] S. Sharma, S. Verma, M. Kumar and L. Sharma, "Use of Motion Capture in 3D Animation: Motion Capture Systems, Challenges, and Recent Trends," 2019 International Conference on Machine Learning, Big Data, Cloud and Parallel Computing (COMITCon), 2019, pp. 289–294, doi:10.1109/COMITCon.2019.8862448

4 Impact of IoT on Big Data Analytics and Applications in Medical Images

Sudhriti Sengupta, Lavanya Sharma, and Mukesh Carpenter

4.1 INTRODUCTION

The Internet of Things (IoT) has become very important in our daily lives and is anticipated to have a significant impact on many aspects of modern society. For instance, immediate traffic flow solutions, reminders about car maintenance, and energy consumption reduction are all possible. Monitoring sensors will identify upcoming maintenance problems and possibly set maintenance worker agendas. Data analysis systems will make it easier for urban areas to manage traffic, waste, pollution, law enforcement, and other essential amenities efficiently. Many apps, from e-mail to e-learning, are popular and have improved otherwise time-consuming processes. Technology is advancing to seamlessly incorporate itself into human routine. The ability to develop a variety of applications that can simplify and facilitate complex operations across multiple sectors has been made possible by the digital environment [1]. The main challenges with the IoT are system complexity, memory usage, volume, integrity, and confidentiality. The complexity of the system is going to rise due to the significant amount of interconnections. The dimensions of the IoT will be an important concern. Directly obtaining sensitive personal data, such as a person's precise geographic location, bank account details, or health information, may put their confidentiality at risk. Big data can be used to leverage this data-driven nature and help with other IoT challenges. The IoT is essentially the result of the fusion of micro-electromechanical systems, microservices, wireless technologies, and the internet. The merger helps to create a bridge between operational and informational technology, allowing for the analysis of data generated by machines on a technological platform. Big data also denotes a significant amount of both structured and unstructured data that is connected to daily living. The amount of data that can be created and preserved globally in this situation is significant. Businesses will keep continuing to receive data, and additional devices will soon merge with the IoT. Therefore, the key to corporate growth will be knowing ways to use IoT app development to harness commercial value and use data to inform decisions [2]. In general, the merging of big data and the IoT has the potential of setting up new commercial opportunities across all sectors of the financial system. This chapter focuses primarily on the impacts on medical images, which helps in providing better healthcare to patients. Medical images are important aspects which help doctors and healthcare providers diagnose diseases timely and correctly. Medical imaging data is collected for a variety of uses, including biomedical research, intraoperative navigation, planned therapies, and post-operative monitoring. Medical images often have poor visual quality, which gives incorrect information and diagnoses for treatment. Images taken during the acquisition process are susceptible to electromagnetic disturbances, have uneven brightness, and produce some artifacts [26–35]. There could be noise, labels, or low-contrast artifacts. This chapter serves as a study of these emerging fields of study by addressing the most recent developments in IoT and big data technology, especially applied to medical images. This chapter is divided into the following sections: Section 4.2 discusses the techniques and application of IoT,

DOI: 10.1201/9781003451846-4

along with connectivity and IoT deployment. Big data analytics and applications are discussed as a part of Section 4.3. Section 4.4 elaborates on the impact of big data in IoT technology consisting of applications and processing. The role of deep learning in medical images to utilize medical images effectively and properly is discussed in Section 4.5. Section 4.6 discusses the various challenges in IoT merged with big data application, followed by a conclusion.

4.2 TECHNIQUES AND APPLICATION USED IN IoT

The IoT is a network of physical items (things) that interact and exchange data with other devices and systems through the internet using software, actuators, sensors, and other technologies. These devices range from domestic equipment to industrial tools. Experts predict that by 2025, there will be an estimated 22 billion connected IoT devices, an increase over the current total, which is approximately 7 billion. The two fundamental components of the Internet of Things are "things," which refers to objects and physical equipment, and "Internet," which serves as the foundation for connectivity. It allows the real-world utilization of physical things to benefit from the potential of the Internet for processing and analyzing data. Wearable health monitors to continually monitor a patient's condition, connected appliances for a better lifestyle, autonomous agricultural equipment introducing precision farming, enhanced energy management systems, and sophisticated surveillance are some of the very common examples of IoT usage [35–44]. The advancement of the use of the IoT in various fields is possible due to low-cost computers, cloud technology, big data, and mobile technologies that enable the sharing and collection of data by tangible things with very little human involvement. Digital systems can record, monitor, and modify every interaction between connected things in today's hyper-connected surroundings [3, 4].

Although the concept of the IoT has been around for a long time, some recent technological advancements have made this concept practical. Some of these are:

1. Low-cost, effective, and reliable sensors.
2. A wide range of network protocols for the internet to enable linking sensors to the cloud and other "things" for effective data transfer.
3. Cloud platforms, which are available to facilitate providing infrastructure for IoT implementation.
4. Different data analytics tools to utilize the IoT.
5. Natural language processing to make IoT devices accessible to general users.
6. Security technology to protect IoT authentication and integrity.

A device that is capable of transmitting data over a network with the least amount of human involvement is the basic component of IoT. These IoT devices can be classified into two distinct categories.

- Devices that collect and send information:
  - A method used for collecting data from non-computer sources is sensors. They convert the physical components of our surroundings into electrical signals that computers are able to comprehend. Examples include motion sensors, radiation sensors, air temperature sensors, and soil moisture sensors. The IoT ensures that the previously disconnected elements are connected in a significant way because of sensors of all varieties.
- Things or devices that receive and utilize data collected by sensors.
  - There are several instances of technological devices that collect data and then respond accordingly. A printer, for instance, accepts a document and prints it. Another is that a door opens when a car gets signals from car keys.

4.2.1 Technological Aspects of the IoT

IoT technology encompasses the devices, applications, tools, sensors, and software essential to facilitate IoT user applications. Anything from medical equipment to smartphones, watches to security cameras, and even factory production lines may be made smart with the help of IoT technology. In order to stop internet-based attacks on networked devices and their applications, IoT technologies also feature security tools. IoT system development is a challenging process. The IoT integrates software and hardware into a simple, unified integration that is ready for implementation or further development to speed up the design process and improve product development [5].

- **Availability of inexpensive, lightweight sensor technology**: More businesses are able to employ IoT technology as a result of reasonably priced and trustworthy sensors.
- **Interconnection**: Using a wide variety of Internet network protocols, sensors can be linked easily to the cloud and other things.
- **Cloud computing:** Organizations and users are able to acquire the infrastructure they need to scale up without having to manage it all as a result of the growing number of cloud platforms.
- **Data analytics and machine learning:** Improvements in machine learning and analytics, as well as access to a wide variety and volume of data stored on the cloud, help organizations to get insights faster and efficiently.
- **Artificial intelligence (AI):** Internet of Things devices, such as digital personal assistants like Alexa, Cortana, and Siri, provide access to natural language processing (NLP). Internet of Things devices are becoming more appealing, useful, and affordable for use at home.

4.2.2 IoT Connectivity

IoT connectivity refers to the process by which an IoT device connects to the cloud and other devices like gateways. Examples of IoT devices can range from a simple sensor in a factory to a self-driving car. There are many different IoT connectivity standards available for businesses to choose from due to the dispersed nature of the Internet of Things implementations. Coverage, energy efficiency, and data throughput are the three key technical requirements for any organization considering Internet of Things connectivity. These are trade-offs that every technology faces, so no particular technology can be the best in every one of these areas. Organizations ought to speculate about where their IoT services will be offered. A connectivity technology that is widely used demands global IoT connectivity. For a comprehensive study, there are three types of IoT connectivity:

1. Traditional cellular technology: Some examples are 2G, 3G, 4G, and 5G. With architectures that are designed for broad consumer voice and data service, its strengths are in data rate (especially 4G, 5G).
2. Short-range technology: Bluetooth Low Energy (BLE) and ZigBee are examples of short-range technologies that value data rate and battery life over connection range.
3. Low power wide area (LPWA): This technology provides better coverage and battery life. However, its main drawback is its lower data transfer rate. Examples are NB-IoT and LTE-M.

IoT connectivity should be selected after carefully analyzing the specifics of each deployment. Very high speed and extremely low latency communication are necessary in some cases. This could result in the adoption of 5G or 4G cellular IoT connectivity. Low-speed connections that are not constantly active may be useful for some modest deployments since they require smaller batteries and provide IoT connectivity at a reasonable cost [6, 7].

4.2.3 Application of the IoT

The Internet of Things is among the most important recent innovations. With its integrated technology, ordinary items like thermostats, baby monitors, and kitchen appliances can link to the internet. Seamless communication between people, processes, and things is now achievable through this technology. Subsequently, there are many domains using IoT in their business processes to streamline productivity and provide better customer satisfaction and feedback [8, 9].

Categorically, applications of the IoT can be divided into consumer, commercial, industrial, and infrastructure spaces. Healthcare is a predominant area of utilization of the IoT. The IoT explores novel aspects of patient care through real-time health monitoring and access to patient health data. Real-time monitoring via connected devices can save lives in the event of a medical emergency such as heart failure, diabetes, or asthma attack. Research in various areas can also be conducted using the IoT. It's because the IoT makes it possible for us to gather vast amounts of data regarding the patient's illness that would have taken many years to gather otherwise. This information can then be used for statistical analysis to aid in the advancement of any kind of research. In case of education, the IoT helps in advancement of teaching and learning skills. Using connected gadgets like digital highlighters and interactive whiteboards, students can now connect with peers, mentors, and educators anywhere worldwide in the comfort of their home or school. QR (quick response) codes have been integrated into textbooks. Students may quickly obtain feedback, assignments, notes, and other knowledge resources by scanning the QR codes with their smart phones. In the field of transportation and logistics, the IoT plays an inevitable role by optimal analysis of the flow of traffic through IoT devices at observation areas in roadways and transit. Improved customer satisfaction by monitoring and observing the pattern in acquiring and purchasing behavior can be analyzed by using IoT devices. This also leads to strategic advertisement to target consumers. Use of the IoT has also increased customer expectations. Users expect that IoT devices will adapt and improve services and abilities based on context from other parts of the world.

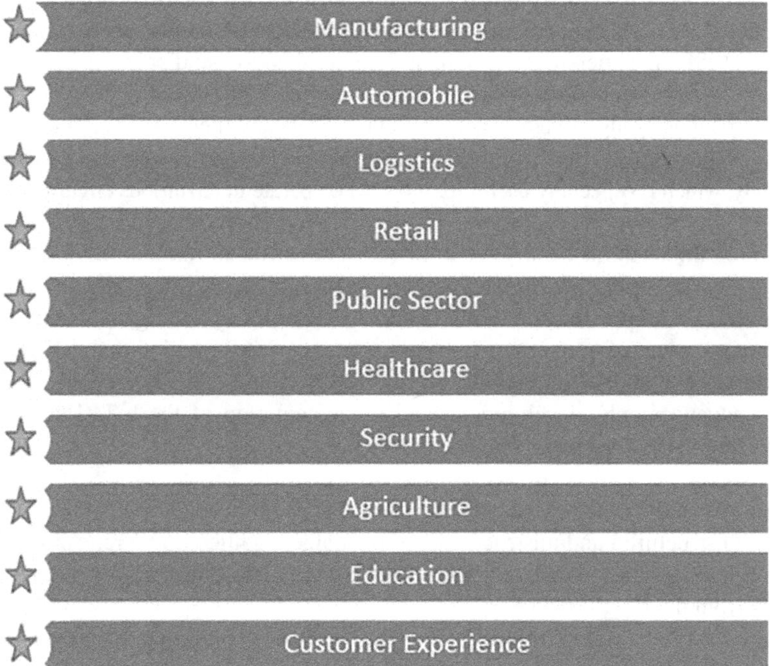

FIGURE 4.1 A range of IoT applications.

The Internet has altered the way people collaborate and interact. However, the advent of the Internet of Things has elevated this to a new level by concurrently connecting a variety of devices to the internet, enabling communication between machines as well as between machines and humans. Four primary components make up an IoT system: sensors/devices, data processing, connection, and a user interface. The device's inbuilt sensors gather data and then upload this data to the cloud using internet connectivity. After that, the software evaluates the data and executes tasks like sending an alert or setting devices autonomously. Finally, we can utilize the user interface to do any necessary modifications or activities per requirements [10].

4.2.4 IoT Deployment

Although acceptance rates for the IoT are increasing rapidly, a lot of businesses continue to find it difficult to deploy, install, and maintain IoT solutions that produce real business results. Many businesses get excited about the IoT's possibility, but many struggle to align their projects with defined business goals like improved operational effectiveness or new revenue-generating service offers. Investments in IoT initiatives that failed to generate profits were left stranded as a result [11]. The following factors must be taken into account in order to prevent wasted funds and negative perceptions toward the IoT inside the business:

- Machines can be monitored continuously to ensure they are working within the specified tolerances.
- Businesses can use tracking to find assets quickly. They can make sure that valuable items are protected from theft and removal.
- An example of the use of the IoT is to improve connected logistics for fleet management in terms of efficiency and safety. IoT fleet surveillance system can help businesses increase productivity by directing vehicles in real time.
- Because of the several layers of complexity at the device, network connectivity, and application levels, as well as the compatibility between each, IoT solution architectures are more complicated than the majority of traditional IT projects. A logical open systems interconnectivity (OSI) stack perspective or an architectural end-to-end perspective can be used to view architectures depending on the nature of applications.
- Internet of Things gadgets help customers better understand their own health and enable clinicians to monitor patients from a distance. Organizations can keep tabs on their employees' health and safety, which is especially useful for those who operate in hazardous circumstances [12].

Accumulation of information from government programs, local vendors, multinational agencies, and consumers led to better and more meaningful information anywhere and anytime, ushering in the era of the IoT. Vast repositories of data require a system for accessing, analyzing, and maintaining an enormous amount of both organized and unorganized information that is highly challenging using conventional methods. Big data and its various tools and techniques work in cooperation to deal with the advancements, development, and implementation of the IoT. The major steps in a workflow of using the IoT with big data are as follows:

1. Businesses install devices with embedded sensors for data collection and transfer.
2. Data, both structured and unstructured, or big data, is gathered in a repository.
3. AI-driven analysis is employed for producing reports, data visualizations, and other insights from data.
4. User devices provide more information through settings, planning, metadata, and various tangible transfers.

The next section aims to provide a detailed discussion on big data, sources of big data and its characteristics and applications [13].

4.3 BIG DATA

A standardized representation of facts, ideas, or instructions is referred to as data. Data is information that is accessible, informative, and usable in some way. Big data is a term used to describe extremely large data collections that can be computationally analyzed to identify patterns, trends, and relationships, especially those that relate to human conduct and interaction. Big data refers to larger, more intricate data sets, particularly from new sources. These data sets are so enormous that they are difficult for traditional data processing tools to handle. However, organizations may make use of these massive amounts of data to solve business problems that were previously impossible. Some instances of companies using big data are helping businesses to improve their advertising and marketing schemes and increase lead sales and consumer engagement, helpful to research how consumer and market behavior changes [14].

The main sources of big data are categorized into three main types, as depicted in Figure 4.2.

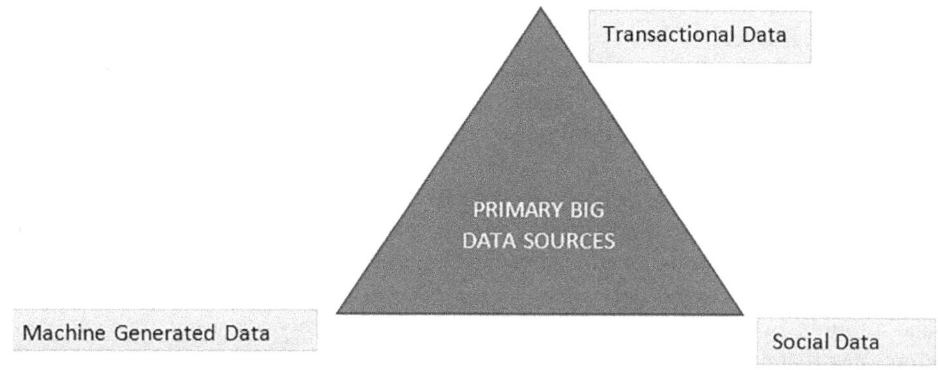

FIGURE 4.2 Sources of big data.

Transactional Data: Information gathered through online and offline transactions at different points of sale is commonly referred to as transactional data. The data comprises important details about transactions such as transaction time, location, products purchased, product pricing, payment methods, discounts/coupons applied, and many more. Some of the common sources of transactional data are payment orders, invoice, receipts, and other data used in transaction. This data is time sensitive; that is, this data will lose its importance with time. Transactional data requires special types of processing, analyzing, interpreting, and managing.

Machine Data: Machine data is information that is generated by a computer process or application activity without human supervision. This type of data is automatically generated as a response to a specific event or schedule. Machine data includes data collected by IoT sensors, surveillance cameras, biometric devices, wearable devices, medical gadgets, satellite and remote sensing data, and geotag data. Generally, this data is used by companies to monitor consumer trends in purchasing and renting. Data derived from automated sources expands exponentially in accordance with the market's changing external environment. If used effectively, machine data can boost profits, increase operational effectiveness, and provide businesses a competitive edge.

Social Data: Users of social media freely exchange social data, which includes metadata such as location, language spoken, biographical information, and shared links. The enormous quantities of data generated through the internet and social media platforms offer both quantitative and qualitative data on every essential aspect of brand–customer involvement. Some common examples of social data include posts on Facebook, tweets on Twitter, stock photos, images shared on social media such as Instagram and Snapchat, and many more.

Big data can be described by the following characteristics, often known as the 5 Vs of big data.

- **Volume:** the scope and volume of big data managed and analyzed by organizations. It addresses how quickly data is generated and moved around. This is a vital element for organizations who need their data to move quickly so that it is available when needed to make the best business decisions.
- **Value:** Value in big data usually derives from pattern recognition and insight identifying, resulting in improved operations. This is a prime example of the benefits that big data could offer, and it impacts what companies can do with the data they obtain.
- **Variety**: Different information, including unstructured, semi-structured, and raw data, is varied and wide ranging. The term "data variety" refers to variations in the formats, departments, and organizational structures used to collect data across an organization.
- **Velocity:** It states how rapidly companies receive, store, and manage data. It describes the rate at which data is generated and transmitted. For organizations who need their data to flow fast so that it is available in order to make the best decisions for their company, this is an essential aspect.
- **Veracity:** It defines the accuracy and quality of the data. The information acquired may be inaccurate, partial, or unable to provide any insightful information. In general, veracity refers to the level of trust that has been placed in the data that has been acquired.

The latest additions to the characteristics of big data in terms of Vs are visualization and veracity. Visualization of information is essential to data analytics since it involves presenting the processed data in a way that is understandable by humans. Fast and informed decision-making is facilitated by successful data visualization. Veracity is concerned with the data's accuracy and validity. In order to guarantee that the data accurately represents critical company procedures and that any data modification, modelling, and analysis do not jeopardize the data's accuracy, the data must go through validation. Before deciding which data should be sent to the data store, big data technologies can be utilized to create a temporary location for new data. A company can unload rarely used data by integrating big data technologies with data storage facilities in this way. Big data offers enhanced customer service, operational efficiency, and decision-making [15].

4.3.1 Big Data Analytics

Big data analytics is the complex procedure of analyzing vast volumes of data to uncover knowledge that could assist businesses in making wise decisions about their operations, such as hidden trends, correlations, market situations, and client preferences. Big data analytics is the application of advanced statistical methods to very large, diverse data sets that comprise structured, semi-structured, and unstructured data from multiple sources and range in size from terabytes to zettabytes. Some of the benefits of big data analysis include quicker and more efficient decision making, reduction of cost, efficiency in operations, usage of varied sources of data, and many more. Big data analysis generally consists of four main steps.

Data is gathered from an extensive variety of sources. In many cases, semi-structured and unstructured data are integrated as data are collected. Some of the common data sources are internet clickstream data, web server logs, cloud applications, mobile applications, social media content, text from customer emails and survey responses, mobile phone records, and machine data captured by sensors connected to the Internet of Things, etc. These data are prepared, cleansed, and analyzed for responding to queries. After the data has been collected and stored in a data warehouse, data experts must properly arrange and segment the data for statistical analyses. Data is filtered in order to enhance its quality. Data cleaning professionals clean the data using scripting tools or data quality software. They clean and organize the data while inspecting it for any possible duplicates or

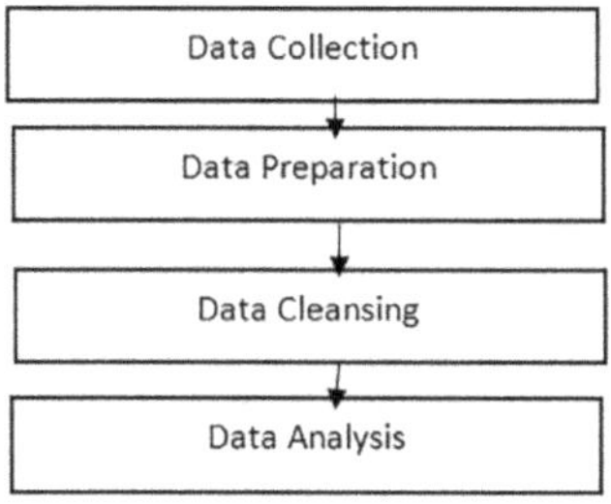

FIGURE 4.3 Steps in big data analytics.

formatting issues. In order to analyze the data that has been collected, prepared, and cleansed, analytics software is used [16]. This may include:

1. data mining: scans through data sets for patterns and trends
2. predictive analytics: develops models to forecast client behavior as well as other upcoming events, circumstances, and trends
3. machine learning: In order to analyze large data sets, it employs a number of algorithms

Data visualization tools for artificial intelligence, text mining software, statistical analysis software, and deep learning are some of the tools used in data analysis. Big Data analytics processes generally involve the use of the following tools and methods:

- The open-source Hadoop framework is used to store and handle large amounts of data. Large volumes of structured and unstructured data can be handled with Hadoop.
- After processing enormous amounts of complicated data, predictive analytics hardware and software utilizes machine learning and statistical algorithms to predict the outcomes of future instances. Businesses employ predictive analytics tools for operations, marketing, risk analysis, and fraud detection.
- Big data is often stored on a variety of platforms or formats. It is cleaned up, assembled, and examined with tools for stream analytics.
- Spark is a cluster computing framework which is open source and used for streaming data and processing.
- Data integration tools are computer programs that intake, combine, transform, and transport data from one location to another while also mapping and cleaning the data. The additional tools you use could make your approach simpler, for example, Microsoft Azure.

4.4 APPLICATION OF BIG DATA

There is a lot of data in the world today. This data is used by large corporations to expand their businesses. The term "big data" has gained a lot of attention. It refers to the massive amount of organized, semi-structured, and unstructured data being exponentially produced by high-performance applications in a variety of fields, including, but not limited to, business, physics, astronomy, genetics, molecular biology, biochemistry, and genetics. Big data analysis and application is built on methodologies such as tagging, filtering, association maps, and adaptable dictionaries. The useful information provided by big data for businesses or organizations can help them become more prosperous and gain deeper insights and a competitive advantage. This demands the most accurate analysis and execution of big data applications [17].

In many situations, as mentioned in the following, useful decisions can be made through analyzing data: The management of large retail stores has to keep information about client spending patterns (including which products they purchased, which brands they preferred, and how frequently they made purchases), shopping habits, and favorite products so they can stock those items in the store. Manufacturing and collection rates for a certain product are fixed based on information about the most popular product that is being searched for and purchased. Big data assists banks in keeping track of out-of-the-ordinary transactions, helps uncover potential fraud before it does significant harm, boosts asset security, and safeguards customer account privacy.

Big data plays a crucial role in the education sector by fostering effective learning, enhancing international recruiting for universities, assisting students in setting career goals, reducing university dropout rates, promoting clear student evaluation, improving the decision-making process, and raising student performance.

It also aids in planning routes according to the user's needs, helping to effectively manage wait times, and detecting accident-prone regions to promote traffic safety. Consequently, big data is important to improving and streamlining the transportation industry.

The use of big data in healthcare is demonstrated by the Mayo Clinic. Big data can significantly improve existing processes in healthcare. Technology has completely transformed the healthcare industry by lowering treatment costs, anticipating epidemic breakouts, avoiding preventable diseases, enhancing life quality, predicting daily patient income to modify staffing, and many more ways. Governments generate and collect huge volumes of data through regular operations, including managing national health systems, collecting taxes, processing payments for pensions and other benefits, monitoring traffic statistics, and creating official documents. The increasing demand for healthcare and social services, as well as standardization and interoperability as crucial prerequisites for public sector technologies and applications and many more [18] necessities the use of Artificial Intelligence and automation in medical industry. The world is experiencing an unprecedented growth in data. Data is being gathered and stored at rates that were previously unthinkable. The challenge lies not only in storing and managing the enormous amount of data ("big data") but also in its analysis and value extraction. There are various methods for gathering, storing, processing, and analyzing big data, which have improved workflow, analysis, and decision-making in a variety of fields. One of the categories of data is unstructured data, where information does not adhere well to relational tables or does not have a predefined data schema. The fastest-growing category of data is unstructured data, which might include imagery, sensor data, telemetry, video, documents, log files, IoT devices, and email data files. To solve this unstructured analytics issue, various strategies might be used [19]. The subsequent section discusses the role of big data in IoT device applications, as shown in Figure 4.4.

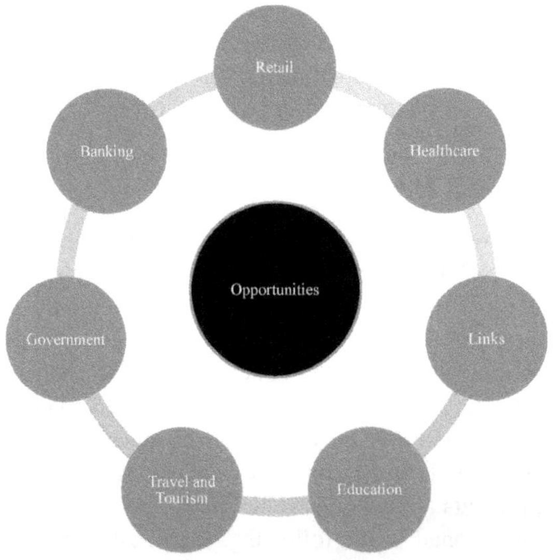

FIGURE 4.4 Applications of big data analytics.

4.5 BIG DATA IN THE IoT

Due to the increasing growth of the IoT, big data technologies have become a vital data analytics tool for bringing information into IoT infrastructures to better match the purpose of IoT systems and enable critical decision-making. The integration of big data and IoT technology has made it possible to provide services for a variety of complex systems, including smart cities. To assist the processing of massive volumes of IoT data that are gathered from various sources in the smart environment, a number of big data technologies have evolved. However, the development of the IoT and its applications in several other fields are leading to a huge rise in the quantity and variety of data. At the same time, big data and related technologies have made it possible for businesses and academic institutions to create innovative IoT solutions. Therefore, the combination of big data and the Internet of Things, as well as the extremely dynamic evolution of the two areas, presents new research issues, which is a challenge to the research and innovation community [20].

In terms of big data, the data generated by IoT devices is valuable data. This is to ensure that businesses may obtain more specific information about their devices and how they are utilized, as they are connected to a physical thing. Machine learning is also widely used by IoT platforms to collect data streams. These data streams will subsequently be correlated and analyzed together. The IoT continuously gathers and processes data. This translates to quicker and more accurate information gathering. Utilizing all the data gathered results in more beneficial and useful conclusions for businesses. In order to take advantage of many of big data's insights, the majority of businesses will need to adapt and develop their technology in order to be able to gather significant amounts of data. IoT devices will be able to communicate with organizations via messages that contain data about activity and behaviors. When the company receives this data, it must be stored on a platform competent of managing such vast and complicated data. Then, businesses may use this information as a reference whether they are creating a product, examining consumer behavior, or thinking back on a product launch. Most importantly, organizations may access this information anytime they need it because it is securely stored [21, 22].

Some factors of Big Data impacted by IoT are as follows:

- **Storage in Big Data**

  The ability to handle extremely large amounts of data, ongoing balancing to keep up with expansion, and the ability to offer the input/output operations per second needed for sending data to analytics tools are the basic needs for big data storage. The facilities used for storing such data must be able to handle the load in adaptive forms because the data comes in many forms and formats. Therefore, the IoT has a direct impact on the large data storage infrastructure. IoT big data collection can be challenging since duplicated data must be filtered. Data must be transferred via a network to a data center and kept after collection. Platform as a Service (PaaS) has become extensively utilized by businesses to manage their IT infrastructure. It supports the creation and operation of web applications. Big data can be managed effectively in this way without the need to significantly expand infrastructure. IoT big data storage is undoubtedly a difficult undertaking because the data is expanding more quickly than anticipated.
- **Security Challenges**

  The IoT has created new security challenges that are unable to be handled by conventional security measures. A change in approach is necessary to address IoT security challenges. Secure computing in distributed environments, secure data centers, secure transactions, secure data filtering, scalable and secure data mining and analytics, access control, and enforcing real-time security are a few security issues. Attacks can be prevented and restrained from propagating to other sections of the network with the use of a multi-layered security system and a proper network infrastructure. IoT systems should adhere to strict network access control standards before being permitted to join.

Big data analytics, such as descriptive analytics, diagnostic analytics, predictive analytics, and prescriptive analytics, can provide numerous kinds of insights when connected with the IoT. Descriptive analytics gives information on how a connected device is currently operating. It can be used for a variety of purposes, such as finding a connected device, deciphering how customers use that device, and spotting irregularities. Machine learning is used in predictive analytics to analyze historical data and generate probability of how the device will perform in the future. When it comes to maintaining IoT devices, this is very helpful. Utilizing this innovation, companies can anticipate issues or maintenance needs before an item faults. Prescriptive analytics provides information on how to influence things that have been seen or projected [23, 24].

4.5.1 IoT Big Data Processing

The function of big data in the IoT is to process enormous amounts of data in real time and store it using various storage methods.

Processing big data for IoT involves four successive steps.

- Big data systems collect a sizable amount of unstructured data that is generated by IoT devices. The IoT's big data is largely influenced by the volume, velocity, and variety.
- The vast volume of data is kept in large data files in the big data system, which is essentially a shared distributed database.
- Utilize analytical technologies like Hadoop MapReduce or Spark to analyze the saved IoT large data.
- Report generation of analyzed data.

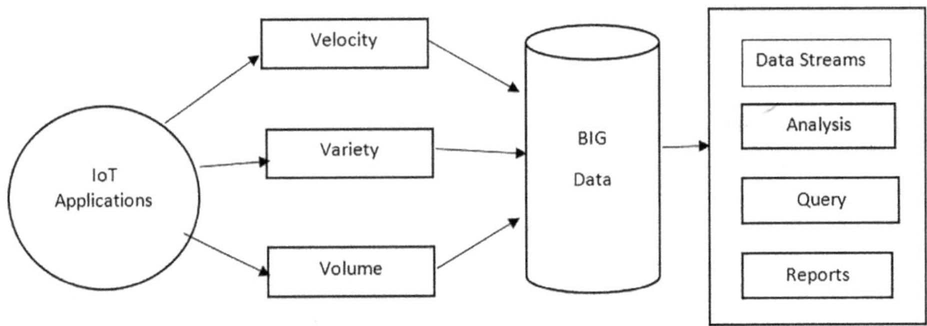

FIGURE 4.5 Big data processing in IoT applications.

Since unstructured data from the IoT is collected through the internet, big data analysis for the IoT is required in order to quickly get insights from the data and make decisions. Big data is therefore critical for the Internet of Things.

4.5.2 Applications of Big Data Integrated with the IoT

Businesses can gain from managing and analyzing massive amounts of IoT big data to determine how they impact operations. As a result, it helps businesses and other organizations acquire greater awareness of the data and make profitable choices. Every business and industry segment can benefit in some way from this. By maximizing information from data to gain more effective business knowledge, IoT and big data analytics are changing how businesses offer value. Businesses now prefer big-data cloud storage because of the rising need for data storage, which ultimately decreases their implementation costs.

- Healthcare

The future generation of e-healthcare systems may change as a result of the IoT and big data's combined features. Big data will result in the shift of hypothesis-driven research into data-driven research. The IoT, on the other hand, will assist in managing and analyzing the various degrees of links between various sensor signals and the already-existing big data. This will make it possible to develop new techniques for remote diagnosis with a deeper understanding of the illness, which will result in the creation of ground-breaking healthcare solutions.

- Smart Cities

The blending of big data and IoT technology has made it possible to provide services for a variety of intricate systems, including smart cities. To assist in the processing of massive volumes of IoT data that are gathered from various sources in the smart environment, a number of big data technologies have evolved. However, the development of the Internet of Things and its applications in numerous fields are leading to a huge rise in the volume and variety of data.

- Transportation

Intelligent transportation systems are now more commonplace as a result of IoT technology. Since transportation is one of the main things humans do, IoT sensors generate a lot of data every day that can be used to develop applications for surveillance, emergency management, traffic control, anomaly detection, situation recognition, and traffic prediction as well as to help with route planning.

- Smart Grids

An evolving intelligent electricity distribution system is the smart grid IoT. This aims to integrate renewable resources in power systems, increase control over the grid for its operators, and engage consumers in efficient power use.

- Industrial Internet of Things (IIoT)

The IoT is associated with a variety of linked devices that assist in duties to regulate the behavior of industrial devices like monitoring, collecting, exchanging, and analyzing, which form a key element of the IIoT with the confluence of the IoT with big data.

- Agriculture

To ensure the quality of products and the satisfaction of end users, agriculture is an essential component of our society that also benefits from IoT technologies. For instance, IoT device monitoring is vital for safeguarding agricultural crops from rodent or insect attacks.

- Military IoT

The IoT is presently utilized in the military, bringing with it a substantial and valuable supply of data that might enhance the intelligence of numerous military applications, including military robots, surveillance, and logistics. Additionally, the use of the IoT in the military is expected to safeguard the lives of civilians by identifying dangerous chemicals or biological weapons.

The confluence of IoT and big data has opened new possibilities and applications across all industries. Additionally, it has the ability to completely transform numerous aspects of the modern world. Big data and the IoT are helping to advance technology and make life faster and more intelligent. In order to collect data, the IoT may connect anything that produces data to the internet, including wearable technology, video games, automobiles, home appliances, and other objects. Big data may help businesses better understand customer preferences and behavior, improving corporate performance while saving time and money.

The merging of IoT and Big data has ushered in an era of automatization in many aspects of human life. However, there are also some challenges in this area, as discussed in the next section [25, 26–43].

4.6 IMPACT OF IoT AND BIG DATA IN MEDICAL IMAGES USING DEEP LEARNING

In many areas, including computer vision, natural language processing, speech recognition, visual object detection, disease prediction, drug discovery, bioinformatics, and biomedicine, deep learning is a popular thing. Healthcare and medical science–related applications are among those that are rapidly expanding. Deep learning is extremely common because of the massive development in large data, the Internet of Things, linked devices, and high-performance computers. The main data sources for deep learning systems for medical application depend on their individual tasks but typically include medical IoT, digital pictures, electronic health record (EHR) data, genomic data, and central medical databases. The requirement for computer-assisted analysis to improve image interpretation has long been a challenge in the field of medical imaging. Recent developments in machine learning, particularly in the form of deep learning, have made significant strides in the area of image understanding by making it easier to recognize, categorize, and quantify patterns in medical images. Deep learning is rapidly establishing itself as an innovative foundation, delivering improved performances in a variety of medical applications. Recently, computer-assisted interventions have started to be advantageous for researchers and physicians due to the wide variances in disease and possible stress of human experts. With the aid of deep learning approaches, computational medical image analysis has been making improvements. For recovery and treatment in today's healthcare environment, a precise and prompt diagnosis is essential. The Internet of Things has undergone a metamorphosis in recent years that makes it possible to analyze historical and real-time data using deep learning techniques. To assist medical diagnostics, the medical IoT blends healthcare infrastructure with AI applications and medical devices. An effective and quick approach that can handle large amount of medical image processing is needed to overcome the contrast and noise issues in magnetic resonance (MR) images. Due to its strong feed-forward algorithms and simple training, Convolutional neural networks (CNNs) have recently become the most promising method for managing large image datasets. They can recreate an image while minimizing the shortcomings of contrast and noise prevalent in medical imaging. Artificial neural networks are further developed by deep learning, which has more layers and allows for higher degrees of abstraction and better data predictions. It is currently establishing itself as a leading tool in the computer vision and general imaging fields. CNNs in particular have proven to be effective tools for a variety of computer vision tasks. Deep CNNs automatically pick up on intermediate and higher-level abstractions derived from unprocessed data (such as pictures). According to recent findings, object localization and object detection in natural images may be accomplished quite effectively using the generic descriptors extracted from CNNs. Medical image analysis experts are rapidly developing a wide range of applications for CNNs and other deep learning techniques.

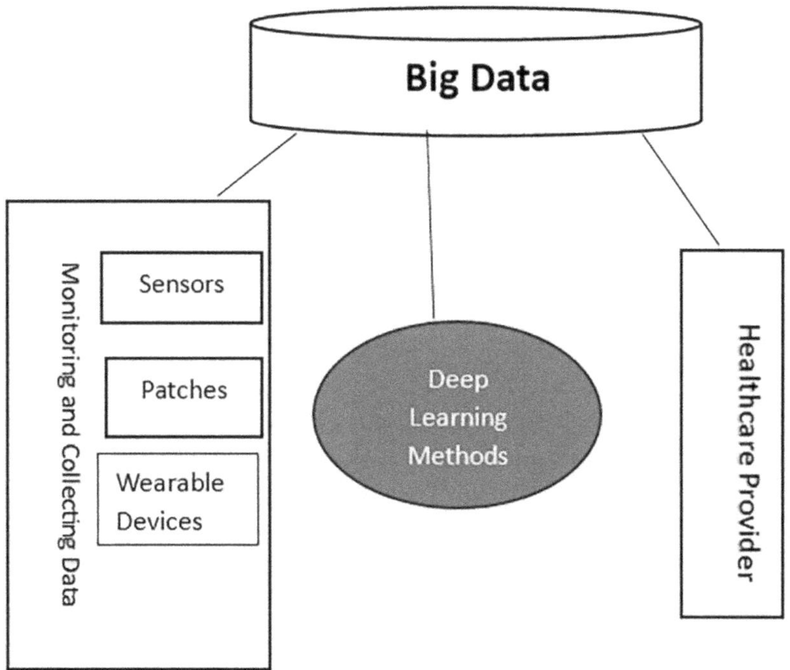

FIGURE 4.6 Schematic flowchart of medical IoT-based information system facilitating doctors.

4.7 CHALLENGES OF THE IMPACT OF THE IoT IN BIG DATA

A large amount of data must be processed to yield something useful; otherwise, these massive amounts of data are completely useless. The gathering, processing, and storing of data also provide some challenges in processing of big data in IoT usage. Prior to data processing, it's crucial to verify that the sensors are in good working order and that the data quality is dependable and unaffected by external circumstances. Terabytes of data are produced by connected devices, making it difficult to decide which data should be kept and which should be deleted. Additionally, certain data may not seem valuable at first, yet one might need it in the future. The problem is to do it at the most affordable rate if one does choose to store the data for the future. Another challenge is determining when rapid analysis is more valuable than comprehensive evaluation. Cybercriminals can link to industries, power plants, and data centers, as well as stealing personal information from telecom companies. For security professionals, IoT big data is a relatively new phenomena, and the absence of pertinent experience raises security vulnerabilities.

4.8 CONCLUSION

This chapter focuses on how the IoT and big data are integrating, as well as the function of real-time analytics in the IoT. The IoT is a developing technology that has the potential to start a fresh wave of analytics applications in human daily life. The IoT's capacity to scale will enable better applications across a variety of industries, from healthcare to safe and secure housing. One of the key advantages of the IoT is the actionable insight that can be obtained by applying real-time analytics to the big data of the IoT. Big data analytics are necessary to make use of the IoT's benefits. Big data produced by the IoT can be used for a variety of purposes, including real-time monitoring, analytics, process optimization, and predictive maintenance. However, it should be remembered that extracting useful insights from vast amounts of data in different forms is not an easy effort. It must be ensured that sensors are functioning well, the data is safely communicated, and the data is processed correctly. IoT development is gaining momentum and assisting businesses from multiple sectors to seize new digital opportunities using big data analytics.

REFERENCES

[1] Cai, H., Xu, B., Jiang, L., Vasilakos, A.V. 2017 IoT-Based Big Data Storage Systems in Cloud Computing: Perspectives and Challenges. *IEEE Internet of Things Journal*, 4 (1): 75–87. doi: 10.1109/JIOT.2016.2619369.

[2] Babar, M., Jan, M. A., He, X., Tariq, M. U., Mastorakis, S., Alturki, R. 2023 An Optimized IoT-Enabled Big Data Analytics Architecture for Edge–Cloud Computing. *IEEE Internet of Things Journal*, 10 (5): 3995–4005. doi: 10.1109/JIOT.2022.3157552.

[3] What Is IoT. 2023 www.oracle.com/in/internet-of-things/what-is-iot (accessed August 5, 2023).

[4] Sengupta, S. 2020 Moving from Cloud to Fog: An Internet of Things Perspective. *Towards Smart World: Homes to Cities Using Internet of Things*, 1: 168–173.

[5] Lee, S., Choi, M., Kim, S. 2017 How and What to Study About IoT: Research Trends and Future Directions from the Perspective of Social Science. *Telecommunications Policy*, 41: 10–30.

[6] The First Choice for IoT. 2023 https://iot.telenor.com/ (accessed August 5, 2023).

[7] Alem, Č., Mesud, H. 2018 Internet of Things (IoT): A Review of Enabling Technologies, Challenges, and Open Research Issues. *Computer Networks*, 144: 17–39.

[8] Nižetić, S., Šolić, P., Diego, L., Patrono, L. 2020 Internet of Things (IoT): Opportunities, Issues and Challenges Towards a Smart and Sustainable Future. Journal of Cleaner Production, 274: 122877.

[9] Mori, H., Kundaliya, J., Naik, K., Shah, M. 2022 IoT Technologies in Smart Environment: Security Issues and Future Enhancements. *Environmental Science and Pollution Research International*, 32: 47969–47987.

[10] Ali Tourani, A.S. 2017 Challenges of Video-Based Vehicle Detection and Tracking in Intelligent Transportation Systems. *2nd National Conference on Soft Computing*, 8:43:23.

[11] Burhanuddin, M., Ismail, R., Basiron, H., Mohammed, A. 2017 Internet of Things Architecture: Current Challenges and Future Direction. *International Journal of Applied Engineering Research*, 12: 11055–11061.

[12] How Big Data Works. 2023 https://mindmajix.com/big-data-in-iot#how-does-big-data-work/ (accessed August 5, 2023).

[13] Cai, H., Xu, B., Jiang, L., Vasilakos, A.V. 2017 IoT-Based Big Data Storage Systems in Cloud Computing: Perspectives and Challenges. *IEEE Internet of Things Journal*, 4: 75–87.

[14] Yusuf, A. 2021 Data Discovery. In *Designing Big Data Platforms: How to Use, Deploy, and Maintain Big Data Systems*, Vol. 1: 179–197. Wiley.

[15] The Seven vs of Big Data Analytics. 2023 www.trigyn.com/insights/seven-vs-big-data-analytics (accessed August 5, 2023).

[16] Sarker, S., Arefin, M.S., Kowsher, M., Bhuiyan, T., Dhar, P.K., Kwon, O.J. 2023 A Comprehensive Review on Big Data for Industries: Challenges and Opportunities. *IEEE Access*, 11: 744–769.

[17] Sagiroglu, S., Sinanc, D. 2013 Big Data: A Review. *International Conference on Collaboration Technologies and Systems (CTS)*, 1: 42–47.

[18] Munné, R. 2016 Big Data in the Public Sector. In *New Horizons for a Data-Driven Economy*. doi: 10.1007/978-3-319-21569-3_11.

[19] Bakshi, K. 2021 Considerations for Big Data: Architecture and Approach. *IEEE Aerospace Conference*, 1: 1–7.

[20] Mouzhi, G., Hind, B., Barbora, B., 2018 Big Data for Internet of Things: A Survey. *Future Generation Computer Systems*, 87: 123–130.

[21] The Big Data-IoT Relationship: How They Help Each Other. www.spiceworks.com/tech/big-data/guest-article/the-big-data-iot-relationship-how-they-help-each-other/ (accessed August 5, 2023).

[22] Mishra, S., Saraswat, R., Sengupta, S. 2023 Role of IoT Enabling Smart Agricultural Society. In *Technological Prospects and Social Applications of Society 5.0*, Vol. 1: 177–184.

[23] Sengupta, S. 2019 IoE: An Innovative Technology for Future Enhancement. *Computer Vision and Internet of Things: Technologies, and Applications*, 1: 19–28.

[24] Sengupta, S. 2019 Role of Image Processing in Artificial Intelligence and Internet of Things. *Computer Vision and Internet of Things: Technologies and Applications*, 1: 63–73.
[25] Internet of Things and Big Data—Better Together. www.whizlabs.com/blog/iot-and-big-data/ (accessed August 5, 2023).
[26] Anand, A., Jha, V., Sharma, L. 2019 An Improved Local Binary Patterns Histograms Techniques for Face Recognition for Real Time Application. *International Journal of Recent Technology and Engineering*, 8(2S7): 524–529 (Indexed in Scopus, DOI: 10.35940/ijrte.B1098.0782S719)
[27] Ayush, Sharma, L., Gupta, D. 2019 Motion Based Object Detection based on Background Subtraction: A Review. In 3rd IEEE International Conference on Electronics Communication and Aerospace Technology, ICECA 2019, Coimbatore, India, 12–14 June.
[28] Chopra, U., Thakur, N., Sharma, L. 2019 Cloud Computing: Elementary Threats & Embellishing Countermeasures for Data Security. *International Journal of Recent Technology and Engineering*, 8(2S7): 518–523 (Indexed in Scopus, DOI: 10.35940/ijrte.B1097.0782S719)
[29] Jha, G., Singh, P., Sharma, L. 2019 Recent Advancements of Augmented Reality in Real Time Applications. *International Journal of Recent Technology and Engineering*, 8(2S7): 538–542 (Indexed in Scopus, DOI: 10.35940/ijrte.B10100.0782S719)
[30] Kumar, A., Jha, G., Sharma, L. 2019 Challenges, Potential & Future of IOT Integrated with Block Chain. *International Journal of Recent Technology and Engineering*, 8(2S7): 530–536 (Indexed in Scopus, DOI: 10.35940/ijrte.B1099.0782S719)
[31] Makkar, S., Sharma, L. 2019 A Face Detection Using Support Vector Machine: Challenging Issues, Recent Trend, Solutions and Proposed Framework. In Singh, M., Gupta, P., Tyagi, V., Flusser, J., Ören, T., Kashyap, R. (eds) *Advances in Computing and Data Sciences. ICACDS 2019. Communications in Computer and Information Science*, vol. 1046. Springer. https://doi.org/10.1007/978-981-13-9942-8_1
[32] Saraogi, G., Gupta, D., Sharma, L., Rana, A. 2021 Un-Supervised Approach to Backorder Prediction Using Deep Autoencoder. *Recent Patents on Computer Science*, Bentham, 14(8) (Indexed in Scopus).
[33] Sharma, L. 2019 *Object Detection with Background Subtraction*. LAP LAMBERT Academic Publishing, SIA OmniScriptum Publishing , European Union (ISBN: 978-613-7-34386-9)
[34] Sharma, L. 2020 *Towards Smart World: Homes to Cities using Internet of Things*. Taylor & Francis, CRC Press (ISSN: 9780429297922)
[35] Sharma, L., Carpenter, M. (Eds.). 2022 *Computer Vision and Internet of Things: Technologies and Applications* (1st ed.). Chapman and Hall/CRC. https://doi.org/10.1201/9781003244165
[36] Sharma, L., Garg, P.K. 2019 *From Visual Surveillance to Internet of Things*. Taylor & Francis, CRC Press. (ISSN: 9780429297922)
[37] Sharma, L., Garg, P.K. 2021a *Artificial Intelligence: Challenges, Technologies and Future*. Wiley (In production).
[38] Sharma, L., Garg, P.K. (Eds.). 2021b *Artificial Intelligence: Technologies, Applications, and Challenges* (1st ed.). Chapman and Hall/CRC. doi:10.1201/9781003140351
[39] Sharma, L., Garg, P.K. (Eds.). 2023 *Technological Prospects and Social Applications of Society 5.0* (1st ed.). Chapman and Hall/CRC. doi:10.1201/9781003324720
[40] Sharma, L., Lohan, N. 2019 Performance Analysis of Moving Object Detection using BGS Techniques in Visual Surveillance. *International Journal of Spatiotemporal Data Science, Inderscience*, 1: 22–53.
[41] Sharma, L., Sengupta, S., Kumar, B. 2021 An Improved Technique for Enhancement of Satellite Images. *Journal of Physics: Conference Series*, 1714: 012051 (Indexed in Scopus, DOI: 10.1088/1742-6596/1714/1/012051)
[42] Sharma, L., Singh, A., Yadav, D.K. 2016 Fisher's Linear Discriminant Ratio based Threshold for Moving Human Detection in Thermal Video. In: *Infrared Physics and Technology*. Elsevier (SCI Impact Factor: 1.58, Published). http://www.inderscience.com/jhome.php?jcode=ijtmcp.
[43] Sharma, L., Yadav, D.K. 2016 Histogram based Adaptive Learning Rate for Background Modelling and Moving Object Detection in Video Surveillance. *International Journal of Telemedicine and Clinical Practices, Inderscience* (ISSN: 2052-8442, DOI: 10.1504/IJTMCP.2017.082107).

5 Geospatial Data Collection Tools in Healthcare

Pradeep Kumar Garg

5.1 INTRODUCTION

The digital technology has brought a revolution to perceptions of data. Geographic information is the collection of geospatial data on places and events on the Earth's surface. This data is geotagged with its location. This property makes it useful for various applications, including healthcare. The combination of communications infrastructure, internet accessibility, sensors, the Internet of Things (IoT), artificial intelligence (AI) and machine learning (ML) technologies, and geospatial data leads to the advancement in the healthcare. Geospatial maps, AI, and sensors are used to prioritize the needs of the population, allocate adequate resources, and make operations efficient (Geraghty, 2022). These advancements, along with the availability of big data, have provided new opportunities that apply to a wide variety of social and health problems (Akter, 2022).

Healthcare has two dimensions (spatial and temporal), considering the dynamics and communication of diseases and distribution of facilities (McLafferty, 2003). The prevention of disease is a priority in developing healthy communities. Policymakers cannot make evidence-informed resolutions without having qualitative or quantitative data. Map data or data on a dashboard helps users visualize and understand the distribution of health issues as compared to tabular data. Location-based data/information allows providers to better understand the risk factors associated with disease or to identify targets for prevention efforts.

The healthcare industry dealing with public medical care is just beginning to realize the potential of geospatial data and its analysis through geographic information systems (GISs) to benefit public medical care (Garg et al., 2022). Healthcare organizations are using GISs to enhance customer service as well as to improve management practices.

Fast and easy access to medical records is crucial to effective treatment. Some hospitals have already integrated geospatial technology into their processes to improve patient care. Electronic health record (EHR) systems along with GIS are used to manage patient data, such as personal records, location, and status, as well as to provide context and analysis on patient flow (Garg et al., 2022). Some hospitals have also introduced GIS-based indoor navigation that helps patients to quickly find the right buildings, parking lots, clinics, testing labs, and offices. Indoor maps have also helped the decision-making authority of the hospital to optimize space planning and facilitate management of patient needs. The patient-centric GIS approach focuses on the development and dissemination of information about the patient. Maps provide geographic information to healthcare practitioners, allowing them to understand the immediate needs of communities and deliver efficient care (Geraghty, 2022). Public health officials can use spatial analysis and predictive modeling to plan and prioritize where and when to allocate resources. Hospital staff can use GIS maps to make operations more efficient and improve patient care. The public health uses of GIS are many, such as tracking child immunizations, conducting health policy research, and establishing service areas.

5.2 GEOSPATIAL DATA COLLECTION DEVICES

Data offers many opportunities in a modern society, especially in the healthcare and medical fields. Geospatial data typically combines the location information of an object (real-world coordinates)

DOI: 10.1201/9781003451846-5

and attribute information (characteristics of the object, event, or time span). The location information provided can be static or dynamic. Governments and commercial organizations both acquire geospatial data and use it for various purposes. More recently, IoT sensors and devices are used in healthcare which generate geospatial big data. This information is very important in control and prevention of various health conditions, such as contagious diseases, non-contagious diseases, and injuries. Geospatial data is most useful in various healthcare activities, as shown in Figure 5.1, when it is discovered, automated, digitized, shared, converted, translated, analyzed, and used in combination with traditional data.

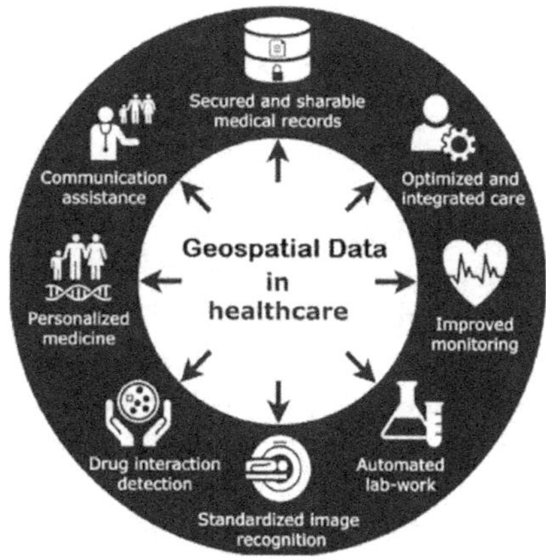

FIGURE 5.1 Use of geospatial data in healthcare (Garg et al., 2022).

With decreases in hardware cost and a rapid increase in computing, collection of geospatial data is becoming easy and faster for the public. Several government and other organizations around the globe have made spatial data publicly available in various forms for the general public to use. Google maps and images and Open Street maps are the best examples to date (Garg, 2020). The Indian website BHUVAN provides various geospatial data of the country. Recently, National Geospatial Policy 2022 was announced in India that aims to create, encourage, and develop a geospatial ecosystem for spatial thinking; strengthen geospatial infrastructure; enhance capacity building; promote the use of geospatial data, services, and solutions; and enhance geospatial entrepreneurship (https://dst.gov.in/news/national-geospatial-policy). It is basically a citizen-centric policy which liberalizes the geospatial domain and democratizes the datasets, generated by public funds. Other examples of spatial data include:

1. Vancouver open data in file formats compatible with the Web, Google Maps and Google Earth, ArcGIS, QGIS, and several other file formats at http://vancouver.ca/your-government/open-data-catalogue.aspx
2. British Columbia open data at www.data.gov.bc.ca/dbc/geographic/index.page?WT.svl=Breadcrumb
3. Canada data in file formats compatible with QGIS and ArcGIS at http://geogratis.cgdi.gc.ca/

There are several options for collecting spatial data which can be done with relatively low-cost resources. Geographic data collection hardware/devices may include maps, photographs, remote sensing images, digitizers, scanners, global positioning system (GPS) units, sensors, light detection and ranging (LiDAR), digital cameras, video cameras, social media data, and mobile devices. Each type of device has its own use cases and benefits, depending on the types of applications, deliverables, and degree of location accuracy required.

5.2.1 Digitization

In view of GIS, digitization mainly refers to converting coordinates, text annotations, or analog maps into digital format so that these can be directly used in GIS software. GIS professionals can use either digitizer tablets or on-screen digitization to easily capture, store, analyze, and manage geospatial data. More details are given in Garg (2020).

5.2.2 Global Positioning Systems

These are devices that receive information from GPS satellites and calculate the geographical position as 3D coordinates (x, y, and z). It is a space-based radio-navigation system consisting of a group of satellites broadcasting navigation signals (Garg, 2020). Currently, there are 31 GPS satellites orbiting the Earth and providing users with precise information on position, velocity, and time any time and anywhere in the world. To get a correct position, at least four visible GPS satellites must be tracked. Using the principle of trilateration, an accurate position can be determined. GPS can also be used for ground truthing of analysis from satellite images.

GPS units fall into three groups: (i) recreation grade (ii) mapping grade, and (iii) survey grade. Recreation-grade GPS units are economical and used mostly by the general public, as these are hand-held. Mapping-grade units are mostly used by government agencies and researchers and provide a significant increase in positional accuracy. They are more expensive than recreation-grade units. Some mapping-grade units offer a high degree of accuracy when augmented with an external antenna. Survey-grade units are often used by professionals and are considered the most accurate. Accuracy ranges from 1 m to within 1 mm. Because they are highly accurate, they are the most expensive.

5.2.3 Mobile Technology

As mobile technology evolved, smartphones and tablets have become useful tools for geospatial data collection. The combination of both mobile communication technologies and a Wi-Fi–based positioning system allows field users to acquire timely location-based information. Location-based information is crucial in case of an emergency (Garg, 2020). Due to the high demand for social networking and location-based services with mobile devices, public participation in geospatial data collection is important, particularly for decision-making processes.

Smartphones are the most available devices for the collection of geospatial data and images, although they don't provide the same level of accuracy as GPS receivers. Tablets are a little bigger in size than smartphones, but they offer one advantage, big screen size. Bigger screen size allows one to view large data sets or detailed maps, which are significant for GIS work. There are various field apps that provide data collection tools to capture field-based information from a mobile device. Depending on the work, each mobile field app will collect information on the ground in different ways. For example, the Field app for Android is a popular open source, whereas ESRI Collector/Survey123 and Fulcrum are commercial data collection tools (GIS Geography, 2023).

5.2.4 Remote Sensing

It is a process of gathering information about the environment, areas, objects, and natural phenomena on the Earth surface. It includes the use of photographs, satellite images, and unmanned aerial vehicle (UAV) images (Garg, 2020). LiDAR is a form of remote sensing that uses laser pulses to measure objects on the ground and provides dense point cloud data. The remote sensing technology is primarily used for mapping and spatial analysis for various applications, including geospatial data visualization.

5.2.5 Sensors

Wearable technology has great potential to provide huge amount of real-time data such as smart watches, which can be used to measure the heart rates and ECGs of patients (Garg et al., 2022). Integrated health devices (IHDs) are also used to check blood sugar levels. People can use wearable sensors to measure their steps, heart rhythms, blood pressure, and so on (Bailey, 2023). Data collected from these sensor-based devices can help patients and clinicals to cross-reference it with geographical information. A public health department can also use this vital information to monitor stress levels, determine an average resting heart rate, conduct age-based blood sugar monitoring, and track cardiac emergencies over time. The Internet of Things provides rapid access, processing, and utilization of big data for various applications, such as disaster management or health monitoring.

5.2.6 Social Media

In the literature, various social media tools are available for healthcare professionals, such as social networking platforms, blogs, wikis, media-sharing sites, and virtual reality and gaming environments. These tools can be used to enhance professional networking, education, patient care and education, and public health programs. Various healthcare providers use social media to improve health outcomes and personal awareness and also provide health information to the community (George et al., 2013). Every sick person will not necessarily consult a doctor; however, they may be willing to share information about their health on social media accounts. They can send a tweet to co-workers informing them about their illness or talk about symptoms on their social media platform. Social media accounts are tied to a location, and GIS technology can track references to an emergency in a particular domain.

5.3 GEOSPATIAL DATA ANALYSIS

Geospatial maps represent various features on the Earth's surface, showing their spatial distribution. The rapid development of information technology and collection of geospatial data have led to the creation of digital maps (Garg, 2020). Digital mapping in healthcare is rapidly changing the way the health sector plans patient care and services. GIS and satellite image data can provide vital information for detection and controlling disease outbreaks (Cromley and McLafferty, 2002). Robust geospatial technologies need to be employed to process and analyze spatial big data in real time.

Patient care within hospitals and medical centers has become a very difficult task, but GISs (spatial data management systems) can be used to integrate, store, adjust, analyze, and organize geographically referenced information. They can be used as decision-making tool for several problems involving spatial data. GISs can also play an vital role for surveillance, management, and disease analysis and their impact on health (Garg et al., 2022). Artificial intelligence, machine learning, deep learning (DL), cloud computing, and data mining are advanced technologies that can be used for geospatial data analysis (GDA) (Garg et al., 2022).

5.4 APPLICATION AREAS OF GEOSPATIAL DATA

Medical practitioners in the public health sector were early users of GIS and continue to find innovative applications of this technology, but in the last decade the use of GIS in the private health sector and patient care has grown significantly. A common theme across geospatial data applications is the utilization of spatial data, such as electronic health records, remote sensing, social media platforms, sensors, location-based data, and maps to advance the science of public health and create new opportunities to more comprehensively answer questions. Data dashboards provide key insights on data to combine maps, plans, lists, and text on a computer screen to present data (Wang, 2020).

Healthcare industries are using geospatial technologies to create analytical and descriptive solutions for various health issues. These have been widely used in health planning such as epidemic disease monitoring, accessibility and healthcare utilization, disease mapping and spread outlines, health information management (HIM), and allocating health resources (Khashoggi and Murad, 2020). GIS has also enhanced the understanding of the spatial relationship between place and health; thus, it is considered a most effective tool to deal with healthcare planning problems (Cromley and McLafferty, 2002).

Health intelligence applications include social media analytics for syndromic surveillance, predictive modelling to classify high-risk disease populations, and medical imaging interpretation. Other application areas include identifying health trends, tracking contagious disease, personal data utilization, service improvement, and disease detection (Richardson et al., 2013).

The COVID-19 pandemic has already highlighted the importance of GIS and spatial analysis to public health. Throughout the pandemic, geospatial data has been utilized in tracking the illness and its spread and impact. This pandemic highlighted the use of GIS in public health needs and deficiencies where GIS can be used in the future. The technology helped create visualizations to make decisions and take action to combat COVID-19. The COVID-19 crisis has shown imbalances between the available services and demands, leading to a variety of crises in many areas/countries (Altaweel, 2020). During the virus outbreak, many governments and health organizations adopted GIS technologies to plan COVID-19 responses and control measures.

5.5 FUTURE SCOPE

There is a strong correlation between healthcare systems and economic growth. When there is an increase in economic growth, governments will provide reasonable and balanced healthcare that meets all the requirements of society. GIS helps in identifying the better requirements of particular healthcare services in a huge region. With the help of GIS, national healthcare services enable developers to work more closely with hospitals. Although GIS has been used for many decades to examine healthcare systems, the contributions of GIS have grown drastically in the last few years.

GIS has helped the healthcare industry manage resources and personnel in the same way as it has helped other consumer service enterprises. In the growing information technology age of healthcare, the role of GIS will have greater importance due to its ability to integrate a wide variety of data and make complex data more quickly and easily understood. Due to rapid advances in real-time technology and affordable sensors, indoor GIS-based mapping applications will be an important part of future healthcare infrastructure (Geraghty, 2022).

The recent Digital Healthcare Ecosystem Market Professional Survey Report 2019 studied the digital healthcare ecosystem market size by players, regions, types and industries, history data 2012–2019 and forecasted data between 2019–2026 (Figure 5.2). It also covers the market drivers and trends, market competition landscape, opportunities and challenging issues, risk factors and entry barriers, sales, and distributors. This information provides a detailed analysis of how the trends could potentially affect the upcoming future of the digital healthcare ecosystem market during the forecast period.

Geospatial data and technology through location-based data analytics can highly benefit governments, healthcare service providers, and end users. Health service planning requires spatial data on health resources, population, consumption, treatments, and results, and data is often not available at both scales (temporal and spatial). The need for geospatial data in the health sector has now clearly been established by the efficient and scientific management of COVID-19. The development of Geospatial Policies 2022 in India has made it easier to acquire, process, and publish geospatial data, and this requires great interaction between businesses, governments, and innovators to develop effective solutions for the benefits of society (Singh, 2022) (https://dst.gov.in/news/national-geospatial-policy). There is also a dire need to modernize the data collection systems at the government and hospital level in order to facilitate faster data exchange when

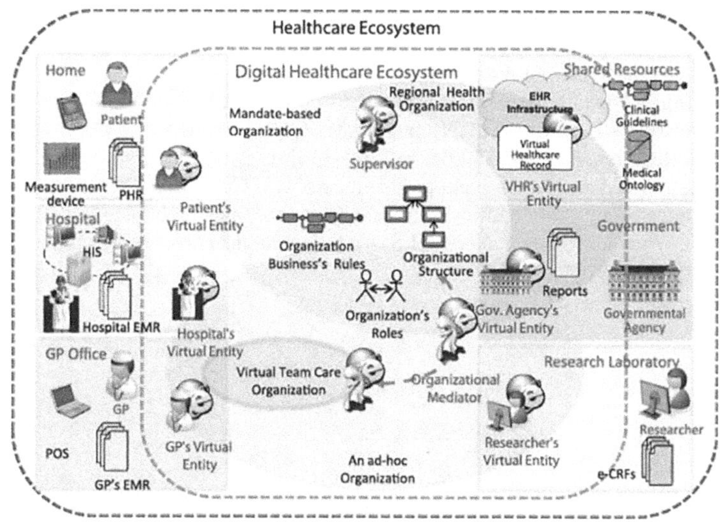

FIGURE 5.2 Digital healthcare ecosystem.

(Source: OpenPR, 2019)

necessary. However, privacy and confidentiality of medical health data of individuals can impose restrictions to access to data about health status and health outcomes (Garg et al., 2022). A modern, well-funded, and data-driven public health system in a country will ensure access to quality healthcare by everyone.

Research areas that can benefit from GIS, such as research on geographic variations in healthcare utilization, have not made full use of the capabilities of GIS (McLafferty, 2003). GIS-based research on service performance and efficiency is still in its infancy. Advances in computing power and the availability of large datasets as well as the development of AI and ML methods have created innovative healthcare applications. Improving healthcare services is the most important advantage of using GIS in this industry. As medical practitioners start to adopt and integrate GIS, the number of advantages is likely to increase, including the relationship between hospitals and communities.

REFERENCES

Akter, Tamanna, (2022), Using Geospatial Technologies in Healthcare, EthicalGEO, https://ethicalgeo.org/using-geospatial-technologies-in-healthcare/.

Altaweel, Mark, (2020), GIS and the Future of Public Health, GIS LOUNGE, July 15, www.gislounge.com/gis-and-the-future-of-public-health/.

Bailey, John, (2023), 6 Transformative Effects GIS Is Having on the Healthcare Industry, www.chetu.com/blogs/healthcare/benefits-of-gis-in-healthcare.php.

Cromley, E. and McLafferty, S., (2002), GIS and Public Health, New York: Guilford Press.

Garg, P. K., (2020), Digital Land Surveying and Mapping, Delhi: New Age International Pvt Ltd.

Garg, P. K., Tripathi, Nitin, Kappas, Martin and Gaur, Loveleen, (2022), Editors: Geospatial Data Science in Healthcare for Society 5.0, Singapore: Springer Nature.

George, D.R., Rovniak, L.S. and Kraschnewski, J.L., (2013), Dangers and Opportunities for Social Media in Medicine. Clin Obstet Gynecol, 56(3):453–462.

Geraghty, Este, (2022), Three Ways GIS Can Modernize Health Infrastructure for Smart Cities, Geospatial World. www.geospatialworld.net/prime/gis-health-infrastructure/.

GISGeography, (2023), 5 Field Apps: Data Collection Tools for Mobile GIS, https://gisgeography.com/field-apps-data-collection-tools/.

Khashoggi, Bandar and Murad, Abdulkader, (2020), Issues of Healthcare Planning and GIS: A Review. ISPRS International Journal of Geo-Information, 9:352. doi: 10.3390/ijgi9060352.

McLafferty, S.L., (2003), GIS and Health Care. Annu Rev Public Health, 24:25–42. doi: 10.1146/annurev.publhealth.24.012902.141012.

OpenPR, (2019), Digital Healthcare Ecosystem Market Professional Survey Report 2019, www.openpr.com/news/1813361/digital-healthcare-ecosystem-market-top-key-players-are-ibm.

Richardson, D.B., Volkow, N.D., Kwan, M.P., Kaplan, R.M., Goodchild, M.F. and Croyle, R.T., (2013), Spatial Turn in Health Research. Science, 339(6126):1390–1392. doi: 10.1126/science.1232257.

Singh, Sakshi, (2022), Transforming the Field of Healthcare with Geospatial Technology, AGI India, https://agiindia.com/transforming-the-field-of-healthcare-with-geospatial-technology/

Wang, Fahui, (2020), Why Public Health Needs GIS: A Methodological Overview. Annals of GIS, 26(1):1–12. doi: 10.1080/19475683.2019.1702099.

6 Geospatial Technology in Healthcare

Prithvi Sai Penumadu

6.1 INTRODUCTION

Since the early 2000s, geographic information system (GIS) technology has increased adoption and acceptance, particularly in the public health sector. The usage of GIS technology in public health applications is expanding rapidly. This chapter summarises the common ways GIS technology is used in public health, specifically focusing on mapping and understanding the burden of diseases [1]. The availability of satellite and remote-sensing data has further broadened the understanding of the spread of diseases and their correlation with external factors like the environment, which is pivotal for studying and analysing the patterns of several communicable and non-communicable diseases. Disease prevention and control strategies, stemming from research conducted within a GIS environment, have demonstrated successful global implementation. Using GIS for geographical analysis has empowered researchers to establish intricate linkages between health, population, and environmental data, enabling quantifying and assessing correlations between environmental risk and health-related factors across diverse demographic groups. Despite the promising results achieved, the broader integration of GIS technology within the Indian public health sector remains impeded by several challenges, including restricted access to GIS infrastructure, inadequate technical and analytical expertise, and disparities in data accessibility. To overcome these limitations, there are opportunities for international collaboration through knowledge sharing and governance efforts. By addressing these challenges collectively, it is possible to enhance the utilisation of GIS technology and its benefits in the public health domain. Additionally, the chapter highlights successful case studies on how India is leveraging GIS technologies to design evidence-based policies to implement various public health schemes seamlessly. Further, a particular emphasis has been placed on the development of AarogyaSetu, a GIS-enabled contact tracing platform during the pandemic, to deliver health services during the first wave of COVID-19 effectively.

6.1.1 The Evolution of the Geospatial Sector

Since the early 19th century, cartography and map making have gained prominence due to the introduction of cartographic machines [1, 2]. With time, computers accelerated geographic information systems and their applications. This section will provide a brief snapshot of the evolution of the geospatial sector from the early 19th century and how the market of GIS systems currently looks in the global landscape.

6.1.2 The Rise of GIS Application in Healthcare

During the initial years, the role of GIS was more towards studying the atmospheric and earth sciences and a few other critical areas of importance. Still, the rapid rise in modern techniques laid a roadmap for applying GIS in disaster management, transportation, and urban planning. Although the application of GIS in healthcare gained prominence in the 1990s, it was during the SARS outbreak that governments and other stakeholders realised the importance of GIS in healthcare. This section highlights how the geospatial sector has gained prominence globally in healthcare. It also

DOI: 10.1201/9781003451846-6

highlights the rise of various health services such as telemedicine and remote patient monitoring, emergency medical services, digital health services, and many others by leveraging GIS systems. Further, this section also highlights how India mainstreamed applications of GIS by implementing various policies and initiatives.

6.1.3 The Role of the Geospatial Sector in Aiding the Delivery of Healthcare Services

Section 6.3 discusses the role of geospatial technologies in developing future platforms or services that can augment the delivery of healthcare services in India. Through geospatial analysis, healthcare providers can identify disease patterns, allocate medical resources efficiently, and assess healthcare accessibility. Geographic information systems further aid in tracking and predicting disease outbreaks, streamlining emergency response, and facilitating the distribution of medical supplies. Moreover, geospatial technologies enable the creation of interactive health maps, supporting informed decision-making and public health communication. This section also highlights three case studies indicating the adoption of GIS technologies that India pioneered in the healthcare sector.

6.1.4 Challenges and Opportunities in Healthcare GIS

This section summarises the key challenges in adopting geospatial technology in the healthcare industry. Further, it emphasises the importance of overcoming these challenges to harness the full potential of geospatial tools for improving healthcare outcomes.

6.1.5 Action Plan and the Way Forward

This section outlines a strategic roadmap for integrating and expanding geographic information systems in healthcare, emphasising the necessary steps, goals, and actions to leverage GIS effectively in the healthcare sector. It further highlights the importance of establishing a nodal agency along the lines of Newspace India Ltd. or NPCI to oversee the entire geospatial ecosystem in the healthcare sector, which focuses on scaling up innovative solutions, forging partnerships, establishing infrastructure, and launching new programs along with supporting stakeholders with policies and regulatory frameworks.

6.2 THE EVOLUTION OF THE GEOSPATIAL SECTOR

Geospatial technologies are modern techniques that encompass a range of tools used for mapping and analysing the Earth's geography and human activities. These technologies have evolved from early cartography and aerial photography to using satellites and computers. In the 19th century, cartography and mapmaking schools were joined by aerial photography in the early 20th century by sending cameras using balloons, pigeons, and airplanes [1, 2]. During the Second World War, with the advent of satellites and computers, the art of map-making and photographic interpretation took a new dimension in an accelerated approach. These techniques include remote sensing, geographic information systems, positioning and navigation systems, and Internet mapping technologies. They enable the collection, storage, and analysis of georeferenced data, allowing complex themes to be examined and communicated through layered maps. Geospatial technologies have become increasingly accessible to various sectors, such as universities, corporations, and non-governmental organisations, informing decision-making in industrial engineering, biodiversity conservation, disaster response, and more. Notably, in the recent past, these technologies have added a new dimension to monitoring and managing resources across various sectors, from agriculture to healthcare, transportation to urban planning.

The geospatial market can be divided into two categories: software and services. Software components include geospatial analytics software for mapping, data management, and spatial analysis, which businesses can deploy to understand business trends with available location information. Services include geocoding and reverse geocoding, data integration, reporting and visualisation, and thematic mapping for creating an inventory of resources, monitoring, and management. As of 2022, the software component makes up 55% of the revenue, with the remaining 45% coming from services. In a recent study conducted in 2021, the North American region has the largest share, with 47% in the global geospatial market, followed by 24% in Europe and 19% in the Asia-Pacific region. India and China dominate the geospatial analytics market in the Asia-Pacific region, which is steered by various government initiatives to improve the ease of governance through evidence-based policies.

6.3 THE RISE OF GIS APPLICATIONS IN HEALTHCARE

One of the critical sectors that rose to prominence is the application of GIS in healthcare. Since 2003, ever since the SARS outbreak, the world has seen a revolution in the application of geographical tools through web-based platforms by ingesting real-time data and displaying results in interactive dashboards built by Johns Hopkins University using ArcGIS and WHO's COVID dashboard [3]. GIS is being extensively utilised in healthcare, with applications falling into two main categories: patient care and operational improvement. GIS is employed in multiple ways in patient care, such as connecting patients with community resources and clinical trials. It also aids medical decision-making by identifying patients at high risk of readmission based on their access to primary or speciality care [4]. On the operational side, healthcare organisations leverage GIS for strategic planning and market development.

The UN Sustainable Development Goals (SDGs) aim to achieve universal health coverage and ensure access to quality healthcare services by 2030 to create a healthier and more equitable world. In line with this vision, India, through its 12th five-year plan, emphasises the provision of high-quality healthcare at affordable costs and addresses disparities in healthcare accessibility among different regions and communities. The focus is on the public provisioning of healthcare services to ensure everyone has access to essential medical care, regardless of their socio-economic background or geographical location. The goal is to bridge the gaps in healthcare services and improve overall health outcomes across the country. In the past three years, GIS technology has played a significant role in India's efforts to manage, respond to, and recover from the pandemic. This technology has empowered healthcare professionals and government decision-makers by providing valuable insights for effective decision-making. Multiple states, cities, and government bodies in India have established GIS-based dashboards to integrate and visualise health data from various sources, facilitating real-time information for better coordination, collaboration, and decision-making among stakeholders managing the pandemic. This extensive use of GIS in the healthcare sector during the COVID-19 pandemic marks a significant milestone for its adoption on a large scale in India. Although the pandemic enabled large-scale adoption, there are several other reasons for the exponential growth of GIS applications in healthcare:

- Digital Health Initiatives: The Indian government's push towards digitalisation in the healthcare sector, such as the National Health Portal and the Digital India campaign, has provided a favourable environment for adopting GIS. These initiatives aimed to improve healthcare delivery, enhance data management, and promote interoperability, creating a platform for GIS integration.
- Public Health Planning and Disease Management: GIS offers powerful tools for analysing spatial data on disease prevalence, healthcare facilities, and population demographics. This has enabled healthcare authorities and policymakers to identify disease hotspots, plan targeted interventions, and allocate resources efficiently.
- Healthcare Infrastructure Development: With India's expanding population and urbanisation, there has been a need for efficient planning and development of healthcare

infrastructure. GIS has been instrumental in site selection for hospitals and healthcare facilities, optimising accessibility, and identifying areas with inadequate healthcare services.

- Emergency Medical Services: GIS has been utilised to improve emergency medical services (EMS) in India. Real-time mapping of ambulance locations, integration with GPS for navigation, and identification of optimal routes have facilitated faster response times and improved patient outcomes. GIS has also been used for efficient resource allocation during disasters and mass casualty incidents.
- Access to Services: The COVID-19 pandemic accelerated the adoption of telemedicine and remote healthcare services in India. GIS has played a vital role in mapping telemedicine providers, connecting patients with remote healthcare facilities, and ensuring access to quality healthcare services, especially in rural and underserved areas.
- Aayushman Bharat Digital Mission: GIS facilitates the integration of health data from multiple sources, such as electronic health records, demographic data, and environmental data. By combining and analysing these datasets spatially, healthcare professionals can gain valuable insights into disease patterns, environmental factors influencing health, and socio-economic determinants of healthcare disparities.

The National Health Policy of 2017 (NHP) outlined the vision of ensuring health and well-being for all individuals across all age groups. It emphasised citizen-centricity, quality care, improved access, universal health coverage, and inclusiveness for all citizens. Recognising the significance of digital technologies in achieving these goals, the government launched the Digital India Program in 2015, promoting technology use in various sectors, including healthcare. In 2020, the National Health Digital Mission (NHDM) became a spin-off from the initiatives to establish an integrated digital health infrastructure and create a national digital health ecosystem. Several new programs were launched to support this mission, including developing a national health stack comprising a health ID system, health data exchange, and personal health record system. Additionally, digital health platforms and registries were established to provide shared digital infrastructure for healthcare services and implement digital health records and telemedicine services.

A significant milestone was achieved in the geospatial industry when the Ministry of Science and Technology formulated the National Geospatial Policy 2022 (NSP) following the removal of restrictions on geospatial data use. The NSP aims to strengthen the geospatial sector to support national development, economic growth, and an information-driven economy. It builds upon guidelines issued by the government of India in 2021 for acquiring and developing geospatial data and services. The policy recognises the wide-ranging applications of geospatial technology across various sectors and emphasises the value of geospatial data as critical national infrastructure. The NSP sets milestones to be achieved in the short term, medium term, and long term by 2035, including liberalising the geospatial sector, enhancing availability and access to location data, establishing geospatial infrastructures, developing a geospatial knowledge infrastructure, conducting surveys, and mapping various areas and infrastructure. It acknowledges the importance of geospatial data in achieving sustainable development goals, emphasises open data and structural reforms, and encourages increased private sector involvement in the geospatial industry. The industry believes that the policy will serve as a catalyst for promoting open platforms, standardised codes and practices, and the democratisation of data. Under this policy, data and other topographic information generated by government departments and other geospatial data financed by public resources will be designated public goods, thereby ensuring open access for all. The Survey of India, a key department within the government of India, will retain a pivotal role in upholding high-resolution standards, spatial accuracy, and the production of ortho imagery, which involves the correction of geographical and optical distortions. However, the collection and compilation of this data will be executed in collaboration with the private sector, marking a significant shift in the dynamics of geospatial data management.

6.4 THE ROLE OF THE GEOSPATIAL SECTOR IN AIDING THE DELIVERY OF HEALTHCARE SERVICES

Since the early 2000s, geographic information systems have played a pivotal role in enhancing the delivery of healthcare services by harnessing spatial data for informed decision-making and resource management. Through GIS, the federal and provincial planning departments strategised the location of healthcare facilities and intervention centres based on the population distribution. Geographic location has become more critical to planning operations, allocating and managing human resources to the established facilities by analysing patient population density and healthcare utilisation rates [5]. In addition, GIS aided in disease surveillance, outbreak management, and public health interventions by mapping the spread of infections and targeting specific areas for interventions. During emergencies and disasters, GIS enables swift response and resource mobilisation, ensuring effective healthcare delivery [6]. Moreover, GIS helps address healthcare access disparities and supports the planning of chronic disease management programs. By exploring the connections between environmental factors and health outcomes, GIS is contributing to gaining insights into public health challenges, enhancing service equity, and improving health outcomes for communities through evidence-based policies besides empowering healthcare organisations [7].

In India, the application of GIS has exponentially increased with the emergence of information technology and remote sensing techniques. Several government schemes that have been initiated in the recent past, such as the Aayushman Bharat Digital Health Mission (ABDM), Malaria Mukt Bharat, National Tuberculosis Elimination Program, and AarogyaSetu during the pandemic, leveraged geospatial data to deliver healthcare services effectively. The successful utilisation of geospatial data in various of government initiatives is described in the following.

6.4.1 Aayushman Bharat Digital Health Mission

As part of the National Health Policy's specific goals and deliverables for adopting digital technologies in the healthcare sector, the Ministry of Health and Family Welfare developed an implementation framework for the National Health Stack [8]. The outcome is to lay out a National Digital Health Blueprint (NDHB) that will become a roadmap and action plan to integrate digital technologies in healthcare. The implementation of the National Digital Health Mission is envisaged to be implemented in Mission mode; hence, the mission is mandated to establish quantifiable objectives and outcomes with interoperable systems that can become a model for adoption by states and other stakeholders in the healthcare sector.

To ensure seamless, interoperable data exchange between various healthcare actors, the mission is envisaged to focus primarily on health data collection and aggregation, creation of health IDs, creation and maintenance of health registries, health data analytics, infrastructure planning, claims, telemedicine, and e-pharmacy networks.

- Healthcare Infrastructure Planning: With the application of GIS, the state health machinery can identify areas with high healthcare demands and underserved regions to establish health centres and pharmacy networks.
- Personal and non-personal health data related to an individual containing detailed information or the number of vector-borne diseases in specific geographies are being collected to map the individual data with the burden of diseases to ensure better health outcomes.
- Electronic records such as medical records and health records ensure interoperability of the patient's data at both intra- and inter-hospital levels, which helps healthcare professionals diagnose better and provide targeted treatment.
- Health ID creation is being done at public hospitals and other health and wellness centres established across the country. The ID can be created for any individual by providing their contact information and demographic details by authenticating their Aadhar credentials.

By authenticating with Aadhar credentials, the health ID can be mapped with Aadhar, which can be used by the government for developing and executing health-related schemes in a targeted approach.

- Health registries contain information regarding various stakeholders of the healthcare ecosystem. It includes public and private doctors and hospitals, nursing staff, medical representatives, community clinics, pathology laboratories, phlebotomists, insurance companies, pharmacies, and district intervention centres, among others. These registries provide accountability and transparency.
- The critical element of NDHM is providing systematic records to disseminate information in an interactive manner for policymakers, researchers, students, and other stakeholders. This information can be represented in the form of charts, maps with GIS layers, tables, and structured data formats for analysis and monitoring.
- Leveraging GIS and private sector participation, the NDHM is expanding access to care services through public and private sector apps. This will provide open access to access pharmacies, healthcare professionals, and other healthcare service providers based on their geospatial coordinates.
- NDHM, in collaboration with Insurance Regulatory and Development Authority of India (IRDAI), is working towards efficient claims processing by leveraging health data, registries, and other relevant information. This eliminates information asymmetry between patients, insurance providers, and hospital administration.

The objective of the mission was to initiate the program in a pilot mode and scale up quickly. This approach is more aligned with the philosophy that revolves around identifying implementation challenges in real time and learning while executing. The implementation of NDHM is structured into three phases: Phase 1 will consist of a pilot in six UTs, and Phase 2 will cover additional states and UTs in pilot mode by expanding the buffet of services, as delineated previously. In Phase 3, the program will be converging with various health schemes across the country by implementing in partnership with the administrative machinery of the states.

Karnataka is one of the states that has been at the forefront of adopting technology into healthcare. The state has rolled out a vision document to aid the healthcare sector by mainstreaming the integration of technology and the healthcare infrastructure. Prior to the pandemic, the state had exponentially scaled up the hospital management information system (HMIS) to initiate the digitisation of healthcare [9]. With the launch of the Ayushman Bharat Digital Mission by the prime minister of India, various states have started to converge their digitalisation efforts with ABDM, and Karnataka also accelerated its adoption. The state has been proactive in implementing the Healthcare Professionals Registry (HPR), and as of June 2023, the state stands at the top with the highest number of registered healthcare professionals on the portal of HPR. Over 90% of the profiles submitted were verified on the portal.

Some of the key strategies that the state executed to attain the top spot in the digitalisation of HPR are:

- Engagement strategy with healthcare professionals and medical councils.
- Building the capacity of state officials and council staff by interacting with NHA and further establishing capacities of district medical and health officers, verifiers, and nodal officers of e-hospitals at the district level.
- Disseminating the benefits of registering on the HPR portal. Historically, the state has been digitally advanced in implementing various public schemes, but the state positioned itself to achieve operational efficiency in the healthcare sector.
- The state converged other public schemes implemented by both the centre and state governments, such as Jeevasarthakathe (state organ and tissue transplantation scheme) and Pradhan Mantri Jan Aarogya Yojana.

- Setting up grievance redressal mechanisms and delegating grievances to district nodal officers.
- Active monitoring of progress—Review meetings under the subject matter division were conducted every week/fortnight.

The success of HPR has led the state to concentrate on registering private healthcare professionals. The state government conducted a massive campaign to create awareness on the importance of HPR. The state has further partnered with various associations, like the Indian Medical Association (IMA), to ensure greater enrolment of doctors in HPR. These GIS-based registries will aid citizens in accessing healthcare services and consulting through a digital application, even at the block level. Further, this registry provides each registered professional with a unique 14-digit healthcare professional ID (HP ID) similar to the UIDAI Aadhar ID, a unique identity helping the public gain trust and confidence in registered professionals. Registered practitioners also benefit from a range of services such as reducing administrative burdens, a wider reach through digital presence, going paperless, and targeted medication through accessing the digital healthcare records of the patient.

6.4.2 Mapping Burden of Diseases

Malaria remains a significant health burden in developing countries, affecting approximately 3.5–5.0 billion people and causing around 1 million deaths annually. The disease's dissemination is influenced by multiple parameters affecting vectors, parasites, and human hosts, with environmental factors contributing to 70–90% of malaria risk. Parameters that are directly related to the environment, such as precipitation, temperature, humidity, and vegetation, significantly influence malaria diffusion. Mapping malaria incidence data is a fundamental tool for analysing regional variation in public health. Map spatial representation and analysis draw attention to locations with higher disease prevalence or patterns. As public health issues become more complex, geospatial visualisation has emerged as a crucial tool in many public health and epidemiology projects. It plays a significant role in planning and managing healthcare facilities and disease mapping. These systems allow for the collection, management, interpretation, integration, display, manipulation, analysis, and utilisation of datasets with spatial and temporal reference, which is vital for malaria research. Further, they become critical in defining the epidemiology of malaria and its relationship to environmental factors by identifying the applicable risk parameters for mapping and estimating the spread of diseases. This technology has facilitated comprehensive studies on the occurrence of the disease and its association with vector distribution, and with the use of spaceborne satellite data, accessing information for large and remote areas has become much more accessible.

Epidemiologists use spatial mapping to analyse correlations between location, environment, and disease. GIS has been extensively used in mapping and monitoring of diseases caused through vectors or water, health situation assessment in specific areas, assessment and analysis of public health situations, identification of high-risk clusters, and intervention monitoring and assessment. Health GIS has become essential for national, regional, town, and village risk assessment in India, where diverse lifestyles, climatic zones, and environmental conditions exist [10]. Several public policy institutions, pressure groups, and government institutions in India are actively advocating the application of health GIS due to the country's vast size and varied conditions. Emphasising the significance of health GIS in India, it enables effective management of malaria and other health-related challenges.

The Uttar Pradesh (UP) state government conducted disease surveillance and mapping of malaria across the state [11]. The health department leveraged GIS to track the spread of disease and map the geographical distribution of reported cases. Using GIS, healthcare authorities identified disease hotspots, analysed patterns, and responded with targeted interventions to control the spread of infections. The mapping is conducted based on multiple factors that contribute to an increase in the transmission of vector-carrying malaria disease [12].

- Rainfall is the primary triggering factor for malaria, leading to soil saturation and increased pore water pressure. This condition creates favourable breeding environments for mosquitoes, the vectors responsible for transmitting malaria.
- Temperature—Various research studies have shown that temperature is a vital factor in the spread of malaria, and the conditions for the development of malaria vectors typically range around a 35-degree profile across tropical regions.
- Population density plays an important role in the prevalence of malaria. In the rural parts of UP, the GIS tools displayed higher pixels, signifying the higher spread, and vice versa when the population density is high.
- Distance to water bodies—The distance to rivers, gullies, and local water bodies is a crucial factor influencing the proliferation of malaria parasites and the prevalence of the disease. The proximity of populated areas to these water bodies is a significant parameter for breeding malaria vectors. In particular, streams can hurt communities residing in low-lying regions, such as villages and settlements near rivers/streams, as they provide conducive breeding sources for malaria-carrying mosquitoes.
- Proximity to roads—This is an essential parameter to measure the accessibility of hospitals or community clinics to the citizens. By creating different buffer areas along the road paths, researchers can assess the impact of road proximity on malaria prevalence. These buffer areas help analyse how the availability and ease of access to healthcare services along the road network influence the prevalence and management of malaria in the region. A differential global positioning system (DGPS) was employed to survey the existing health facilities, allowing for precise geographic mapping.
- Land use/cover and natural vegetation—Land cover and information on vegetation also play a critical role in developing a susceptibility map to track vector-borne diseases. The government has created a land cover map of Uttar Pradesh using a GIS platform with an image processing layer, focusing on five main classes: agricultural and fallow lands, community settlements, and forest and water resources. It has been identified that naturally occurring resources, such as forests and water bodies, play crucial roles as breeding grounds for malaria vectors. Areas with dense tree cover provide conducive conditions for the proliferation of malaria-carrying mosquitoes. Additionally, crop fields, particularly in regions dominated by rice cultivation, are vital, as they serve as a breeding source for various disease-causing vectors.

The core objective of mapping malaria susceptibility across Uttar Pradesh is to correlate malaria occurrence in UP with the parameters that are known to cause malaria. This exercise has enabled the health department to improve access to healthcare facilities and provide targeted delivery of services in areas affected by malaria. Prior detection through improved surveillance and expediting measures taken in a timely manner can contain the spread of diseases in the hot spots.

6.4.3 AarogyaSetu—A Digital Initiative to Fight the Pandemic by Leveraging GIS Technology

In recent times, geospatial techniques have gained significant prominence in technology and science. Amidst the global outbreak of COVID-19, researchers and policymakers pondered how to leverage these technologies for social good. The pandemic caused by the novel coronavirus has posed grave threats to human health, livelihoods, social functioning, and international relations. In dealing with infectious disease outbreaks, especially pandemics like COVID-19, geographic understanding is crucial in detection, comprehension, and response. Geospatial technology emerged as a powerful tool for preventing the spread of the pandemic rather than solely focusing on treatment. Multiple holistic strategies emerged due to innovations in big data and GIS technologies to contain the spread of COVID-19. Several global dashboards have come into existence to monitor and anticipate the diffusion rate of the virus. Various nations are engaged in the development of contact-tracing methodologies aimed at identifying individuals suspected of being infected. For instance, in South Korea, governmental authorities maintain an extensive database containing pertinent information about confirmed patients, including age, gender, and occupation.

Similarly, the Israeli government has developed strategies to monitor the data of individuals suspected of harbouring the infection through their mobile phones [13]. Meanwhile, Singapore has introduced a mobile application named TraceTogether, which leverages Bluetooth technology to detect proximity between users of the application. Should an individual's COVID-19 diagnosis be confirmed, human contact tracers can initiate appropriate follow-up measures. Similarly, India has also developed a mobile-based tracing application known as AarogyaSetu. This application functions by notifying users as soon as they are in proximity with an individual known to be infected, utilising a combination of Bluetooth and positioning coordinates. Notably, the information collected through the application remains confidential and is exclusively employed by the government for COVID-19 tracing, monitoring, and control.

These details help to find if individuals are positioned within a safe vicinity. In international travel history situations, the application cross-references the user's history with the government's database to identify and correlate with those who tested positive for COVID-19. While developing any comprehensive data analytics system, the development integrates the following systems: an edge sensor, an intermediate data aggregation mechanism, and cloud-based analytics. This intricate development task necessitates meticulous consideration of many aspects, including the societal implications surrounding deploying the system.

In the context of the AarogyaSetu application, a systematic approach is employed to record and transmit symptoms. The acquisition of latitude and longitude coordinates is crucial for ensuring the prompt accessibility of the nearest COVID care facility for the afflicted individual. The application's utilisation of Bluetooth technology enables the tracking of contacts [14]. Through the allocation of distinct device identifiers to the mobile devices of individuals A and B, reciprocal storage of these identifiers occurs within each other's devices. If individual A receives a positive diagnosis, the cloud system retrieves the pertinent data from mobile device A. This dataset encompasses mobile identifiers, temporal durations, and proximity details about all individuals who have had contact with individual A. Drawing upon these data points and employing guidelines formulated by virologists, alert notifications are dispatched to the mobile device identifiers associated with those who have come into contact with individual A. The development cycle encompassed various stages, commencing with the installation of software requirement specifications. This was followed by phases such as functional testing, performance testing, and security testing. Subsequently, the system underwent deployment, culminating in end-user acceptance assessments. The subsequent phases involved user engagement, utilisation, drawing inferences, and a detailed examination of the application's implementation through a designated case study.

Several criticisms have arisen regarding the rationale behind gathering location information. Those overseeing the tracking of disease transmission find it impractical to contact each person individually. Nevertheless, the initiation of any practical measures hinges on the acquisition of location data. The question then emerges: How can this approach be expanded on a larger scale? Establishing a high level of trust with end users is paramount when designing such systems. The gauge of success hinges on the user engagement rate, reflecting the extent to which the system is embraced. During the formulation of software requirement specifications (SRSs), user perception assumes great significance. It becomes imperative to offer transparent explanations for the necessity of specific data. While dealing with such systems, the criticality revolves around two core factors: privacy and security. A noteworthy accomplishment of the application is its ability to safeguard the anonymity of individuals in contact with a COVID-positive person. The app has effectively ensured that the information identifying the intermediary individual remains undisclosed.

The mobile application is integrated with the cloud for storing the data in a secured and encrypted form. The cloud automatically removes data that is obsolete, as the impact of virus typically stays for a period of two weeks as scientific evidence. Additionally, the application enables every user to upload information relating to the symptoms notified by the government of India, which is eventually stored in the cloud. This information will only be triggered when the individuals test positive for COVID-19. This data serves as the foundation for a comprehensive contact-tracing process, where associations with COVID-19–positive individuals are extracted. A sophisticated epidemiological model meticulously evaluates the contact trace information, assigning risk classifications—ranging from high to low risk—to each contact. These risk assessments are communicated back to traced device IDs via mobile devices. Furthermore, users receive supplementary information encompassing infection spread within their proximity and the locations of available test centres.

An IT-enabled Telco information-based hotspot analysis system (ITIHAS) is the underlying framework for predictive hotspot analysis. Properly harnessed and analysed, the data embedded within ITIHAS yields invaluable insights [15]. The system processed over 200,000 self-assessments and traces daily. A crucial realisation emerged that the system's efficacy hinges entirely on effective follow-up procedures. Thus, comprehensive considerations spanning states, districts, pin codes, and sub-post offices are imperative. Each sub-post office is meticulously geotagged with latitude and longitude coordinates, allowing precise alignment between queries on geographical coordinates and corresponding sub-post offices.

The operational framework of ITIHAS operates using information pertaining to COVID-positive individuals within a specific area over a 15-day window. Self-assessment data is amalgamated with latitude and longitude coordinates, adding a spatial dimension to the analysis. Based on the synthesised data, regions are categorised into distinct zones, differentiated by colour codes. These zones include immediate security areas (pink), scrutiny areas (amber), watchlist areas (light blue), and immediate watchlist areas (dark blue). The central goal of this classification is to detect, alert, and categorise potential infection-prone areas drilled down to the pin-code sub-post office level.

Furthermore, the system aims to identify specific sub-areas within these zones. Follow-up actions are prescribed for mobile numbers within these designated areas, contingent upon their reporting of symptoms through the self-assessment feature. State-wise reports are generated, facilitating the identification of district-wise hidden COVID-19 spots that may have evaded the spotlight in previous hotspot assessments.

To summarise, the application served as a valuable tool for government agencies, effectively monitoring individuals who tested positive for the virus. It fulfilled a dual role, offering users insights into localised infection cases while alerting them if they had inadvertently encountered a COVID-19–positive individual. Leveraging its API, the application employs periodic exchange of tracing keys among smartphones, thus facilitating the local storage of contact information while maintaining privacy and security through cryptographic techniques.

Beyond reporting user self-assessment results and positive cases, the application has the potential to display a geographical map highlighting areas with confirmed COVID-19 cases nearby. Swift notifications via email and SMS are feasible upon entering designated red zones or containment areas. The lessons and insights garnered from this study offer a valuable roadmap for other countries and regions to develop similar contact-tracing applications tailored to their unique circumstances.

By showcasing the application's multifaceted utility, which was developed in less than 21 days, the platform catalysed the advancement of contact-tracing technologies in various communities and regions, fostering collective efforts to combat the challenges of infectious diseases.

6.5 CHALLENGES AND OPPORTUNITIES IN HEALTHCARE GIS

By adopting GIS technologies in the healthcare industry, there are a variety of challenges. The first and foremost is related to data quality, integration, and governance, which leads to concerns regarding privacy and security aspects. Further, the technical expertise regarding the methodologies adopted for data collection and analysis is critical for improving the decision-making and delivery of services. Some of the key challenges include:

- **Data Integration and Quality**: Healthcare data is often dispersed across various systems and formats in India due to the lack of standardised systems. Integrating data from different sources into a cohesive GIS platform can be complex, affecting data quality and accuracy.
- **Privacy and Security:** Healthcare data is sensitive and subject to strict privacy regulations (such as the DPDP Act, 2023). Implementing GIS solutions while maintaining patient confidentiality and data security is challenging, considering India's demography.
- **Interoperability:** Integrating GIS with existing healthcare systems (electronic, etc.) can be difficult due to differences in data formats, standards, and protocols.
- **Technical Expertise:** Implementing and maintaining GIS technologies require specialised skills and expertise. Healthcare professionals might lack the necessary training to utilise these tools effectively.
- **Cost:** GIS implementation involves costs associated with software, hardware, training, and maintenance. These expenses can be significant, particularly for smaller healthcare facilities.
- **Change Management:** Introducing new technologies often requires a cultural shift within an organisation. Resistance to change from staff accustomed to traditional methods can hinder adoption.
- **Data Governance:** Establishing clear data governance policies is essential to manage data sharing, access, and usage within the GIS framework, especially in collaborative healthcare settings.
- **Regulatory Challenge:** The difficulty in integrating the CORS network with the India Health stack and the need for adequate protocols and guidelines can hinder the adoption of GIS technologies.
- **Licensing and Accreditations:** The absence of a nodal entity to define protocols, standards, guidelines, and accreditation may create a lack of trust in adopting the developed technologies.

While there are multiple challenges to address, the classification of the geospatial sector as a Sunrise sector in the 2022–23 budget by the government of India has created many opportunities in the healthcare sector for improved decision-making, disease surveillance, resource allocation, and community engagement.

- **Disease Surveillance and Analysis:** India experiences a high rate of burden of diseases such as tuberculosis, malaria, and cancer, among others. Adopting GIS can track the spread of diseases, analyse hotspot areas, and support epidemiological research. This is particularly relevant during outbreaks or when studying the impact of environmental factors on health.
- **Public Health Initiatives:** The Indian government spends over 2.1% of its GDP on healthcare. GIS can assist in planning healthcare facilities by identifying underserved areas, predicting patient demand, and optimising resource allocation for better patient care. Further, GIS can have a huge impact on developing targeted interventions by mapping disease distribution, vaccination coverage, and other factors impacting community health.
- **Emergency Response:** With the growing impact of climate change, disasters, and emergencies, GIS can provide real-time data on healthcare facility locations, available resources, and affected areas, enabling efficient response and resource deployment.
- **Telemedicine and Digital Interventions:** In India's digital initiatives and Ayushmann Bharat Mission, GIS can be integrated into the health stack, telemedicine applications, and

other digital interventions to provide patients with location-specific healthcare resources, nearby providers, and appointment scheduling.

- **Environmental Health:** Geospatial technologies can be used to quantify the impact of environmental factors on public health, such as air and water pollution, and access to green land and blue spaces, such as open areas, parks, and waterbodies.

6.6 ACTION PLAN AND THE WAY FORWARD

The integration of GIS interventions within India's healthcare system offers a promising trajectory for the future. The healthcare landscape in India stands on the cusp of a profound transformation, propelled by technological strides, amplified cooperation between public and private entities, and encouraging policy measures. Pivotal advancements, exemplified by the expansion of the Ayushman Bharat Digital Mission and strategic endeavours aimed at alleviating disease burdens through AI/ML-integrated surveillance, mapping, and digital health solutions, are poised to redefine the country's healthcare landscape. These technological enablers will usher in remote healthcare provisions, facilitate seamless patient-provider communication, and revolutionise healthcare delivery paradigms. Their significance extends to bridging healthcare access gaps in rural and remote precincts, augmenting health outcomes, and curtailing healthcare expenditures.

Concurrently, the assimilation of cutting-edge technologies, like drones for mapping and advanced data collection techniques, possesses the potential to revolutionise India's geospatial framework, engendering swifter response times and augmented care accessibility. The imperative lies in surmounting current system challenges—resource limitations and inadequate infrastructure for integrating mapping algorithms, ensuring the efficacious roll-out of technology-enabled GIS solutions. Collaboration between public and private stakeholders and supportive policy initiatives emerge as linchpins in shaping India's healthcare trajectory.

Furthermore, establishing a central agency akin to New Space India Ltd or NPCI assumes pivotal significance, tasked with catalysing GIS technology adoption in healthcare. This institution could undertake the formulation of apt regulatory and legal frameworks—data privacy, security, licensing, and incentivising policies—that promote the deployment of innovative healthcare solutions and public–private collaborations. As technological horizons broaden and India's healthcare ecosystem evolves, the landscape for pioneering healthcare solutions and public–private synergies is primed for innovation and advancement.

REFERENCES

[1] Fletcher-Lartey, S.M. and Caprarelli, G. (2016) Application of GIS Technology in Public Health: Successes and Challenges. Cambridge University Press.

[2] Blossom, J.C., Finkelstein, J.L., Guan, W.W. and Burns, B. (2011) Applying GIS Methods to Public Health Research at Harvard University. J. Map Geog. Lib., 7(3): 349–376.

[3] Balamurugan, G., Roy, N., Samrat, S., Kurne, V.N., Purwar, D. and Siddarth, D.D. (2011) *Applications of GIS in Public Health Risk Reduction—ArcGIS Approach*, 12th Esri India User Conference.

[4] Brooker, S. (2010). Estimating the Global Distribution and Disease Burden of Intestinal Nematode Infections: Adding Up the Numbers—A Review. Int. J. Paras., 40: 1137–1144.

[5] Chang, A., Parrales, M., Jimenez, J., Sobieszczyk, M., Hammer, S., Copenhaver, D. and Kulkarni, R. (2009). Combining Google Earth and GIS Mapping Technologies in a Dengue Surveillance System for Developing Countries. Intern. J. Health Geog., 8: 49.

[6] Beale, L., Hodgson, S., Abellan, J. J., Lefevre, S. and Jarup, L. (2010). The Rapid Inquiry Facility Evaluates Spatial Relationships Between Health and the Environment. Environ. Health Persp., 118: 1306.

[7] Mullner, R.M., Kyusuk, C., Croke, K.G. and Menash, E.K. (2004). Geographical Information Systems in Public Health and Medicine. J. Med. Sys., 28(3): 215–221.

[8] Making India a Digital Health Nation Enabling Digital Healthcare for All, Strategy Overview. (2020). National Health Authority, Ministry of Health & Family Welfare.

[9] Ayushman Bharat Digital Mission, Healthcare Professional Registry: National Health Authority—Karnataka a Case Study. Available at: https://hpr.abdm.gov.in/en
[10] Rai, P. and Nathawat, M. (2013). Application of GIS and Statistical Methods to Select Optimum Model for Malaria Susceptibility Zonation: A Case Study. Analele ştiinţifice ale Universităţii "Al. I. Cuza" din Iaşi. Secţiunea IIIc, Ştiinţe economice, 1976: 73–94.
[11] Rai, P.K., Nathawat, M.S. and Onagh, M. (2012). Application of Multiple Linear Regression Model Through GIS & Remote Sensing for Malaria Mapping in Varanasi District, India. Health Sci. J., 6(4): 731–749.
[12] Rai, P.K., Nathawat, M.S., Mishra, A., Singh, S.B. and Onagh, M. (2011). Role of GIS and GPS in VBD Mapping: A Case Study. J. GIS Trend. Acad. Sci., 2(1): 20–27.
[13] Devasia, E. and Joshi, P. (2023). A Study on the Awareness of and Overall Brand Perception of Contact Tracing App for Covid 19—The Case of AarogyaSetu App. Acad. Mark. Stud. J., 27(4).
[14] Gupta, R., Bedi, M., Goyal, P., Wadhera, S. and Verma, V. (2020). Analysis of COVID-19 Tracking Tool in India: Case Study of AarogyaSetu Mobile Application. Digit. Gov. Res. Pract. 1(4), Article 28.
[15] AarogyaSetu—A Case Study of a Large-Scale Data-Driven System for Pandemic Control. Available at: https://eecs.iisc.ac.in/aarogya-setu-a-case-study-of-a-large-scale-data-driven-system-for-pandemic-control/

7 Advancement of Geospatial Technology in Healthcare Systems

Yaman Hooda and Haobam Derit Singh

7.1 INTRODUCTION TO GEOSPATIAL TECHNOLOGIES

The term used for describing the contribution of modern tools to geographic mapping and its analysis is geospatial technologies. These technologies are used to gather data from any part of the Earth with the help of different equipment. The foundation of the evolution of geospatial technologies was the development of maps by gathering data in primeval times. In the late 19th century, the schools and institutions of map-making and cartography collaborated with the process of making maps with the help of aerial photographs (a concept termed aerial photogrammetry). With ongoing incidents of world wars, industrial revolutions, and cold wars, the process of map-making took on a fresh dimension due to the advent of technological advancements in the form of computers and satellite systems.

One of the main functions of satellites in geospatial technologies is to take images of the surface of the Earth and activities of the human race, with certain well-defined shortcomings. Computer systems were designed to store and analyse the data captured by the satellite systems. The final results obtained in the form of images were put together, and with other technological developments, a digitised map was created. GIS is a term to designate the expansion of digitised mapping and datasets based on environmental as well as socio-economic domains, cooperatively. The capability to assemble a wide range of geospatial data for a layered–structured set of maps analysed on the basis of specific themes and then re-communicated to society is the most significant characteristic of GIS. The term "geospatial" applies because the layering of the data was enabled by the information gathered at different locations precisely on the earth's surface [1].

Considering the advancements in the past decade, applications of geospatial technologies have developed a wide network of satellites accompanied by controlling GIS hardware tools in the disciplines of scientific research and security. Moreover, GIS found its place in aerial remote sensing, such as unmanned aerial vehicles for non-military applications [6–24]. Also, the data captured/final output is available to researchers of non-governmental organisations, corporations, and universities. The sectors and areas that are implementing geospatial technologies are reported to be growing at a rapid rate: apprising decision makers in the domains of humanitarian relief, conversation of biodiversity, monitoring of agriculture, industrial engineering, and suppression of forest fires are a few.

Geospatial technologies include (Figure 7.1) the following.

1. *Remote Sensing:*

   Geospatial technology aims to study surfaces or objects at distant locations with the help of images, and collection of data done either from space or aerial photogrammetry and sensor-based stations is known as remote sensing. With the help of data collected at sensor-based stations and its analysis, concerned personnel are able to evaluate the properties of the target and thus present corresponding conclusions. Different options for the

DOI: 10.1201/9781003451846-7

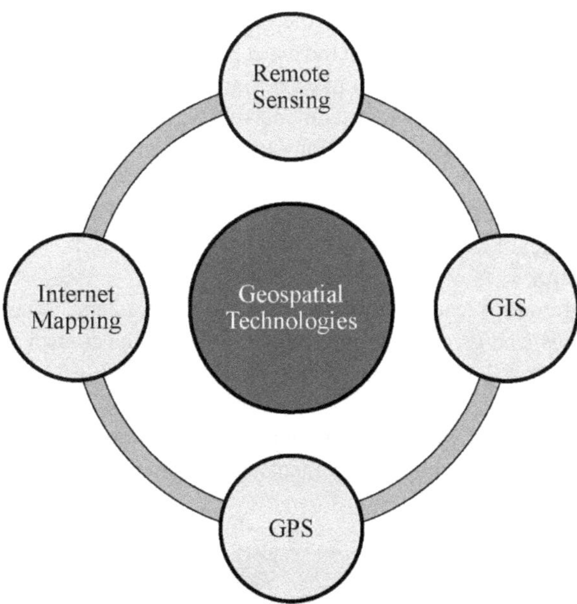

FIGURE 7.1 Types of digital transformation in a society.

source location and procedures of geospatial technologies had been used for the generation of images with the help of satellites orbiting the Earth. They may include:

a. Electromagnetic impulses with the channels of visible, microwave, and infrared.
b. Digitised aerial images captured from drones and aircraft.
c. Light detection and ranging (LiDAR) and radar (radio detection and ranging) for evaluating distance with the help of light or radio signals.

In current scenarios, the application of artificial intelligence (AI) and the Internet of Things (IoT) is being blended with the concept of remote sensing to increase the efficiency in the process of data collection, processing, and transmission with less time.

2. *Geographic Information Systems:*

Geographic information systems are systems of collection of data, with management or storage, mapping, and analysis of the physical available data located at a specific point or area on the surface of the Earth. GIS systems consider the geographic data available in the form of layers for conducting spatial analysis and the production of imitative maps. This geospatial technology discloses the insights of the data deeply, which consists of data patterns and the relationship between them and their surrounding environment, helping users in making smart conclusions. With technological advancements, GIS systems have found application in the domain of disaster response and mitigation, engineering, astronomy, criminal justice and law enforcement, environmental conservation, business, sociology, transportation, travel and tourism, ecology, marketing, demography, healthcare, and news media.

3. *Global Positioning Systems:*

Global positioning systems (GPSs) are navigational systems built of various components such as satellites or networks of satellites, a receiver, and wide range of data algorithms for proper synchronisation of the location and its related characteristics such as time and velocity data of wind and ocean currents. The mathematical practice of trilateration is the working principle of GPS systems. The technique of trilateration requires three satellites for the determination of an accurate position of the data point under consideration, as a single satellite is used to provide a general position of the point under consideration when a larger circular area on the surface of the earth is considered [2]. The second satellite enables the GPS system to converge to the exact location of the designated point. The third satellite is thus able to provide the accurate designated location of the point on the surface of the Earth. There are three separate segments of a typical GPS system (Figure 7.2), which work together to provide exact information of the location on the Earth's surface:

- *Satellite:*
  The application of satellites is in the transmission of signals to different users on their geographical location.
- *Ground Control:*
  A ground control system consists of three components: monitor stations, master control stations, and ground antenna. The function of the control system is monitoring the signal transmissions and operating and tracking satellites.
- *User Equipment:*
  User equipment for a GPS system includes devices used for receiving and transmitting signals, such as telematic instruments, smartphones, and smart watches.

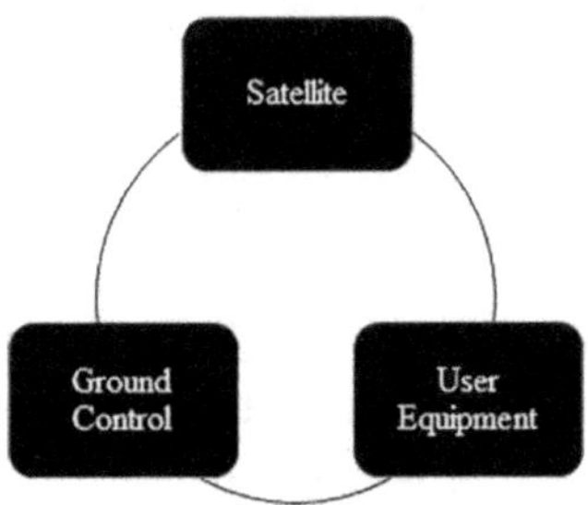

FIGURE 7.2 Distinguished segments of a typical GPS system.

4. *Internet Mapping Technologies:*
   Internet mapping technologies include advanced web features and software programs through which geospatial data can be easily observed, assessed, and circulated. With the changing trends of technology, major progressive expansions are even observed in user-interface devices, making the geospatial data available with ease and higher accuracy.

7.2 APPLICATION OF GEOSPATIAL TECHNOLOGY IN PUBLIC HEALTH SYSTEMS

The application of geospatial technologies has already begun and is increasing, both in central and state government bodies. Specifically in India, the application of geospatial technologies is playing a vital role in e-governance systems and digital reformation systems such as the Smart Cities Mission, Sarv Shiksha Abhiyaan, Digital India, R-APDRV, and Swachh Bharat Mission. Currently, the effective implementation of geospatial technologies can be seen across India in large healthcare programs like Pradhan Mantri Jan Arogya Abhiyan and Ayushman Bharat. For both developing and developed nations worldwide, it is a must to set up a healthcare system and healthcare initiatives that feature geospatial technologies. The priorities and objectives of setting up a geospatial healthcare system at district, state, and national levels are different, but they will be complementary to each other. A holistic picture of the collected information connected to the infrastructure, resources, and asset availability of healthcare systems at the district level will be helpful in detecting situations at ground level. The data or information so obtained at the district level is helpful at the state level in understanding and determining the gaps in the availability of resources and assets so as to meet the requirements of the healthcare systems at the state level. The information so obtained is then visualised, understood, and analysed and becomes a critical resource at the national level for efficient planning and responses, and thus necessary decisions and actions are taken into consideration for the implementation of healthcare systems and policies at the national level.

Geospatial-based data collection, data mapping and data analysis were considered significant technologies at the beginning for international health bodies and international agencies such as the World Health Organisation (WHO), United Nations International Children's Emergency Fund (UNICEF), Centers for Disease Control and Prevention (CDC), United Nations Development Programme (UNDP), and United Nations Office for Disaster Risk Reduction (UNDRR) for understanding the cause of events and controlling the spread of diseases such as Zika, Ebola, and SARS. In the Indian context, healthcare-related institutions such as the Indian Council of Medical Research (ICMR) and National Institute of Malaria Research (NIMR) had been using geospatial technologies in the detection of outbreaks of waterborne diseases such as dengue and malaria.

The coronavirus of 2019, commonly known as COVID-19, had a drastic worldwide impact and left a lesson that the ability for response in critical healthcare systems will remain inhibited unless a proper understanding of spatial data is established. Geospatial technology, such as remote sensing and GIS, allows one to collect and store data, whether in the form of spatial or non-spatial, from variable sources. This data is used for further analysis and thus yields improved insights towards an actionable intelligence. The combined outcomes of all the insights ensure a system of better efficiency and improved understanding, transmission (or communication), and collaboration. The application of geospatial technologies has given enormous access to professionals and personnel related to healthcare systems and also aids in decision making in regard to the following situations:

1. Determination of the location and area of the provision of healthcare facilities, such as testing centres.
2. Evaluation of the location and area of the setting up of quarantine centres.
3. Demography of the impacted population.
4. Classification of the affected population into students, senior citizens, and migrants.
5. Zoning of areas on the basis of the active cases of COVID-19.
6. Availability of needed items such as ventilators and personal protective equipments (PPEs).
7. Responsive strategies to cope with the increasing trend of epidemic.
8. Re-opening measures in predicting the worst-case scenarios.

The application of geospatial technologies was used by all the nations worldwide in developing a dashboard which helps in communication and getting information on integrated health data obtained from different healthcare facilities at various levels. The very efficient and effective method of communication amongst various agencies involved in the management of the epidemic proved to be maps or digital imagery.

7.3 ADVANCEMENTS IN GEOSPATIAL TECHNOLOGIES IN PRIVATE HEALTHCARE SYSTEMS

As technology advances, modifications in healthcare systems need to be incorporated for better treatment of society. The technological boon lies in the fact that this must be focused on saving the lives of people rather than comforting patients. Fascinatingly, the technological boom that is becoming a vital, effective, and efficient tool in the modern healthcare domain is the relationship between geospatial technologies and the Internet of Things. The application of geospatial technologies in the public domain is not a new concept, but its adoption in the private healthcare sector has been observed to be growing substantially in the last decade. Private healthcare systems are using the concept of geospatial technologies in curtailing costs related to healthcare and thus improving the quality of the system with efficient operational and management systems.

Geospatial technologies have been utilised by global healthcare organisations and institutions, making an effort in improving the health of the population at all levels of society. Geospatial technological applications were focused on strategic planning and marketing purposes in the private sector. However, reform in the healthcare system had a noteworthy influence in the amount of private-domain institutions and organisations that are focusing on this technology for providing support to the health of the population and thus for initiatives towards community benefit. Taking a step towards value-based payment and accountable care, service providers are using geospatial technologies for assessment of risk on the basis of geography and its associated population by considering the fact that healthcare facilities must be provided to those desired locations where the reported cases of affected population are highest, thus prioritising the areas for the purpose of interventions [3–5].

As stated by one of the leading healthcare professionals, "Location-based intelligence is critical. Everything happens somewhere. Insight into 'where' makes all the difference in access to care, quality of care delivered, and the opportunity to achieve a positive healthcare outcome". With the conjunction of the IoT with geospatial technologies, travel time has been cut to reach a nearby medical service if a person is suffering from a disease or has even been wounded in an accident. Emerging technologies are even making possible the delivery of emergency resuscitation kits and equipment to patients with heart-related issues by using spatial intelligence technology with the help of smart drone systems.

All healthcare issues have an intrinsic geospatial characterisation. When the healthcare sector is considered an industry, the most common issues that are considered taken care of are directly or indirectly linked to medical establishments such as hospital structures, doctors' offices, and medical facilities. The geospatial domain of remote sensing is closely related to the medical analysis of imagery, as both are related to finding remotely sensed digital imagery for any kind of abnormality and pattern. Geospatial technologies in the healthcare system are often termed health geoinformatics, considered an emerging domain which utilises geospatial technologies for investigation of issues related to health. Health geoinformatics permits analysis and displays multipart statistics in a stimulating format visually by presenting the ability to uncover patterns which may not have been apparent to the interpreter.

The various application domains of geospatial technologies in private healthcare systems includes (Figure 7.3) the following.

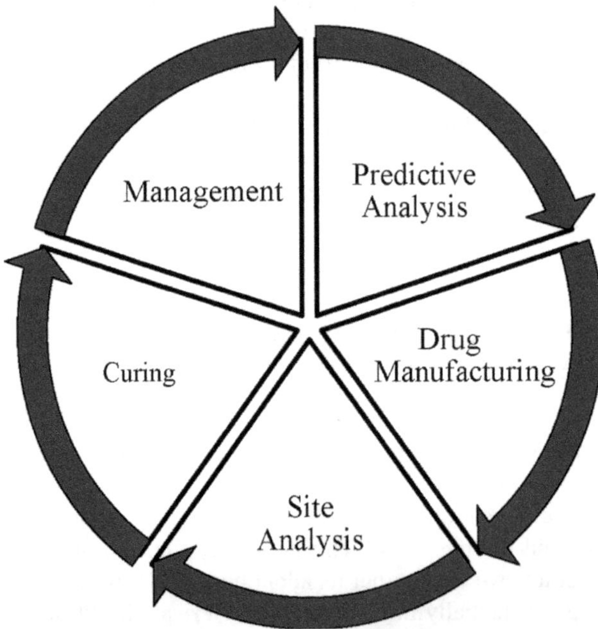

FIGURE 7.3 Application domains of the geospatial technologies in private healthcare systems.

1. *Management:*

Insufficient information regarding the number and demography of patients, availability of healthcare equipment, number and demography of hospital staff, and their status directly increases the mean duration of the patient stay and medical procedure completion time, which directly affects the overall efficiency of the hospital system. One of the major solutions to this issue is a geospatial-based analytical solution. In this solution, the data gathered/stored is envisaged as a hotspot analysis. The dashboard of the system provides a series of reporting tools in the form of key performance indicators (KPIs); this enables management of the hospital system to dramatically improve in determination and understanding of the demand status by allowing them to break down the information stored in different categories such as case numbers and wait time of patients and then split the information into easily understandable figures with different time frames. This solution provides an enhanced process of resourcing, appointing a good number of medical support staff to meet the requirements of increased demand on critical days and thus lighten the resource pressure, diminishing the cost of keeping healthcare standards at optimum performance. Another solution is to develop a database at the community level for supporting health initiatives. The analytical tool application of StreetMap Premium for ArcGIS provides a solution for validation or decoding of data from the existing location of the data point of interest rather than searching and scrubbing different websites for months in an effort to locate the data. The team not only used for locating the positions of community clinics, hospitals, schools, and pharmacies on the map, it also focused on the identification and mapping of the locations that showcased the lacking of necessary assets. Some of the common health-related issues that are easily mapped with higher concentrations of patients include diabetes, asthma, and heart-related issues. Also, the team of management focuses on the identification of areas that are lacking in providing health-related resources for people suffering from mental health issues, obesity, and respiratory illness. Thus, by implementing the geospatial technological domain of GIS, hospital management can dedicate more time to improving the healthcare system of the community rather than worrying about validation of the quality and quantity of the data.

Geospatial technologies allow healthcare systems to develop location-based strategies for keeping a record of the health of the population of a particular community. Both facets of the analytic tools—temporal and spatial—need a strong database management system for the determination of the rate of refresh of the data and to establish a standard coding system for location and time. The various stakeholders associated with the system can perform retrospective analysis easily in discovering patterns once the data is maintained and managed properly. Once the relation between the healthcare and location establishes a particular stature in receiving the recognition, the service providers will develop methods in integrating community-specific information and social determinants into their healthcare-based management approaches and policies. Currently, healthcare service providers are using geospatial technologies as a stage for the purpose of integration and analysis of clinical data, with its effect on behavioural data, socio-economic data, and environment data in gaining a holistic, complete interpretation and understanding the requirements of the patients. Also, these technologies have been used to assess non-clinical factors which impact health outcomes poorly and such locations that must be helped with interventions at community level.

Real-time location systems (RTLS) deliver contextual operational intelligence and awareness to the systems of the IoT for the purpose of increasing efficiency, improving quality management, and effective economy. Medial devices enabled with the technologies of AI and the IoT are able to monitor the health parameters of the patient and help health service providers make decisions on the basis of analysis, prognosis, and health remedies for the ailing patient. Considering developing nations, setting priorities is considered a vital issue faced by the management of healthcare systems, affecting the requirement of health services depending on the availability of health resources. The geospatial technologies used by the healthcare systems of developing nations are only focusing on developing a centralised network system for the assessment of medical records of patients rather than finding their applicability for building an infrastructural networking system. One of the biggest reasons for this is the interest of investors in such an infrastructure which focuses on creating a networking system that enables the patient's data to be transferred as and when required by the concerned personnel. The next concern is how the patients are going to access such a network and networking system. In developing nations like India, where health services are cost restrained, the investment in this system may not be able profitable but legible. The issue in developing nations may get worse as the number of network providers shrinks in the domain of data management and application of geospatial technologies in building networks for healthcare providers.

2. *Site Analysis:*

   Doctors and practitioners working at hospitals and clinics want to get information about their surrounding communities for determination of the nature of the patients to deal with as a whole. To carry out such an analysis, geospatial technological-based data analysis tools are found to be a notable development in the process of decision-making. Geospatial services help healthcare systems to determine which population needs private healthcare facilities and services. The system provides an appreciated visual presentation of the different types of people living in a community, their opinions on private healthcare services, and the existing healthcare facilities and systems available in the area of concern. Such analytical tools are able to provide information regarding the demography of the data collected and thus allow a database management system to be built, revealing the critical locations that need an increase in healthcare facilities and hospital networking systems. With the application of geospatial technologies in the domain of the public health sector, the private health sector is finding its way using the different domains of geospatial technologies in the process of planning and managing healthcare services.

3. *Manufacturing of Drugs:*

   With the emerging applications of AI and the IoT in the domain of drug manufacturing companies, the rate of the production of drugs can be increased with the help of increasing applications of sensor technology at the manufacturing phase. The term for determining the sensor networks that are useful in improving the outcomes of patients radically is the Internet of Things for pharmaceutical manufacturing (IoT-PM). The beginning stage focused on three parameters:

   - Condition Monitoring
   - Predictive Maintenance
   - Analytics

   Some of the important applications of the IoT-PM in healthcare systems include remote diagnostics, supervision on production of drugs, and effective management of drug flow. With the increasing application of internet in everyday devices, an exclusive opportunity was created for getting a better analysis of the frequency and location of healthcare issues. It can be understood in two ways: (1) faster access to the response mechanism of health outbreaks and (2) getting an improved glimpse of the needs and requirements of every community to provide better healthcare services and facilities to people such as pharmaceuticals and medical materials and equipment. Better decisions can be taken once the data is visualised and analysed in meaningful ways by the application of sophisticated yet simple and fast IoT-enabled tools. The application of the IoT in geospatial technologies provides an opportunity to build a connection between sensors and equipment at the time of manufacturing and thus aggregate the information collected over manifold layers in and across production plants worldwide. This technology allows a suitable supervision of the production actions at any time, from any location. The life quality of healthcare customers can be improved with the help of real-time monitoring systems. Exemptions may be expressed in minimisation of waste, reducing production costs, and improvement in utilisation of equipment. An improved pharmaceutical procedure confirms that manufactured drugs are reasonably priced for patients. With the advancements in the technologies such as Big Data technologies, cloud computing, and mobility and sensor technology, a systematic and advanced sensor network system can be created; thus, the potential of the application of the IoT-PM can be further enhanced in different domains of healthcare systems.

4. *Predictive Analysis:*

   As observed in the change of the landscape for healthcare facilities and services, most management systems in the healthcare sector are looking for the application of geospatial technologies to implement the correct infrastructure for the generation of actionable understanding from a batch of fresh sources. The implementation of big data in this category proves beneficial in most healthcare services and facilities. The application of big data in healthcare systems follows the principle in geospatial technologies where the information or data of every patient is stored in a private account and can be accessed by both the patients and hospital management as and when required. By avoiding the carrying of reports in hard copy, the application of geospatial technologies allows storage of data of higher size, such as the results of x-rays, CAT scans, and MRIs. Moreover, healthcare management as well as staff can access the data for analytical purposes in an efficient, repeatable, and intuitive manner. The ability to string together a huge number of analytical procedures and represent them in a user-friendly manner is one of the keys to the communication of complex information in a simple manner. With the application of geospatial technologies, data can be stored and preserved efficiently, as such technological-based databases have the ability to establish a relationship between different patterns, which is obsolete in traditional IT-based healthcare systems. With the present scenario of the variance of unstructured data in healthcare systems, the application of predictive analytical software tools can be helpful in structuring the data stored for proper understanding as well as assessing it when needed to improve the quality and condition of the healthcare facilities provided to patients.

5. *Curing:*

   One emerging technological advancement playing a vital role in healthcare transformation systems for patients is wearable technology. The advancements in wearable technology are becoming more mobile and thus creating fresh replacements for the traditional methods of the facilities provided to patients, including interaction, performing medical tests, collection of data, and delivering treatments. Geospatial technological devices are becoming a lifesaver to patients suffering with disorientation, autism, memory loss, and specific dementias such as Parkinson or Alzheimer's. With the application of GPS tracking services, wearables are allowing senior citizens to be located in a quicker and safer manner. Some emerging solutions for addressing wandering and helping to keep patients suffering from dementias secure and safe are Mindme, Safe Link, Project Lifesaver, and GPS Shoe.

   With its increasing applications, governments of some developed nations are covering the cost related to services and hardware installations for GPS tracking devices designed for severely autistic children and others in similar circumstances. Geospatial technologies are also playing an important role in curing children on the autism spectrum, a condition where the children are unable to recognise basic facial emotions. Leading research organisations around the world are using Google Glass to helping children distinguish between the seven various types of facial expressions.

Healthcare services and facilities are distributed around the world unevenly. The most common challenges faced by healthcare services are topography and infrastructure. Under such circumstances, geospatial technology in form of drone technology plays a major role. Major health organisations/institutions and technology-based companies are using the application of unmanned aerial vehicles (UAVs) worldwide to get information from island-based nations for isolating the population from Nepal to South American jungles.

The positive impact of the collaboration between health organisations/institutions and technology-based companies is the invention of prototypes or models used for the benefit of society. For example, a prototype of a drone was developed for delivery of life-saving equipment. The drone, equipped with emerging technological advancements in the domain of AI and the IoT, a video screen, sensor system, separate camera device, and two-way radio system, was used in reaching out to victims during emergency scenarios until the proper healthcare facilities were provided. Also, instructions for emergency treatment can be easily relayed by doctors from hospitals/clinics to the victims via signal transmission through drones.

The major application of drone technology is mostly seen during post-disaster recovery scenarios. Drones were utilised for delivery of small aid parcels after the 2012 Haitian seismic event. Also, drones were used by doctors for transporting medical equipment to areas of concern. For developing nations like India, it has been reported that people needing organ transplants are increasing with an alarming rate, and drone technologies can be considered lifesavers in such scenarios.

The application of geospatial technologies can increase its domain to a larger global patient-based network and provide facilities and services that are impossible physically. For the success of such a technological amalgamation in the current healthcare system, a proper system must be developed, installed, and most importantly maintained for improving the quality of health standards and for individualising and standardising the quality of care provided in larger patient-based networking systems.

7.4 CHALLENGES IN APPLICATION OF GEOSPATIAL TECHNOLOGIES IN HEALTHCARE SYSTEMS

The robustness of any complex relation between two or more phenomena depends upon blending the phenomena together. In search of positive applications of geospatial technologies in healthcare systems, one must also focus on the challenges that will be occurring at different levels during their adaptation at the societal as well as global level. With some recent studies, it had been observed that there can be uncertainty in the process of application of geospatial data in the healthcare system, which may propagate in the spatial analysis. Some of the challenges that cause uncertainty in the application of geospatial technologies in healthcare systems are (Figure 7.4) as follows.

1. *Geocoding:*

   "Geocoding" is defined as "The process by which an entity on the earth's surface, a household, for example, is given a label identifying its location with respect to some common point or frame of reference". These are computer documents that consist of geographic features, including information regarding rail lines, roads, and railroads. For a better understanding of the files, the feature of "road" is considered a "centre-line", and other relevant information is geocoded, such as the name of the street, number or range of the street, nature of the street, and directional data. The efficiency of the application of geodata in geospatial technologies is based on the accuracy of choosing the reference point, and then all other relevant information are being determined and stored for the analysis purposes. Thus, it's a must that the information stored in a geo-dataset be updated as and when required and geocoded effectively for its application in determination and access of feature points to increase the overall efficiency of the healthcare system worldwide.

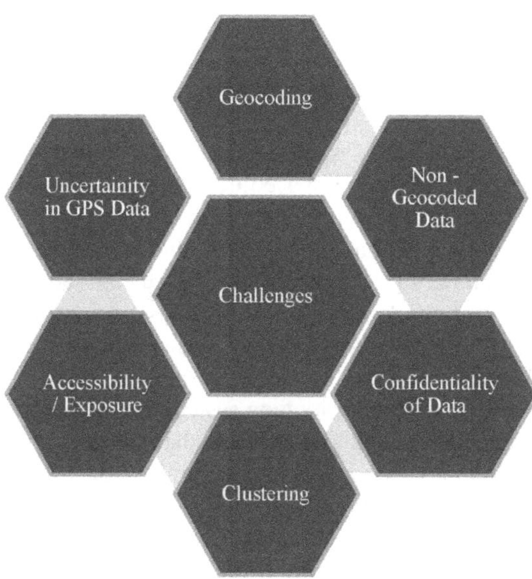

FIGURE 7.4 Approaches for digitisation in natural disaster management.

2. *Non-Geocoded Data:*

   In situations of an unidentified location, incomplete address, or outdated reference database, there may be a higher chance of geocoding of all the addresses. For example, the data of any historical street may become obsolete after fresh residential constructions in urban regions of a country. Non-geocoded data were identified and eliminated from analysis traditionally. Researchers are addressing concerns regarding the availability of non-geocoded data and questioning its influence in dealing with databases made for healthcare policies and programmatic intercession implications. The majority of the data that falls under this category belongs to rural areas, where the general addresses of households and routes are not geocoded. This becomes a challenge while performing sampling analysis and designing for case-controlled experiments.
3. *Confidentiality Issues:*

   One of the most common yet least discussed challenges for the application of geospatial technologies in healthcare systems is the issue of confidentiality. In the sectors of public health, privacy and confidentiality are significantly considered. A breach in confidentiality increases the risk of spreading the information of every individual unknowingly, including their personal information as well as all the database formed regarding one's health conditions. When geocoding datasets, researchers have to be very attentive and focused.
4. *Clustering:*

   Errors may be generated regarding false positions of addresses, resulting in either over-estimation or under-estimation of any risk at all levels of society, which will potentially lead to an increase in both false negatives and false positives. With the studies conducted earlier, even a small error in geocoding the data obtained from geospatial technologies can result in discernible outcome on the analytical results and negatively affect all the clusters of healthcare units. An error in determination of information regarding the cluster of any location affected the overall efficiency of the healthcare unit; for example, if that particular area need medical services and facilities for different reasons and there was an error in the stored information, there would be a high chance that the healthcare facilities delivered would either be more or less than the desired quantity. The former case is not objectionable, but the latter would be critical, as it affects the lives of people directly.

5. *Accessibility/Exposure:*

   Earlier studies in the domain of spatial epidemiology attempted quantification of the exposure of a case-based study via spacetime and space analysis, including different sources of varying geometrical identities, such as point, line, area, and volume. With the application of the geospatial technologies of GIS and GPS, measurements regarding an individual's residential proximity to environment-based exposed sources can be achieved. However, errors in exposure of individuals and areas, not accounting for mobility, and variation in the accessibility measure lead to misclassification of the geo-database.

6. *Uncertainty in GPS Data:*

   The data obtained from global positioning system tracking services in cellular devices is extensively used in studies related to health. The data obtained from GPS software applications is used in addressing geographical context issues. Such datasets provide a precise demarcation of specific surroundings, resulting in a truly relevant geographical context rather than static geographical areas. However, the data obtained from GPS software applications has its own spaciotemporal uncertainties due to the following reasons:

   - Satellite clock drift
   - Satellite location error
   - Receiver clock drift
   - Multipath effects
   - Atmospheric effects
   - Geometric dilution of precision
   - Unpredictable human or system errors

   Such errors are classified as critical when they are combined with reference datasets in the case of intelligent transportation systems. Accurate determination of activity positions is becoming a clear concern for all the research studies based on data derived from GPS systems.

7.5 FUTURE OF GEOSPATIAL TECHNOLOGIES IN HEALTHCARE SYSTEMS

The future of the application of geospatial technologies in healthcare systems is even more promising as compared to its current scenario. One of the most prominent applications would be providing assistance in reaching out to weighted decisions and thus allowing more accurate analysis of storing and maintaining data in healthcare databases. These applications tend to be economical for a wider range of audience and thus their real-time use will inspire a huge spectrum of applications in the future. The reason behind the popular demand for geospatial technologies in healthcare systems lies in the accurate determination of essential data, leading to better decision making and thereby enhancing the productivity and effectiveness of the healthcare system.

REFERENCES

1. Yongwan Chun, Mei-Po Kwan, Daniel A. Griffith (2019) Uncertainty and Context in GIScience and Geography: Challenges in the Era of Geospatial Big Data. International Journal of Geographical Information Science, 33(6), 1131–1134. https://doi.org/10.1080/13658816.2019.1566552.
2. Alan T. Murray, Tony H. Grubesic, Ran Wei, Elizabeth A. Mack (2015) A Hybrid Geocoding Methodology for Spatio-Temporal Data. https://doi.org/10.1111/j.1467-9671.2011.01289.x.
3. Y. Hooda (2022) "IoT and Remote Sensing," in *Computer Vision and Internet of Things*. Chapman and Hall/CRC, pp. 111–140.
4. Yaman Hooda, Haobam Derit Singh (2023) "Digital Reforms in Public Services and Infrastructure Development & Management," in *Technological Prospects and Social Applications of Society 5.0*. Chapman and Hall/CRC, pp. 219–237.

5. Haobam Derit Singh, Yaman Hooda (2023) "Resilience of Digital Society to Natural Disasters," in *Technological Prospects and Social Applications of Society 5.0*. Chapman and Hall/CRC, pp. 185–199.
6. Akshit Anand, Vikrant Jha, Lavanya Sharma (2019) An Improved Local Binary Patterns Histograms Techniques for Face Recognition for Real Time Application. *International Journal of Recent Technology and Engineering*, 8(2S7), 524–529 (Indexed in Scopus, DOI: 10.35940/ijrte.B1098.0782S719) ISSN: 2277-3878
7. Ayush, Lavanya Sharma, Deepa Gupta (2019) "Motion Based Object Detection based on Background Subtraction: A Review", in 3rd IEEE International Conference on Electronics Communication and Aerospace Technology, ICECA 2019, Coimbatore, India, 12–14 June.
8. Ujwal Chopra, Naman Thakur, Lavanya Sharma (2019) Cloud Computing: Elementary Threats & Embellishing Countermeasures for Data Security. *International Journal of Recent Technology and Engineering*, 8(2S7), 518–523 (Indexed in Scopus, DOI: 10.35940/ijrte.B1097.0782S719)
9. Gauri Jha, Pawan Singh, Lavanya Sharma (2019) Recent Advancements of Augmented Reality in Real Time Applications. *International Journal of Recent Technology and Engineering*, 8(2S7), 538–542 (Indexed in Scopus, DOI: 10.35940/ijrte.B10100.0782S719
10. Anubhav Kumar, Gaurav Jha, Lavanya Sharma (2019) Challenges, Potential & Future of IOT Integrated with Block Chain. *International Journal of Recent Technology and Engineering*, 8(2S7), 530–536 (Indexed in Scopus, DOI: 10.35940/ijrte.B1099.0782S719)
11. S. Makkar, L. Sharma (2019) "A Face Detection Using Support Vector Machine: Challenging Issues, Recent Trend, Solutions and Proposed Framework," in M. Singh, P. Gupta, V. Tyagi, J. Flusser, T. Ören, R. Kashyap (eds) Advances in Computing and Data Sciences. ICACDS 2019. Communications in Computer and Information Science, vol. 1046. Springer. https://doi.org/10.1007/978-981-13-9942-8_1
12. Gunjan Saraogi, Deepa Gupta, Lavanya Sharma, Ajay Rana (2021) Un-Supervised Approach to Backorder Prediction Using Deep Autoencoder. *Recent Patents on Computer Science, Bentham*, 14(8) (Indexed in Scopus).
13. Lavanya Sharma (2019) *Object Detection with Background Subtraction*. LAP LAMBERT Academic Publishing, SIA OmniScriptum Publishing, European Union (ISBN: 978-613-7-34386-9).
14. L. Sharma, M. Carpenter (Eds.) (2022) *Computer Vision and Internet of Things: Technologies and Applications* (1st ed.). Chapman and Hall/CRC. https://doi.org/10.1201/9781003244165
15. L. Sharma, P.K. Garg (Eds.) (2021) *Artificial Intelligence: Technologies, Applications, and Challenges* (1st ed.). Chapman and Hall/CRC. https://doi.org/10.1201/9781003140351
16. L. Sharma, P.K. Garg (Eds.) (2023) *Technological Prospects and Social Applications of Society 5.0* (1st ed.). Chapman and Hall/CRC. https://doi.org/10.1201/9781003324720
17. Lavanya Sharma (2020) *Towards Smart World: Homes to Cities using Internet of Things*. Taylor & Francis, CRC Press (ISSN: 9780429297922).
18. Lavanya Sharma, Pradeep K. Garg (2019) *From Visual Surveillance to Internet of Things*. Taylor & Francis, CRC Press (ISSN: 9780429297922).
19. Lavanya Sharma, Pradeep K. Garg (2021) *Artificial Intelligence: Challenges, Technologies and Future*. Wiley (In production).
20. Lavanya Sharma, Annapurna Singh, Dileep Kumar Yadav (2016) *Fisher's Linear Discriminant Ratio based Threshold for Moving Human Detection in Thermal Video, Infrared Physics and Technology*. Elsevier. (SCI impact factor: 1.58, Published)
21. Lavanya Sharma, Dileep Kumar Yadav (2016) Histogram Based Adaptive Learning Rate for Background Modelling and Moving Object Detection in Video Surveillance. *International Journal of Telemedicine and Clinical Practices, Inderscience* (ISSN: 2052-8442, DOI: 10.1504/IJTMCP.2017.082107).
22. Lavanya Sharma, Nirvikar Lohan (2019) Performance Analysis of Moving Object Detection using BGS Techniques in Visual Surveillance. *International Journal of Spatiotemporal Data Science, Inderscience*, 1, 22–53.
23. Lavanya Sharma, Sudhriti Sengupta, Birendra Kumar (2021) An Improved Technique for Enhancement of Satellite Images. *Journal of Physics: Conference Series*, 1714, 012051 (Indexed in Scopus, DOI: 10.1088/1742-6596/1714/1/012051)
24. Supreet Singh, Lavanya Sharma, Birendra Kumar (2021) A Machine Learning Based Predictive Model for Coronavirus Pandemic Scenario. *Journal of Physics: Conference Series*, 1714, 012023 (Indexed in Scopus).

8 Implementation of Deep Learning in Assessment of Health-Hazardous Air Pollutants

Nishi Srivastava and Nisheeth Saxena

8.1 INTRODUCTION

The contamination of air with different polluting airborne substances and gaseous pollutants is called air pollution. Extended exposure to this contaminated air can cause severe harm to human health and ecosystems. The major way that humans are exposed to air pollution is through their respiratory system. Inhalation of these pollutants causes severe damage to human organs such as the lungs, heart, brain, and other organs. These pollutants are harmful for all the organs but especially attack the respiratory and cardiovascular systems. According to their aerodynamic sizes, the suspended particles can reach different depths in the respiratory system. They can be blocked in the upper part of the respiratory system or can go deep into the lungs. They can even enter the bloodstream through these organs and can reach all other parts of the body, causing infection and carcinogenicity.

Air pollution can be a cause of various diseases and can even be lethal in cases of severe exposure. The term "hazardous air pollutants," sometimes known as "toxic air pollutants" or "air toxins," refers to airborne contaminants that are known or strongly suspected to be responsible for respiratory diseases, cardiovascular disease, cancer, and other severe health issues. There is a possible link between air pollution exposure and a higher risk of miscarriage, various malignancies, diabetes, cognitive decline, and neurological disorders.

People may be more likely to get cancer or suffer severe health problems if exposed to harmful air pollution for long enough periods. Air pollution can damage the human immune system, nervous system, and reproductive system and also can affect physical growth. These air pollutants are sometimes deposited in soil or dissolved in various water bodies and thus indirectly affect humans, other living things, and ecosystems through various food chains. This is in addition to exposure through breathing intoxicants. If exposed to enough air toxins over an extended period, animals may suffer from health issues similar to those that affect humans. Various toxic substances are suspended in the atmosphere, and the primary pollutants measured by the pollution monitoring authority in India (Central Pollution Control Board, CPCB) are suspended particulate matter (PM), nitrogen dioxide (NO_2), sulfur dioxide (SO_2), carbon monoxide (CO), and ozone (O_3). All these pollutants significantly affect human health and the ecosystem in many ways. These pollutants can penetrate to different depths in the respiratory system depending on their sizes. They can also enter the blood and cause significant damage to tissues and cells. Particulate matter primarily infects the respiratory system at different levels. Very small particles can go deep into the system and can cause severe damage.

The health impact varies according to the exposure time to polluted air. According to the exposure, these impacts are classified as short- and long-term exposure. Exposure time decides the severity of the impact of pollution on the receptor's health. The range of allowable exposure times and levels vary with different pollutants, and accordingly, health impact also varies. However, it isn't easy to

DOI: 10.1201/9781003451846-8

quantify the health impact in exact terms of exposure time and amount of pollutants. In general, even a small percentage of pollutants and very short exposure will also have some negative impact but may not be measurable. Different time exposure causes different levels of damage to human organs and the entire body. For example, short exposure to particulates can affect lung functioning and enhance asthma frequency and severity, which may damage the respiratory system. Cardiovascular diseases, cancer, and pulmonary disease can be caused by extended exposure to pollutants. Children, elders, and pregnant women are more vulnerable groups that are affected severely by pollution.

However, due to their comparable composition, ambient and domestic air pollution exposure often shares the same health hazards and disease pathways. There are various air pollutants, and their health impact depends mainly on the pollutant concentration, type of pollutant, and exposure time to outdoor and indoor polluted air. As an illustration, fine particulate matter is a frequent and significant contributor to indoor and outdoor air pollution.

Various techniques are implemented to estimate and monitor the air pollutants in the air. With the advancement of computational skills, new computation techniques have been developed and employed to estimate air pollution. Artificial intelligence is one of these technologies.

The term artificial intelligence (AI) refers to the intelligence demonstrated by a system that humans have created. Natural language processing, healthcare, marketing, robotics, finance, e-commerce, agriculture, social media, analytics, geosciences, and other research fields are the areas where AI applications are widely used (Zhu et al., 2020). Machine learning (ML) and deep learning (DL) are both subsets of artificial intelligence. Algorithms for machine learning examine how computers imitate or apply the potential for automatic improvement that characterizes human learning behavior. Through additional abilities, this improved the already existing understanding of learning algorithms. Deep learning technology is a critical area of AI research and has been developed to address the fundamental problems associated with machine learning models (Mitchell, 2007). The health and environmental pollution disciplines utilize the most recent advancements in AI approaches as research tools. The ecological processes incorporate various features ranging through different temporal and spatial scales. Thus, AI approaches are found computationally efficient for this study and incorporate different details of the environment. AI approaches can improve the accuracy of real-time analysis and forecasting of weather and environmental phenomena. These techniques are also helpful for urban planning, land mapping, variation in land cover, and surface properties.

This chapter provides a comprehensive view of the major concepts in the quickly evolving field of artificial intelligence use in evaluating various contaminants that represent a risk to human health. First, we briefly discuss the various air pollutants usually present in the air. Then, we concentrate on the fundamental principles and methods of machine learning, deep learning, various pollutants, and the use of AI, ML, and DL in their estimation. This chapter presents a general description of air pollution, its impact on health, details of AI techniques, and their applications in pollution research.

8.2 AIR POLLUTION AND ITS IMPACT ON HEALTH

Air pollution is an important issue that affects both developed and developing nations, but underdeveloped countries are more impacted. Since there are so many diverse causes of air pollution and their individual impacts are cumulative and synergistic, their health impact is more complex. Concerns are being raised about indoor and outdoor air quality in both rural and urban locations. In actuality, indoor environments in developing countries are where people are exposed to the most air pollution. Inhalation of air pollutants causes harm to respiratory systems, and their traces have also been found in the blood. Thus, the contaminants reach each body organ, causing severe damage.

Additionally, these contaminants are deposited on plants, soil, and water, adding to human exposure. The ability of a material to have harmful effects on living things is known as toxicity. This relative aptitude depends on several factors. These factors are:

- Entry pathways

- Whether a chemical's effects are poisonous, nontoxic, or positive depends on the amount or dose of the substance
- Exposure length and frequency
- How the pollutant's environmental concentrations are actually measured
- Differences within a single species and between distinct species (interspecies and intraspecies differences)

Understanding the pathway from the source to the site is essential for understanding and efficiently controlling the effects of pollutants since monitoring and management can take place anywhere in the trajectory. However, only at the source can accurate control measures be done. The environmental exposure pathway offers a conceptual framework for describing, in general, the relationships between pollutant sources and their effects on human health. The pollutants from an emitter can be released into the atmosphere, water bodies, and soil as well. After release of these pollutants into various essential components for life, they can easily reach human bodies through organs like the nose, mouth, and skin. Therefore, after the level of exposure has been established, it is easy to estimate the dosage, or how much of the pollutant is ingested during a certain time. The result on health is thus determined by the dose.

The pollutant source can also be natural and anthropogenic. The sources can be classified based on their nature of origin, source variability in space, and span of the region associated with emission. Summarizing these quantities regarding the nature of pollution sources, they can be classified as natural, area, mobile, and stationary. Figure 8.1 provides an overview of the different sources of air pollution.

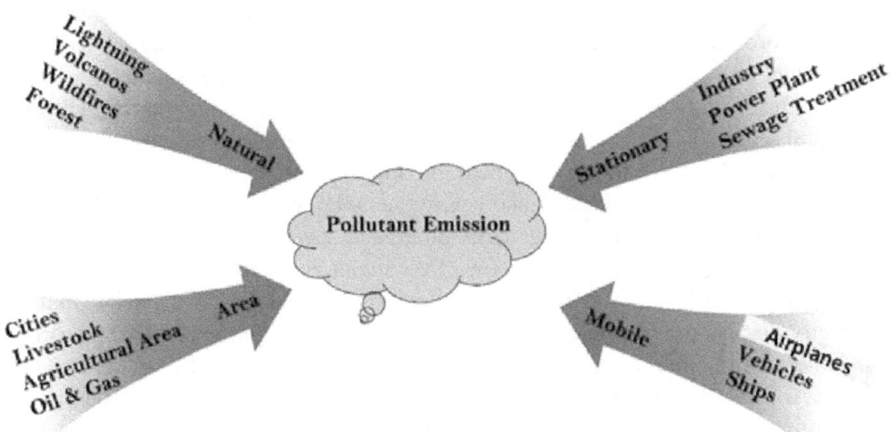

FIGURE 8.1 Overview of the different sources of air pollution.

8.3 HEALTH HAZARDOUS POLLUTANTS

Various pollutants are listed as health hazardous pollutants on the global level. The Indian pollution monitoring/control authority (Central Pollution Control Board, CPCB) monitors various pollutants such as particulate matter (suspended particulate matter, SPM and respiratory suspended particulate matter, RSPM), oxides of nitrogen, ammonia, sulfur dioxide, carbon monoxide, ozone, benzene, toluene, xylene, arsenic, nickel, and benzopyrene particulate phases. Table 8.1 provides revised National Ambient Air Quality Standards (NAAQS) for these pollutants. These pollutants are briefly discussed in the following.

8.3.1 Particulate Matter

Liquid and solid particles suspended in the air are called particulate matter. Particles that are big or dark and can be seen by the naked eye include dust, dirt, soot, and smoke. These are called suspended particulate matter or coarse particulate matter. The suspended particles could also be microscopic in size; thus, they are visible only through specific instruments, such as an electron microscope, due to their tiny size. These particulate matter particles are called fine particles. Particles less than 10 μm in size are called PM_{10}, and particulate matter particles less than 2.5 μm are called $PM_{2.5}$. There are numerous sources of these particles in the environment, including forest fires, anthropogenic activities, construction activities, farming, industrial emissions, power plants, and dust events. Breathing in these fine particles can seriously harm a person's health, as they can reach different depths in the respiratory system and cause moderate to severe damage to respiratory organs depending on their exposure amount and time. Finer particles are more dangerous than coarse ones in terms of health aspects.

8.3.2 Sulfur Dioxide

Sulfur dioxide is a gaseous air pollutant measured as a primary pollutant by the CPCB. Various burning activities, vehicular emissions, industrial emissions, and fossil fuel burning cause emissions of SO_2 in the ambient air. In the atmosphere, sulfur dioxide also changes into sulfates. Emissions from diesel-based vehicles cause significant concentrations of SO_2 in the atmosphere. The conditions of vehicle engines also govern the emissions of SO_2 from them, and old vehicles emit more than new ones. Atmospheric inversion causes the confinement of pollutants in the atmosphere. Power plants running on coal may cause significant amounts of SO_2 in atmospheric inversion conditions. High emission amounts from sulfur dioxide are also produced near ports, smelters, and other sources.

The highest SO_2 exposure is experienced by those who live and work close to these massive sources. After entering the atmosphere, SO_2 undergoes a chemical transformation that produces sulfate particles that can travel hundreds of miles.

Sulfur dioxide has a variety of negative consequences on the lungs, including chest tightness, wheezing, shortness of breath, and other issues, particularly during physical exertion or exercise. Enhanced exposure time to SO_2 may cause respiratory illness, including lung dysfunction. Mouth respiration causes increased inhalation of SO_2 in the human body and can reach deep into the lungs. Exposure to high SO_2 concentrations harms all, but even a tiny amount can cause breathing difficulty in asthmatic patients.

8.3.3 Oxides of Nitrogen

Nitrogen and oxygen-containing gases are combined to form oxides of nitrogen. Nitric oxide (NO), nitrogen dioxide (NO_2), nitrogen monoxide, and nitrogen pentoxide are primarily included in this group. Nitric acid is created by producing nitrogen dioxide. The majority of nitric acid is used to make fertilizers, although it is also used to make explosives for both mining and military applications.

Exposure to low amounts of these gases may cause infection in eyes and respiratory organs. As a result of prolonged exposure, fluid might build up in the lungs. High quantities of nitrogen oxides in the air can result in fast burning, upper respiratory tract spasms and swelling, and fluid accumulation in lungs, which may cause death. Severe burns are likely to result when coming into contact with excessive concentrations of nitrogen dioxide liquid or nitrogen oxide gases on the skin or in the eyes.

People in urban areas and near industrial areas are prone to exposure to high-concentration NOx. Vehicular emission is the prime cause of elevated levels of NOx in cities, while coal-based power plants, wood burning, and fossil fuel burning cause its emission. During the course of their employment, employees who operate in environments that make nitric acid, use welding materials, or use specific explosives may breathe in nitrogen oxides.

8.3.4 Ammonia

Ammonia is a very pungent-smelling gas without any color and is nonflammable. It is a water-soluble gas, causing irritation to the contact area. Ammonia is primarily used as a fertilizer; thus, agricultural activities generate a significant amount of it in the atmosphere. It is also generated in various textiles, chemicals, dyes, pesticides, and other industries. Industrial cleaning products include higher ammonia concentrations, which can quickly irritate skin and result in burns.

Ammonia is typically inhaled as a gas or vapor, which exposes most humans to it. Ammonia can be exposed from these sources because it is found in cleaning supplies and in nature. Due to the widespread use of ammonia in agriculture, industry, and commerce, exposure might also result from an unintentional release.

The physical mass of ammonia is less than the dry air; thus, following the laws of physics, it will float above dry air. But in the presence of moisture, its behavior changes and its weight is higher than moist air, thus settling near the ground in the presence of moist air. The presence of ammonia in lower levels is very harmful for inhabitants.

8.3.5 Carbon Monoxide

Carbon monoxide is an odorless, tasteless, and colorless gas. Carbon monoxide is produced through various anthropogenic activities. Burning with low oxygen levels causes carbon monoxide emissions in the atmosphere. Multiple appliances can also generate it due to inadequate ventilation. The concentration of CO can also rise in a very crowded place.

Excessive consumption of CO causes blood poisoning as red cells absorb CO in place of oxygen and cause severe tissue damage, leading to death. CO poisoning affects the whole body with a primary attack on the heart and brain. Frequent exposure to CO causes flu symptoms.

8.3.6 Ozone

Tropospheric ozone (O_3) is a well-known global air contaminant and the primary index substance of the phenomena of photochemical smog. Ozone formation in the troposphere is caused by photochemical reactions, where nitrogen oxides, volatile organic compounds (VOCs), and carbon monoxide reach each other in the presence of solar radiation (Özbay et al., 2011). In the troposphere, the presence of ozone acts as an air pollutant and is also called bad ozone. Nowadays, due to the increase in precursor gases of ozone formation in the atmosphere, the concentration of the tropospheric ozone is increasing significantly (MEEC, 2021; USEPA, 2021). Emergency response systems exist in several developed nations, which act in various ways to reduce high ozone levels and also issue health advisories in cases of forthcoming high ozone concentration incidence (MEPPRC, 2015; USEPA, 2015). Anthropogenic pollutant emissions and tropospheric ozone levels are connected (Alvim-Ferraz et al., 2006). Lowered pulmonary functions and cardiovascular illnesses are linked to long-term exposure to high amounts of O_3 (Zhan et al., 2018). According to Hayes et al. (2010), elevated ground-level O_3 harms vegetation by causing leaf damage and reduced development. Ozone in the troposphere act as a greenhouse gases and thus has significant potential to raise global temperature (Sharma et al., 2017). Indeed, as O_3 concentrations rise, the severity of the effects mentioned previously also does as well.

One of the primary greenhouse gases and air pollutants, ground-level O_3 has detrimental consequences on both human health and climate change. According to epidemiological research, ground-level ozone has a negative impact on human health (Liu et al., 2020). Significant checks on the emission of precursor gases of ozone may cause notable reductions in ozone levels, and various cities have observed this by creating strict emission norms (Cheng et al., 2019).

8.3.7 Benzene

Benzene is an air pollutant emitted from various sources, primarily from fossil fuel burning. Along with air, it also causes water pollution. The origins of benzene in the environment can be natural (i.e., volcanoes and forest fires) or anthropogenic (i.e., vehicular exhaust, emissions from natural gas and oil industry, and cigarette smoke).

With the increase in industrial activities and vehicular concentrations, the ambient concentration of benzene is increasing. Benzene is an indoor air pollutant as well. Mostly, the indoor concentration of it is higher than the outdoor concentration. Various sprays, paint, and chemicals (as different types of cleaning agents and detergents) contribute to the increased indoor concentrations of benzene. Its concentration can be significantly high near the dumpsites of city waste and gas stations.

8.3.8 Toluene

Toluene is primarily an indoor air pollutant that is emitted from various paints and other sprays. It is also used as a solvent in making benzene, which is also a pollutant. One can be exposed to toluene by breathing ambient or indoor air that has been influenced by such sources. Both acute (short-term) and chronic (long-term) toluene exposures in humans and animals primarily target the neurological system. When exposed acutely to high amounts of toluene in the air, people commonly experience symptoms like lethargy, sleepiness, headaches, and nausea.

Along with household painted items, cigarette smoke is also a potential contributor of toluene to indoor air. Besides the smoker, the surrounding persons are also exposed to high levels of toluene in such indoor air pollution conditions. Workers who work in industries where toluene is regularly used as a solvent, including printing or painting, are more likely to be exposed to the chemical. The primary source of toluene in the air is from automobile emissions. When toluene-containing industrial and consumer products are produced, used, and disposed of, toluene may also be emitted into the surrounding atmosphere (Kishimoto et al., 2006; Irvani et al., 2018).

8.3.9 Xylene

Xylene is a harmful VOC to the environment. It serves as a solvent for dyes, paints, polishes, medical technologies, and other sectors. When exposed to sunshine, xylene readily vaporizes and breaks down into other safe compounds. High doses and amounts of xylene injure the liver, and even its byproducts affect hepatocytes. Different factors, such as the exposure route, length, and how each person reacts to varying degrees of exposure, influence the kind and severity of the health impacts induced by xylene (Niaz et al., 2015).

8.3.10 Arsenic

High-temperature processes spew arsenic into the atmosphere, including volcanism, burning vegetation, and coal-fired power plants. Long-term consumption of arsenic-contaminated water causes arsenic poisoning, also known as arsenicosis, which can result in serious diseases, including cancer.

8.3.11 Nickel

Nickel, a transition metal, is widely found in the air, water, and soil pollution. Natural and anthropogenic sources are responsible for its emission in the environment. Various types of urban solid waste and industrial waste cause nickel pollution in the environment (Genchi et al., 2020). Fossil fuel burning primarily contributes to its release into the atmosphere. It causes various types of allergies, lung infections, and heart diseases and may also be cancerous in cases of severe exposure (Genchi et al., 2020).

TABLE 8.1
National Ambient Air Quality Standards

			Concentration in Ambient Air	
Sr. No.	Pollutants	Time-Weighted Average	Industrial, Residential, Rural, and Other Areas	Ecologically Sensitive Area (Notified by Central Government)
1.	Sulfur Dioxide (SO_2), µg/m^3	Annual*	50	20
		24 Hours**	80	80
2.	Nitrogen Dioxide (NO_2), µg/m^3	Annual*	40	30
		24 Hours**	80	80
3.	Particulate Matter (Size <10 µm) or PM10 µg/m^3	Annual*	60	60
		24 Hours**	100	100
4.	Particulate Matter (Size <2.5 µm) or PM2.5 µg/m^3	Annual*	40	40
		24 Hours **	60	60
5.	Ozone (O_3), µg/m^3	8 Hours**	100	100
		1 Hours **	180	180
6.	Lead (Pb), µg/m^3	Annual *	0.50	0.50
		24 Hour**	1.0	1.0
7.	Carbon Monoxide (CO), mg/m^3	8 Hours **	02	02
		1 Hour**	04	04
8.	Ammonia (NH_3), µg/m^3	Annual*	100	100
		24 Hour**	400	400
9.	Benzene (C_6H_6), µg/m^3	Annual *	05	05
10.	Benzo(a)Pyrene (BaP): Particulate Phase Only, ng/m^3	Annual*	01	01
11.	Arsenic (As), ng/m^3	Annual*	06	06
12.	Nickel (Ni), ng/m^3	Annual*	20	20

(*Source:* NAAQS Notification dated 18 November 2009)

* Annual arithmetic mean of minimum 104 measurements in a year at a particular site taken twice a week 24-hourly at uniform intervals.

** 24-hourly, 8-hourly, or 1-hourly monitored values, as applicable, shall be complied with 98% of the time in a year. 2% of the time, they may exceed the limits, but not on two consecutive days of monitoring.

8.4 NEW TRENDS IN COMPUTING

Artificial intelligence, machine learning, and deep learning techniques have piqued the interest of both scientists and ordinary people for many years. The capacity of computers to think, make decisions, and behave like humans would have been one of the most significant and prominent advancements in computer science. AI, ML, and DL have been known for quite a few decades and have been applied or thought to be implemented several times to make machines conceivably achieve anything that humans are capable of doing without being explicitly directed or programmed. There is a fundamental difference between conventional and artificial intelligence (machine learning) programming. In conventional programming, we have manually formulated programming along with the data to generate desired outcomes, but coding rules are personalized. In machine learning programming, the outputs and available data are used to formulate the algorithm's rules. Figure 8.2 shows a schematic representation of the difference between conventional and artificial intelligence (machine learning) programming.

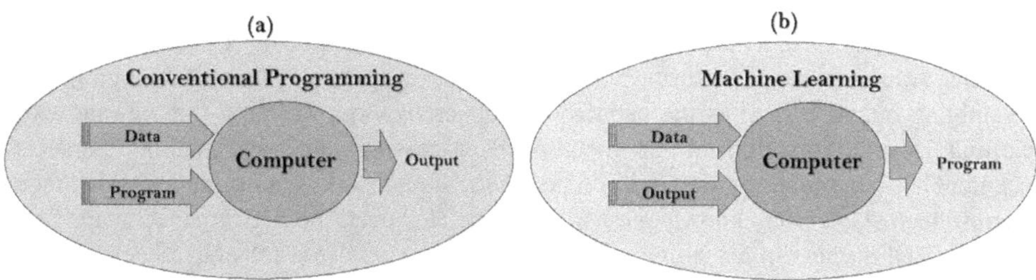

FIGURE 8.2 Conventional programming vs. machine learning.

8.4.1 Artificial Intelligence

Digital computers were developed in the 1940s, and since then, it has been shown that computers can be trained to carry out exceptionally challenging tasks, such as uncovering theorem proofs or growing into masters at the games of Go and Chess. AI refers to the intellect manifested by a machine created or designed by humans. AI is a revolutionary technology swiftly altering our society, economy, and jobs. Popular AI applications include social networks, autonomous automobiles, chatbots, robot stock traders, voice and personal assistants, and internet search engines. In contradiction to the natural intelligence exhibited by humans and other animals (only to some extent), artificial intelligence, or the intelligence of machines, is displayed by machines. It strives to do functions such as speech recognition, learning, planning, and problem-solving, to name a few. AI is a branch of computer science that entails designing computer programs to achieve tasks that would otherwise need human intelligence and reasoning abilities. AI algorithms may tackle challenges related to learning, perception, problem-solving, language comprehension, rational thinking, and several other areas. AI is rapidly evolving, and science fiction frequently depicts AI as robots and humanoids that are as human-like as possible.

8.4.1.1 Some Standard Definitions

In this section, we present several definitions of AI, ML, and DL, as suggested by the best researchers in the field.

8.4.1.1.1 Copeland and Proudfoot (2007)

The ability of a digital computer or computer-controlled robot to perform tasks commonly associated with intelligent beings.

8.4.1.1.2 John McCarthy (Andresen, 2002)

The science and engineering of making intelligent machines.

8.4.1.1.3 Haugeland (Andre, 1986)

The exciting new effort to make computers think . . . machines with minds, in the full and literal sense.

8.4.1.1.4 Rich and Knight (1991)

The study of how to make computers do things at which, at the moment, people are better.

8.4.1.1.5 Winston (1992)

The study of the computations that make it possible to perceive, reason, and act.

8.4.1.1.6 Luger and Stubblefield (1993)

The branch of computer science that is concerned with the automation of intelligent behavior.

AI refers to a computer's or a machine's capacity to command other devices, such as robots, to carry out activities similar to those performed by humans. AI refers to a system with cognitive properties resembling humans, such as the capacity for generalization, meaning-finding, and experiential learning. Despite exceptional gains in computer processing power and memory, no substantial advancement has been achieved that can compete with human skills over more extensive regions or tasks requiring vast everyday knowledge and memory. However, the performance levels of human professionals and masters in executing specific repetitive specialized jobs have been surpassed by computer programs, commonly called expert systems. Figure 8.3 is a pictorial representation of AI evolution progress from the present to the future.

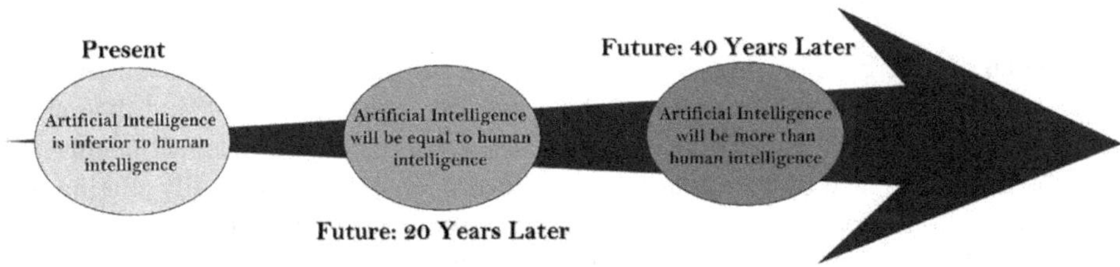

FIGURE 8.3 Future evolution of artificial intelligence.

8.4.1.2 Traits of AI

- AI can anticipate and adapt because it employs algorithms that detect patterns in massive volumes of data.
- AI can augment human intelligence, deliver insights, and improve efficiency.
- AI employs algorithms to build analytical models through continual learning. AI technology will learn how to do tasks from these algorithms through several rounds of trial and error.
- AI is a technology capable of perception and sense, enabling people to reevaluate how they analyze data, combine information, and make better judgments after applying these realizations.

8.4.2 Machine Learning

AI and ML are closely connected disciplines, and ML focuses on computer-aided predictions. ML is basically an optimization problem that addresses problems using tools, theories, and algorithms. ML trains a computer to learn from its data inputs and develop artificial intelligence without explicit programming.

Arthur Samuel pioneered machine learning research and proposed the term "machine learning" in 1959. In machine learning, algorithms examine and interpret data to train themselves and produce best results for new datasets (Li et al., 2020b). To help in the acquisition of AI, ML trains a computer program to learn from labeled and unlabeled input datasets without the need for explicit programming.

Machine Learning (Samuel, 1967):

> Field of study that gives computers the ability to learn without being explicitly programmed.

ML algorithms investigate ways computers replicate or utilize the learning process of human conduct, which is defined by the capacity to automatically improve with experience, increasing the knowledge of learning algorithms through novel traits. The fundamental goals of machine learning are to categorize and regress information using already found, well-known qualities from training data. Machine learning develops a model that can be trained, tested, and validated from sample data to enhance its performance over time.

Machine learning (Mitchell, 2007) is:

> A computer program is said to learn from experience E with respect to some class of tasks T and performance measure P, if its performance at tasks in T, as measured by P, improves with experience E.

This implies that a computer can learn and gain expertise by doing specific tasks and enhance its performance while performing similar tasks in the future. The data is fed into the system from a source. Algorithms used in ML train computers to perform daily tasks in a way that comes naturally and with no work, which includes analyzing an email and determining whether to flag it as spam or ham, looking at the weather to decide whether to bring an umbrella when going outside, or simply recognizing the distinctive features of a fruit to figure out if it is an apple or an orange. Classification, regression, similarity or anomaly detection, ranking systems, and sequence prediction are among the challenges that ML can address. Classification is used to establish the category to which an object belongs, for example, determining if a tumor is malignant or benign. Regression is used for predicting a continuous numeric-valued characteristic of an item, for example, the likelihood of a person clicking on an advertisement or stock price forecast. Similarity detection or anomaly revelation is utilized to find comparable entities or differences in behavior, for example, looking for similar photographs or detecting abnormality in user behavior. A ranking system, such as Google Page Rank, sorts relevant data based on specific input. Sequence prediction is used to predict the next data point in a series, in natural language processing (NLP), for example, predicting the following word in a phrase.

ML has been active in developing several innovative technologies as a particular type of AI. It provides an immediate, meaningful, and continuous contribution. It has spawned multiple innovative applications in various industries, accelerated countless advances, and will continue progressing technology.

Machine learning algorithms may be categorized into one of three distinct groups: supervised learning, unsupervised learning, and reinforcement learning.

8.4.2.1 Supervised Learning

It utilizes a method that requires the use of a labeled dataset. There are two sets of data in the tagged input database: training and testing. In order to determine the accuracy of outcome predictions, supervised algorithms first attempt to identify patterns in a collection of training data before validating these patterns using a testing dataset. The supervised ML algorithm is trained repeatedly until it achieves the desired accuracy. It is common practice to utilize supervised learning to resolve classification issues because one of its purposes is teaching the computer a categorization system. The most popular algorithms in this domain include linear regression, support vector machines (SVMs), k-nearest neighbor (k-NN), naive Bayes and decision trees, and artificial neural networks (ANNs).

8.4.2.2 Unsupervised Learning

It handles unlabeled datasets. The program attempts to construct clusters based on the input dataset's characteristics or attributes. It identifies the data class setter using previously learned attributes.

Clustering and association problems can be one of the critical areas on which unsupervised learning systems focus. In order to separate datasets into discrete clusters, the unsupervised machine learning algorithm looks for concealed characteristics based on patterns, similarities, and differences in the datasets.

The machine's ability to accurately identify the structure has not been evaluated. The k-means method for clustering and the a priori algorithm for association problems are two examples of notable unsupervised learning algorithms.

8.4.2.3 Reinforcement Learning

It is a reward and punishment system for action-based learning. Activities in this sort of learning are motivated by rewards and punishments system; thus the outputs have a higher value in the desired favorable circumstance since the reward reinforces the outcomes (Sutton and Barto, 1998). The learner's decision or activity affects current and future situations.

A machine is exposed to an environment in which it makes trial-and-error judgments and learns from its actions and prior experiences in reinforcement learning. The machine receives reward signals from the environment for each successful decision, which works as a reinforcement signal, and the knowledge about the rewarded state-action combination is recorded.

When confronted with a similar scenario, the machine iterates the rewarded action. Reinforcement learning algorithms, such as in self-driving cars, are utilized in fields where strategic decision-making is critical to success. Q-learning and Markov decision processes are the most frequently used reinforcement learning algorithms. Many parts of modern life and modern civilizations are made possible by machine learning, including web searches, content screening on social networks, and suggestions on e-commerce platforms. Growing consumer goods like cameras and smartphones also use machine learning techniques for better image capturing and modifications. Machine learning techniques are utilized in areas such as recognizing objects in photos; converting speech to text; matching news stories, blog posts, or goods with users' interests; and choosing appropriate search results.

8.4.3 Deep Learning

Deep learning, a machine learning subfield, evaluates the learning process using deep neural networks. In a hierarchical approach, DL permits independent learning of input properties and their representations at many levels. Deep learning is a machine learning component consisting of techniques that let software train itself to carry out tasks like voice and picture recognition by being exposed to a large quantity of data. This technique is crucial in AI research for overcoming machine learning bottlenecks such as many model types, extended training, difficulty calculating parameter weights, and various parameters (Mitchell, 2007).

Deep learning's robust approach makes it more resilient than traditional machine learning models. The complete architecture of DL is used for extraction of attributes and customization procedures. The initial layers do little more than analyze new raw data or learn superficial traits. Their combined output is then sent to the subsequent layers, which learn sophisticated attributes. Consequently, deep learning is ideally adapted to processing vast volumes of complex data (Zhang et al., 2017). Robust DL techniques do not need one-of-a-kind design components. Instead, they are powerful owing to their self-directed learning approach and depiction of the best attributes for each job.

As we approach the present day, a new era of artificial neural networks called deep learning has begun to emerge. Various researchers contributed to deep learning and started the next phase of the neural network's growth in 2005 (Goodfellow et al., 2016). The first computer model based on neurons was proposed by McCulloch and Pitts in 1943. Deep learning is a broad technique. Therefore, transfer learning, the act of using it on other datasets and applications, is easily possible.

It is advantageous when there is insufficient data to solve the issue at hand (Ackley et al., 1985; He et al., 2016). The ability to grow and to create critical data when relevant information for system learning is unavailable are fundamental key obstacles for DL techniques. Deep learning methods employ several layers of representation while learning representations. They are constructed by assembling specified but non-linear modules that turn a representation at one level, beginning with the raw input, into a representation at a higher, somewhat more abstract level. If enough of these changes are coupled, it is possible to learn extremely complicated functions (LeCun et al., 2015). The critical attribute of deep learning is that the layers of features are learned from data using a general-purpose method rather than being composed by human scientists. Deep learning usage is presently being pushed by enhanced computational capabilities, especially as GPU units, low-cost computer hardware, and current machine learning project successes (Marko, 2012; Minsky and Papert, 2017).

Deep learning scalability increases in hardware and software and may be handled by high-performance computing/supercomputing. The relationship between AI, ML, and DL can be seen in Figure 8.4. Deep learning is expected to accomplish many more victories soon since it requires no manual engineering and can readily benefit from technological breakthroughs in the number of accessible computers and data. Deep neural network learning methods and architectures now being created will serve to accelerate this advancement.

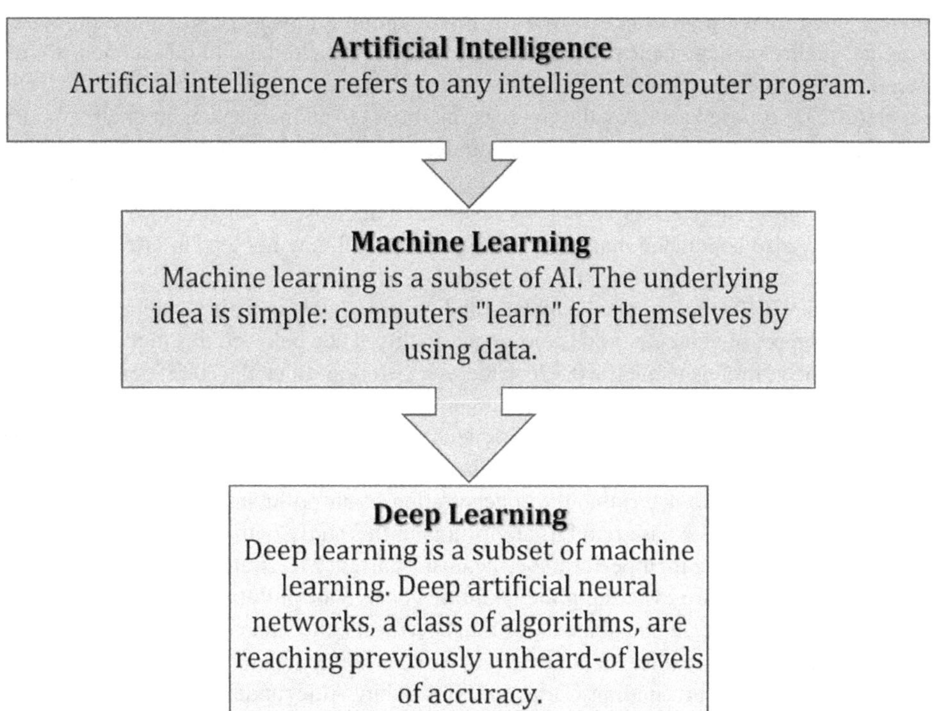

FIGURE 8.4 Interconnection of artificial intelligence, machine learning, and deep learning.

8.5 APPLICATION OF AI/ML/DL IN ESTIMATION OF HEALTH-HAZARDOUS POLLUTANTS

With evolution in computation power, artificial intelligence techniques (ANN/ML/DL) are becoming more important in tackling massive data sets and various research issues. Supervised learning techniques, including ANN, random forests (RFs), and support vector machines, are the most widely used machine learning algorithms. Computer modeling of classification and regression primarily relies on sample data (Zhong et al., 2021). ML techniques are used to improve prediction accuracy and resilience while working with massive data sets to reduce the outlier's impact on the information to be extracted from these data (Yuchi et al., 2019; Ucun Ozel et al., 2020; Chen et al., 2022). As various ecological processes are nonlinear, they attempt to find the solution with minimum error estimators (Feng et al., 2011; Zimmerman et al., 2018; Chen et al., 2022). Additionally, when building a model, several forms of data, such as strings and integers, can be included. The new computation techniques have been found more cost-effective, quicker, and simpler compared to traditional numerical models. Due to these benefits, ML/DL models are becoming more and more common in the fields of environmental and geosciences (Liao et al., 2021; Zheng et al., 2021). In air pollution studies, these models are frequently used for forecasting pollutants and their health and climatic impacts and mapping the chemical behavior of pollutants (Huang et al., 2021; Yan et al., 2021; Lv et al., 2023).

ML/DL are becoming popular due to their strength in predicting air pollutants with good accuracy and short duration. At the same time, these technologies are capable of handling the enormous amount of data coming from Earth observations. Four key areas of study emerged from cluster analysis for using these techniques: forecasting, enhancement in monitoring, air pollutant categorization, and improved emission techniques. The capacity to investigate the chemical properties of various contaminants, examine chemical reactions and the forces that drive them, and model scenarios have improved by using these algorithms. Future research should pay more attention to ML/DL models since they are an effective tool for investigating atmospheric chemical processes and assessing air quality management when combined with multi-field data. In this section, we discuss AI's recent development/use in assessing various air pollutants.

Fu et al. (2023) proposed an air quality forecasting model to address actual air quality monitoring challenges in environmental protection. Their model was based on an improved AI techniques to reduce errors. Their model incorporated a meteorological model with spatio-temporal information to predict air pollution more effectively. They observed a decrease in performance with an increase in step size. They also concluded that using a single AI model may not lead to effective forecasting of air pollution.

Suleiman et al. (2019) incorporated sophisticated AI techniques in their machine-learning model to estimate the impact of vehicular emissions on air quality. They believed this model did a great job of predicting concentrations using the 0.8 *R*-value as a criterion. Li et al. (2023) performed a review of the application of AL/ML in solving environmental problems.

Various methods, including these computing techniques, are employed to assess the impact of lockdown owing to COVID-19 on air quality (Chau et al., 2022). Weather models developed using these techniques are used to determine the concentration of air pollutants. They suggested weather normalized models (WNMs) based on DL algorithms in this study with the goal of testing five DL architectures and evaluating their performance against a current ML strategy. In the Ecuadorian capital of Quito, researchers are examining the quantities of five air pollutants (CO, NO_2, $PM_{2.5}$, SO_2, and O_3). The findings indicate that some algorithms perform better than others, and as a result, they have suggested a suitable weather model to assess lockdown impact on air quality.

In a metropolitan area surrounding Cartagena, Colombia, Aldegunde et al. (2022) identified the optimum spatial representation of $PM_{2.5}$, relative humidity, temperature, and wind speed. The empirical regression prediction method was used to accommodate the wind effects. These interpolation techniques identified the areas of the city where $PM_{2.5}$ concentrations were above the allowable limits and characterized three important meteorological variables continuously on the surface. To determine visitor exposure to mine aerosols, Bralewska et al. (2022) estimated particulate matter concentrations in southern Poland and compared them to the concentrations of the same particulate matter concentration fractions in the atmosphere.

Various relationships, including linear and nonlinear, are assumed between $PM_{2.5}$ and predictors by traditional statistical models (Lee et al., 2016a; You et al., 2015) or other models (Breiman, 2001), and these predictions sometimes resulted in high accuracy. There are studies which connected the particulate matter concentration with aerosol optical depth (AOD) using ANN, ML, and DL techniques (Srivastava et al., 2021). Simplification of complicated nonlinear relationships between particulate matter and AOD results in the underestimation of particulate matter concentrations (Reid et al., 2015; Zhan et al., 2017; Zheng et al., 2016). The relationship between particulate matter and AOD is very complicated and governed by numerous factors and parameters; thus, all these factors and relationships should be adequately described while using machine learning techniques (Lary et al., 2014). With moving towards the core techniques of AI, the simulation capabilities of the model increase progressively, and these models are much more efficient than the basic models (Li et al., 2017). Thus, the evolved model simulates the complex nonlinear relationship between parameters more efficiently, and the same is true for the case of $PM_{2.5}$ concentration and AOD. According to Chudnovsky et al. (2013) and Li et al. (2015), there is not a direct correlation between AOD values and $PM_{2.5}$ concentrations. When AOD is the only input to the model, there is a great deal of uncertainty in particulate matter concentration and AOD (Saunders et al., 2014). On inclusion of other parameters, such as meteorological elements as predictors, the model's output, that is, particulate matter concentration estimation, improved significantly (Paciorek et al., 2008; Tian and Chen, 2010).

These computational techniques are very effective in replicating the nonlinear relationships between different parameters, and thus $PM_{2.5}$ simulation based on AOD information is done very efficiently with the help of these models. AOD gives information regarding the total load of aerosols in the atmosphere and thus is used as an indirect estimator for $PM_{2.5}$. PM2.5 contributes only a fraction of the total aerosol load; therefore, it is difficult to find the exact relation between AOD and PM2.5, leading to inaccurate predictions of $PM_{2.5}$. To reduce these inaccuracies, various other information regarding gaseous pollutants and secondary aerosol is included in the model, and this improves the underestimation of particulate matter concentrations based on AOD and climatic parameters. Researchers produced a daily continuous $PM_{2.5}$ spatial distribution, projected the $PM_{2.5}$ concentration in the missing AOD areas, and minimized the estimated bias brought on by the absence of AOD.

In the Libyan city of Tripoli, Esager and Ünlü (2023) investigated particulate matter concentration prediction. Using a univariate time series approach along with three core AI models, they anticipated $PM_{2.5}$ levels. This study used the long short-term memory (LSTM), gated recurrent unit and a convolutional neural network approach with the best performance of convolutional neural networks with the maximum accuracy and least error. The conclusions from the study have vital information about how deep learning algorithms can estimate $PM_{2.5}$ and help with managing air quality decisions.

As the human population of the planet grows dramatically, carbon dioxide (CO_2) levels are increasing day by day, which causes the atmosphere to heat up to an extreme point and contributes significantly to climate change. Global attempts to slow down climate change are concentrated on reducing the number of days in the future when the environment will be extremely hot. Numerous studies about the causes of the high CO_2 emissions in various nations have been carried out by scientists, students, and other officials. The majority of empirical investigations use parametric modeling to examine the variables that cause and sustain CO_2 emissions. The conventional parametric approach, on the other hand, uses a set of finite and predetermined parameters to optimize a function to a given form. The parametric models' predictive ability is constrained by this rigidity. Nonparametric machine learning techniques have dominated the improvement of the forecast in recent years.

Surface ozone concentration is another important air pollutant which has been estimated using ANN, ML, and DL. The most notable advantages of deep learning techniques over traditional neural networks can be categorized as the need for fewer computer units and automated learning with enhanced efficiency (Wu and Lin, 2019). Consequently, these advanced computational techniques are considered a potential approach for predicting ground-level O_3 concentrations since they give enough accuracy in addressing complicated issues even in the presence of massive datasets (Wang et al., 2020). It is necessary to examine the effectiveness of various techniques with single-use and hybrid approaches to estimate pollutants, including ozone. Wu and Lin (2019) attempted to estimate the hourly ozone concentration in their work with few parameters.

Initially, ozone concentration was predicted with statistical and deterministic techniques. The foundation of linear and non-linear statistical methods is the analysis of monitored records to predict ozone concentration. On the contrary, deterministic chemistry-transport techniques like Eulerian, Lagrangian, and Gaussian are utilized to predict atmospheric phenomena. These techniques are available to generate forecast time- and space-resolved concentrations for ground-level ozone and to learn how ground-level ozone is formed. Emerging techniques for effective modeling of various air contaminants use deep learning technologies (Li et al., 2016; Zhang et al., 2016a).

In a work by Ekinci et al. (2021), hourly ozone levels during a pandemic lockdown for an industrialized region of Turkey were predicted using deep learning techniques. In this process, they evaluated various advanced AI techniques in terms of minimum error estimators to check the effectiveness of the model. While major pollutant species have decreased, higher ground-level ozone levels have been seen in numerous nations. The surface ozone concentration can be forecast well with the help of an ensemble forecast system for surface ozone, similar to contemporary ensemble prediction systems for the weather (Zhang et al., 2023). By focusing on the spatial patterns of weather, deep learning approaches significantly reduced the computation cost of the problem.

Yafouz et al. (2021) performed their study based on the modeling of nonlinear interactions of ozone with other pollutants and meteorological data. As a result, six artificial intelligence techniques were examined in this research. This study used seven combination scenarios to focus on six input parameter datasets from three air quality monitoring stations. This paper aimed to thoroughly examine the accuracy of O_3 concentration prediction utilizing individual machine learning models, deep learning models, and hybrid models. The model was trained and tested for different input parameters to predict O_3 concentration and evaluated with different time lags.

A deep learning model approach was proposed by Wang et al. (2022) to estimate the daily maximum 8 h average of O_3 concentrations over fine grids in eastern China. Long short-term memory was enabled with an attention mechanism and residual connection to improve this model's temporal processing ability. Other air pollutants can also be estimated with the help of this model, as the model showed a good performance and applicability to be employed on other air pollutants.

New computation techniques have also been employed in estimating gaseous pollutants. The risks associated with various hazardous pollutants and their detection can be reduced by utilizing innovative gas-sensing systems. Nevertheless, the fabrication of robust sensors requires a time-consuming and expensive process of synthesizing functional nanoparticles. At the same time, toxic gas sensors always come with a hefty price tag and a danger of hazardous gas leaks during operation.

Information on meteorological variables and nitric acid concentrations are used to simulate the ground NO_2 concentration levels (Li et al., 2020a). The regression neural network was fed with the raster layers, normalized difference vegetation index (NDVI) data from satellite data, and a digital elevation model. In a different study, Ghahremanloo et al. (2021) used interpolated population data and deep learning techniques with satellite observations and simulated meteorological parameters to predict NO_2 concentrations. In another work, Beloconi and Vounatsou (2020) also examined using ML/DL techniques to estimate the daily NO_2 concentration. In this model, other predictors included vegetation coverage and NDVI, nighttime radiation, land use information along with terrain height, and meteorological information.

Using machine learning, Gheibi et al. (2023) assessed NO_2 content. They optimized NO_2 sensing utilizing the response surface technique (RSM) in their study by using three different parameters. The Jacobson model can be used in the control unit of a sensor system for better implementation. Various numerical techniques are used to implement the machine learning computations in these models. The results showed that a decision support system could be offered for the NO_2 gas sensor system by hybridizing various techniques as a controller.

Next, we studied biogenic aerosol estimation through artificial neural techniques. Exposure to bioaerosols poses a serious risk to the public's health, especially in crowded public areas with insufficient ventilation (Huffman et al., 2020; Tian et al., 2018). Estimation and prediction of bioaerosols are still tedious tasks. Historically, culture-based techniques have been used to estimate bioaerosol concentrations (Schäfer et al., 2017; Duquenne, 2018). However, they cannot provide real-time data because they call for off-site processing. Furthermore, adopting this method often results in underestimating bioaerosol concentrations, as a specific lab setting is required for estimation of many microorganisms (Chi and Li, 2006; Lloyd et al., 2018). However, they can only be used as proxies. Bioaerosol concentration can be predicted based on information associated with occupancy and CO_2 concentration (Hospodsky et al., 2012; Peng and Jimenez, 2021). On the other hand, fluorescence technique-based devices can do real-time estimation of bioaerosol concentration (Hernandez et al., 2016; Li et al., 2022; Nieto-Caballero et al., 2022).

Artificial intelligence-based approaches have been also used to predict indoor air pollutants with the help of observed data from real-time sensors (Wei et al., 2019). Using these techniques, researchers could forecast the CO_2 concentration's high correlation with observed data (Putra and Safrilah, 2018; Ahn et al., 2017). In another instance, a multi-linear regression model was fitted with pollutants and meteorological parameters to predict bioaerosols.

In their work, Lee et al. (2023) developed AI models using information from indoor sensors and physical information of observed bioaerosols. As a result, they could accurately predict biological aerosols and particulate matter (10 and 2.5 μm) in a short-time real forecast (within 60 min). Several AI models were constructed and validated using the observed data from various public places. A deep learning model approach based on observed time-series data from a few sites was trained and tested in significantly low time. It provided very high accuracy in the prediction of bioaerosols and particulate matter. Thus, researchers have shown the superiority of new computation techniques in order to enhance the real-time forecasting of indoor air pollutants, including bioaerosols.

8.6 CONCLUSIONS

This chapter began with a fundamental overview of modern computational techniques, their basic methodology and structure, and their application to environmental research. In the present chapter, we have discussed the application of artificial intelligence in assessing air pollution. First, we've given a concise overview of vital air contaminants, their means of dispersal, and their effects on human health. These new computational approaches have several research applications in the environmental research field.

This chapter examined the use of machine learning and deep learning to evaluate air pollution around the globe. This chapter discussed advanced AI methods and their applications in analyzing environmental data for pollution and air quality research.

REFERENCES

Ackley, D.H., Hinton, G.E., Sejnowski, T.J., 1985. A learning algorithm for Boltzmann machines. Cogn. Sci. 9(1), 147–169.

Ahn, J., Shin, D., Kim, K., Yang, J., 2017. Indoor air quality analysis using deep learning with sensor data. Sensors 17, 2476. https://doi.org/10.3390/s17112476.

Aldegunde, J.A.Á., Sánchez, A.F., Saba, M., Bolaños, E.Q., Palenque, J.Ú., 2022. Analysis of PM2.5 and meteorological variables using enhanced geospatial techniques in developing countries: a case study of Cartagena de Indias City (Colombia). Atmosphere 13, 506.

Alvim-Ferraz, M., Sousa, S., Pereira, M., Martins, F., 2006. Contribution of anthropogenic pollutants to the increase of tropospheric ozone levels in the Oporto Metropolitan Area, Portugal since the 19th century. Environ. Pollut. 140(3), 516–524.

Andre, V., 1986. Artificial intelligence: the very idea: J. Haugeland, (MIT Press, Cambridge, MA, 1985); 287 pp. Arti. Intell. 29, 349–353.

Andresen, S.L., 2002. John McCarthy: father of AI. IEEE Intell. Syst. 17, 84–85. doi: 10.1109/MIS.2002.1039837.

Beloconi, A., Vounatsou, P., 2020. Bayesian geostatistical modelling of high-resolution NO_2 exposure in Europe combining data from monitors, satellites and chemical transport models. Environ. Int. 138, 105578.

Bralewska, K., Rogula-Kozłowska, W., Mucha, D., Badyda, A.J., Kostrzon, M., Bralewski, A., Biedugnis, S., 2022. Properties of particulate matter in the air of the Wieliczka salt mine and related health benefits for tourists. Int. J. Environ. Res. Public Health 19, 826.

Breiman, L., 2001. Statistical modeling: the two cultures. Stat. Sci. 16, 199–215. https://doi.org/10.1214/ss/1009213726.

Chau, P.N., Zalakeviciute, R., Thomas, I., Rybarczyk, Y., 2022. Deep learning approach for assessing air quality during COVID-19 lockdown in Quito. Front. Big Data 5, 842455. https://doi.org/10.3389/fdata.2022.842455.

Chen, X., Zheng, H., Wang, H., Yan, T., 2022. Can machine learning algorithms perform better than multiple linear regression in predicting nitrogen excretion from lactating dairy cows. Sci. Rep. 12, 12478.

Cheng, N., Li, R., Xu, C., Chen, Z., Chen, D., Meng, F., Cheng, B., Ma, Z., Zhuang, Y., He, B., Gao, B., 2019. Ground ozone variations at an urban and a rural station in Beijing from 2006 to 2017: Trend, meteorological influences and formation regimes. J. Clean. Prod. 235, 11–20. https://doi.org/10.1016/j.jclepro.2019.06.204.

Chi, M.C., Li, C.S., 2006. Analysis of bioaerosols from chicken houses by culture and non-culture method. Aerosol Sci. Technol. 40, 1071–1079. https://doi.org/10.1080/02786820600957408.

Chudnovsky, A., Tang, C., Lyapustin, A., Wang, Y., Schwartz, J., Koutrakis, P., 2013. A critical assessment of high resolution aerosol optical depth (AOD) retrievals for fine particulate matter (PM) predictions. Atmospheric Chem. Physics, 13, 10907–10917. https://doi.org/10.5194/acp-13-10907-2013.

Copeland, B.J., Proudfoot, D., 2007. Artificial Intelligence: History, Foundations, and Philosophical Issues, in: Philosophy of Psychology and Cognitive Science. North-Holland: Elsevier, 429–482. https://doi.org/10.1016/B978-044451540-7/50032-3.

Duquenne, P., 2018. On the identification of culturable microorganisms for the assessment of biodiversity in bioaerosols. Ann. Work Expo. Health 62, 139–146. https://doi.org/10.1093/annweh/wxx096.

Ekinci, E., Omurca, S.İ., Özbay, B., 2021. Comparative assessment of modeling deep learning networks for modeling ground-level ozone concentrations of pandemic lock-down period. Ecol. Modell. 457, 109676. https://doi.org/10.1016/j.ecolmodel.2021.109676.

Esager, M.W.M., Ünlü, K.D., 2023. Forecasting air quality in Tripoli: an evaluation of deep learning models for hourly PM2.5 surface mass concentrations. Atmosphere 14, 478. https://doi.org/10.3390/atmos14030478.

Feng, Y., Zhang, W., Sun, D., Zhang, L., 2011. Ozone concentration forecast method based on genetic algorithm optimized back propagation neural networks and support vector machine data classification. Atmos. Environ. 45, 1979–1985.

Fu, L., Junlong, L., Yifei, C., 2023. An innovative decision making method for air quality monitoring based on big data-assisted artificial intelligence technique. J. Innov. Knowl. 8, 100294.

Genchi, G., Sinicropi, M.S., Lauria, G., Carocci, A., Catalano, A., 2020. The effects of cadmium toxicity. Int. J. Environ. Res. Public Health 7(11), 3782. https://doi.org/10.3390/ijerph17113782.

Ghahremanloo, M., Lops, Y., Choi, Y., Yeganeh, B., 2021. Deep learning estimation of daily ground-level NO_2 concentrations from remote sensing data. J. Geophys. Res. Atmos. 126, e2021JD034925.

Gheibi, M., Taghavian, H., Moezzi, R., Waclawek, S., Cyrus, J., Dawiec-Lisniewska, A., Koci, J., Khaleghiabbasabadi, M., 2023. Design of a decision support system to operate a NO_2 gas sensor using machine learning, sensitive analysis and conceptual control process modelling. Chemosensors, 11, 126. https://doi.org/10.3390/chemosensors11020126.

Goodfellow, T., Bengio, Y., Courville, A., 2016. Deep Learning. MIT Press. www.deeplearningbook.org.

Hayes, F., Mills, G., Jones, L., Ashmore, M., 2010. Does a simulated upland grassland community respond to increasing background, peak or accumulated exposure of ozone? Atmos. Environ. 44(34), 4155–4164.

He, K., Zhang, X., Ren, S., Sun, J., 2016. Deep Residual Learning for Image Recognition, in: Proceedings of the IEEE Conference on Computer Vision and Pattern Recognition, Las Vegas, NV, pp. 770–778.

Hernandez, M., Perring, A.E., McCabe, K., Kok, G., Granger, G., Baumgardner, D., 2016. Chamber catalogues of optical and fluorescent signatures distinguish bioaerosol classes. Atmos. Meas. Tech. 9, 3283–3292. https://doi.org/10.5194/amt-9-3283–2016.

Hospodsky, D., Qian, J., Nazaroff, W.W., Yamamoto, N., Bibby, K., Rismani-Yazdi, H., Peccia, J., 2012. Human occupancy as a source of indoor airborne bacteria. PLoS One 7, e34867.

Huang, G., Li, X., Zhang, B., Ren, J., 2021. PM2.5 concentration forecasting at surface monitoring sites using GRU neural network based on empirical mode decomposition. Sci. Total. Environ. 768, 144516.

Huffman, J.A., Perring, A.E., Savage, N.J., Clot, B., Crouzy, B., Tummon, F., Shoshanim, O., Damit, B., Schneider, J., Sivaprakasam, V., Zawadowicz, M.A., Crawford, I., Gallagher, M., Topping, D., Doughty, D.C., Hill, S.C., Pan, Y., 2020. Real-time sensing of bioaerosols: review and current perspectives. Aerosol Sci. Technol. 54, 465–495. https://doi.org/10.1080/02786826.2019.1664724.

Irvani, H., Pour, M.N., Vahidi, A., Arezoomandan, S., Abady, H.S., 2018. Removal of toluene vapors from the polluted air with modified natural zeolite and titanium dioxide nanoparticles. Med. Gas Res. 8(3), 91–97. https://doi.org/10.4103/2045-9912.241074.

Kishimoto, A., Cao, H., Gamo, M., 2006. Assessment of exposure to and risk posed by toluene in Japanese residents: Combining exposure from indoor and outdoor sources. Environ Sci. 13(1), 31–42.

Lary, D.J., Faruque, F.S., Malakar, N., Moore, A., Roscoe, B., Adams, Z.L., Eggelston, Y., 2014. Estimating the global abundance of ground level presence of particulate matter (PM2.5). Geospatial Health 8, S611. https://doi.org/10.4081/gh.2014.292.

LeCun, Y., Bengio, Y., Hinton, G., 2015. Deep learning. Nature 521(7553), 436–444.

Lee, H., Ahn, Y., Lee, H., Ha, S., Lee, S.G., 2016a. Quote Recommendation in Dialogue Using Deep Neural Network, in: Proceedings of the 39th International ACM SIGIR Conference on Research and Development in Information Retrieval, pp. 957–960.

Lee, J.Y.Y., Yanhao, M., Ricky, L.T.C., Mark, H., Patrick, K.H.L., 2023. Artificial intelligence-based prediction of indoor bioaerosol concentrations from indoor air quality sensor data. Environ. Int. 174, 107900.

Li, J., Zuraimi, S., Schiavon, S., Wan, M.P., Xiong, J., Tham, K.W., 2022. Diurnal trends of indoor and outdoor fluorescent biological aerosol particles in a tropical urban area. Sci. Total Environ. 848, 157811 https://doi.org/10.1016/j. scitotenv.2022.157811.

Li, M., Zhang, Z., Jiang, S., Liu, Q., Chen, C., Zhang, Y., Wang, X., 2020a. Predicting the epidemic trend of COVID-19 in China and across the world using the machine learning approach. medRxiv. 1, 17–34. https://doi.org/10.1101/2020.03.18.20038117.

Li, R., Gong, J., Chen, L., Wang, Z., 2015. Estimating ground-level PM2.5 using fine-resolution satellite data in the megacity of Beijing, China. Aerosol. Air Qual. Res. 15, 1347–1356. https://doi.org/10.4209/aaqr.2015.01.0009.

Li, T., Shen, H., Chao, Z., Yuan, Q., Zhang, L., 2017. Point-surface fusion of station measurements and satellite observations for mapping PM2.5 distribution in China: methods and assessment. Atmos. Environ. 152, 477–489. https://doi.org/10.1016/j.atmosenv.2017.01.004.

Li, T., Wang, Y., Yuan, Q., 2020b. Remote sensing estimation of regional NO_2 via space-time neural networks. Remote Sens. 12, 2514.

Li, X., Peng, L., Hu, Y., Shao, J., Chi, T., 2016. Deep learning architecture for air quality predictions. Environ. Sci. Pollut. Res. 23(22), 22408–22417.

Li, Y., Zhipeng, S., Aohan, T., Keith, G., Xuejun, L., 2023. The application of machine learning to air pollution research: a bibliometric analysis. Ecotoxicol. Environ. Saf. 257, 114911.

Liao, K., Huang, X., Dang, H., Ren, Y., Zuo, S., Duan, C., 2021. Statistical approaches for forecasting primary air pollutants: a review. Atmosphere 12(6), 686.

Liu, R., Ma, Z., Liu, Y., Shao, Y., Zhao, W., Bi, J., 2020. Spatiotemporal distributions of surface ozone levels in China from 2005 to 2017: a machine learning approach. Environ. Inter. 142, 105823. https://doi.org/10.1016/j.envint.2020.105823.

Lloyd, K.G., Steen, A.D., Ladau, J., Yin, J., Crosby, L., 2018. Phylogenetically novel uncultured microbial cells dominate earth microbiomes. mSystems 3, e00055–e00118. https://doi.org/10.1128/mSystems.00055-18.

Luger, G.F., Stubblefield, W.A., 1993. Artificial Intelligence: Structures and Strategies for Complex Problem Solving (3rd edition). USA: Addison-Wesley.

Lv, Y., Tian, H., Luo, L., Liu, S., Bai, X., Zhao, H., Zhang, K., Lin, S., Zhao, S., Guo, Z., Xiao, Y., Yang, J., 2023. Understanding and revealing the intrinsic impacts of the COVID-19 lockdown on air quality and public health in North China using machine learning. Sci. Total. Environ. 857, 159339.

Marko, J., 2012. Scientists See Promise in Deep Learning Programs, New York Times. Retrieved from https://www.nytimes.com/2012/11/24/science/scientists-see-advances-in-deep-learning-a-part-of-artificial-intelligence.html.

McCulloch, W.S., Pitts, W., 1943. A logical calculus of the ideas immanent in nervous activity. Bull. Math. Biophys. 5, 115–133.

Ministry of Ecology and Environment of the People's Republic of China (MEEC), 2021. Report on the State of the Ecology and Environment in China 2021. Retrieved from www.gov.cn/xinwen/2022-05/28/5692799/files/349e930e68794f3287888d8dbe9b3ced.pdf.

Ministry of Environmental Protection of the People's Republic of China (MEPPRC), 2015. Emergency Management Methods for Environmental Emergencies. Retrieved from www.mee.gov.cn/gzk/gz/202112/P020211211513660082369.docx.

Minsky, M., Papert, S.A., 2017. Perceptrons: An Introduction to Computational Geometry. Cambridge, MA: MIT Press.

Mitchell, T.M., 1997. Machine Learning. New York: McGraw-Hill Science/Engineering/Math.

Mitchell, T.M., 2007. Machine Learning (Vol. 1). New York: McGraw Hill.

National Ambient Air Quality Status (NAAQS), 2009. National Ambient Air Quality Standards Central Pollution Control Board Notification New Delhi, November 18. Retrieved from https://cpcb.nic.in/openpdffile.php?id=UHVibGljYXRpb25GaWxlLzYzMF8xNDU3NTA2Mjk1X1B1YmxpY2F0aW9uXzUxNF9haXJxdWFsaXR5c3RhdHVzMjAwOS5wZGY=.

Niaz, K., Bahadar, H., Maqbool, F., Abdollahi, M., 2015. A review of environmental and occupational exposure to xylene and its health concerns. Excli J. 14, 1167–1186. https://doi.org/10.17179/excli2015-623.

Nieto-Caballero, M., Gomez, O.M., Shaughnessy, R., Hernandez, M., 2022. Aerosol fluorescence, airborne hexosaminidase, and quantitative genomics distinguish reductions in airborne fungal loads following major school renovations. Indoor Air 32. https://doi.org/10.1111/ina.12975.

Özbay, B., Keskin, G.A., Doğruparmak, C.C., Ayberk, S., 2011. Predicting tropospheric ozone concentrations in different temporal scales by using multilayer perceptron models. Ecol. Inform. 6 (3–4), 242–247.

Paciorek, C.J., Liu, Y., Moreno-Macias, H., Kondragunta, S., 2008. Spatiotemporal associations between GOES aerosol optical depth retrievals and ground-level PM2.5. Environ. Sci. Technol. 42, 5800–5806. https://doi.org/10.1021/es703181j.

Peng, Z., Jimenez, J. L., 2021. Exhaled CO_2 as a COVID-19 infection risk proxy for different indoor environments and activities. Environ. Sci. Technol. Lett. 8, 392–397. https://doi.org/10.1021/acs.estlett.1c00183.

Putra, J.C.P., Safrilah, Ihsan, M., 2018. The Prediction of Indoor Air Quality in Office Room Using Artificial Neural Network, in: AIP Conference Proceedings. Presented at the Human-Dedicated Sustainable Product and Process Design: Materials, Resources, and Energy: Proceedings of the 4th International Conference on Engineering, Technology, and Industrial Application (ICETIA), Surakarta, p. 020040. https://doi.org/10.1063/1.5042896.

Reid, C.E., Jerrett, M., Petersen, M.L., Pfister, G.G., Morefield, P.E., Tager, I.B., Raffuse, S.M., Balmes, J.R., 2015. Spatiotemporal prediction of fine particulate matter during the 2008 Northern California wildfires using machine learning. Environ. Sci. Technol. 49, 3887–3896. https://doi.org/10.1021/es505846r.

Rich, E., Knight, K., 1991. Artificial Intelligence. New York: McGraw-Hill.

Samuel, A.L., 1967. Some studies in machine learning using the game of checkers. IBM J. Res. Dev. 44, 206–227.

Saunders, R.O., Kahl, J.D., Ghorai, J.K., 2014. Improved estimation of PM2.5 using Lagrangian satellite-measured aerosol optical depth. Atmos. Environ. 91, 146–153. https://doi.org/10.1016/j.atmosenv.2014.03.060.

Schäfer, J., Weiß, S., Jackel, U., 2017. Preliminary validation of a method combining cultivation and cloning-based approaches to monitor airborne bacteria. Ann. Work Expo. Health 61, 633–642. https://doi.org/10.1093/annweh/wxx038.

Sharma, S., Sharma, P., Khare, M., 2017. Photo-chemical transport modelling of tropospheric ozone: a review. Atmos. Environ. 159, 34–54.

Srivastava, N., Vignesh, D., Saxena, N., 2021. Investigation of artificial neural network performance in the aerosol properties retrieval. J. Water Clim. Chan. 12(6), 2814–2834. https://doi.org/10.2166/wcc.2021.336.

Suleiman, A., Tight, M.R., Quinn, A.D., 2019. Applying machine learning methods in managing urban concentrations of traffic-related particulate matter (PM10 and PM2.5). Atmos. Pollut. Res. 10, 134–144.

Sutton, R.S., 1992. Introduction: The Challenge of Reinforcement Learning, in: Machine Learning, 8. Boston, MA: Kluwer Academic Publishers, 225–227.

Sutton, R.S., Barto, A.G., 1998. Reinforcement Learning: An Introduction. Cambridge: MIT Press.

Tian, J., Chen, D., 2010. A semi-empirical model for predicting hourly ground-level fine particulate matter (PM2.5) concentration in southern Ontario from satellite remote sensing and ground-based meteorological measurements. Remote Sens. Environ. 114, 221–229. https://doi.org/10.1016/j.rse.2009.09.011.

Tian, Y., Liu, Y., Misztal, P.K., Xiong, J., Arata, C.M., Goldstein, A.H., Nazaroff, W.W., 2018. Fluorescent biological aerosol particles: concentrations, emissions, and exposures in a northern California residence. Indoor Air 28, 559–571. https://doi.org/10.1111/ina.12461.

U. S. Environmental Protection Agency, 2015. Air Quality Guide for Ozone. Retrieved from www.epa.gov/sites/production/files/2017-12/documents/air-quality-guide_ozone_2015.pdf.

U.S. Environmental Protection Agency, 2021. Our Nation's air: Trends through 2021. Retrieved from https://gispub.epa.gov/air/trendsreport/2022.

Ucun Ozel, H., Gemici, B.T., Gemici, E., Ozel, H.B., Cetin, M., Sevik, H., 2020. Application of artificial neural networks to predict the heavy metal contamination in the Bartin River. Environ. Sci. Pollut. Res. Int. 27, 42495–42512.

Wang, H.-W., Li, X.-B., Wang, D., Zhao, J., Hong-di, H., Peng, Z.-R., 2020. Regional prediction of ground-level ozone using a hybrid sequence-to-sequence deep learning approach. J. Cleaner Prod. 253, 119841.

Wang, S., Mu, X., Jiang, P., Huo, Y., Zhu, L., Zhu, Z., Wu, Y., 2022. New deep learning model to estimate ozone concentrations found worrying exposure level over eastern China. Int. J. Environ. Res. Public Health 19, 7186. https://doi.org/10.3390/ijerph19127186.

Wei, W., Ramalho, O., Malingre, L., Sivanantham, S., Little, J.C., Mandin, C., 2019. Machine learning and statistical models for predicting indoor air quality. Indoor Air 29, 704–726. https://doi.org/10.1111/ina.12580.

Winston, P.H., 1992. Artificial Intelligence (3rd edition). Reading, MA: Addison-Wesley.

Wu, Q., Lin, H., 2019. A novel optimal-hybrid model for daily air quality index prediction considering air pollutant factors. Sci. Total Environ. 683, 808–821. https://doi.org/10.1016/j.scitotenv.2019.05.2885.

Yafouz, A., Ali, N.A., Nur'atiah, Z., Mohsen, S., Ahmed, S., Ahmed, E.-S., 2021. Hybrid deep learning model for ozone concentration prediction: comprehensive evaluation and comparison with various machine and deep learning algorithms. Eng. Appl. Comput. Fluid Mech., 15(1), 902–933. https://doi.org/10.1080/19942060.2021.1926328.

Yan, R., Liao, J., Yang, J., Sun, W., Nong, M., Li, F., 2021. Multi-hour and multi-site air quality index forecasting in Beijing using CNN, LSTM, CNN-LSTM, and spatiotemporal clustering. Expert Syst. Appl. 169, 114513.

You, W., Zang, Z., Pan, X., Zhang, L., Chen, D., 2015. Estimating PM2.5 in Xi'an, China using aerosol optical depth: a comparison between the MODIS and MISR retrieval models. Sci. Total Environ. 505, 1156–1165. https://doi.org/10.1016/j.scitotenv.2014.11.024.

Yuchi, W., Gombojav, E., Boldbaatar, B., Galsuren, J., Enkhmaa, S., Beejin, B., Naidan, G., Ochir, C., Legtseg, B., Byambaa, T., Barn, P., Henderson, S.B., Janes, C. R., Lanphear, B.P., McCandless, L.C., Takaro, T.K., Venners, S.A., Webster, G.M., Allen, R.W., 2019. Evaluation of random forest regression and multiple linear regression for predicting indoor fine particulate matter concentrations in a highly polluted city. Environ. Pollut. 245, 746–753.

Zhan, Y., Luo, Y., Deng, X., Chen, H., Grieneisen, M. L., Shen, X., Zhu, L., Zhang, M., 2017. Spatiotemporal prediction of continuous daily PM2.5 concentrations across China using a spatially explicit machine learning algorithm. Atmos. Environ. 155, 129–139. https://doi.org/10.1016/j.atmosenv.2017.02.023.

Zhan, Y., Luo, Y., Deng, X., Grieneisen, M.L., Zhang, M., Di, B., 2018. Spatiotemporal prediction of daily ambient ozone levels across China using random forest for human exposure assessment. Environ. Pollut. 233, 464–473.

Zhang, A., Fu, T.-M., Feng, X., Guo, J., Liu, C., Chen, J., Mo, J., Zhang, X., Wang, X., Wu, W., Hou, Y., Yang, H., Lu, C., 2023. Deep learning-based ensemble forecasts and predictability assessments for surface ozone pollution. Geophys. Res. Lett. 50, e2022GL102611. https://doi.org/10.1029/2022GL102611.

Zhang, C., Yan, J., Li, C., Rui, X., Liu, L., Bie, R., 2016a. On Estimating Air Pollution From Photos Using Convolutional Neural Network, in: Proceedings of the 24th ACM International Conference on Multimedia, pp. 297–301.

Zhang, L., Wang, S., Liu, B., 2017. Deep Learning for Sentiment Analysis: A Survey. National Science Foundation (NSF), Huawei Technologies Co. Ltd.

Zheng, L., Lin, R., Wang, X., Chen, W., 2021. The development and application of machine learning in atmospheric environment studies. Remote Sens-Basel 13, 4839.

Zheng, Y., Zhang, Q., Liu, Y., Geng, G., He, K., 2016. Estimating ground-level PM2.5 concentrations over three megalopolises in China using satellite-derived aerosol optical depth measurements. Atmos. Environ. 124, 232–242. https://doi.org/10.1016/j.atmosenv.2015.06.046.

Zhong, S., Zhang, K., Bagheri, M., Burken, J.G., Gu, A., Li, B., Ma, X., Marrone, B.L., Ren, Z.J., Schrier, J., Shi, W., Tan, H., Wang, T., Wang, X., Wong, B.M., Xiao, X., Yu, X., Zhu, J.J., Zhang, H., 2021. Machine learning: new ideas and tools in environmental science and engineering. Environ. Sci. Technol. 55, 12741–12754.

Zhu, Y., Tao, G., Lifeng, F., Siyuan, H., Mark, E., Hangxin, L., Feng, G., Chi, Z., Siyuan, Q., Ying, N.W., Joshua, B.T., Song-Chun, Z., 2020. Dark, beyond deep: a paradigm shift to cognitive AI with humanlike common sense. Engineering, 6(3), 310–345. https://doi.org/10.1016/j.eng.2020.01.011.

Zimmerman, N., Presto, A.A., Kumar, S.P.N., Gu, J., Hauryliuk, A., Robinson, E.S., Robinson, A.L., 2018. A machine learning calibration model using random forests to improve sensor performance for lower-cost air quality monitoring. Atmos. Meas. Tech. 11, 291–313.

9 Technological Interventions in Healthcare

Sonal Agrawal, Himanshu Kumar Agrawal, and Naman Kumar Agrawal

9.1 INTRODUCTION

In recent years, technological interventions have emerged as a game-changer in various industries, including healthcare. In India, where access to healthcare services in rural and remote areas is often limited, drones have the potential to revolutionise the delivery of medical supplies, diagnostics, and emergency care.

This chapter will explore the various applications of technological interventions in healthcare, focusing on the Indian context, and discuss the challenges and opportunities associated with their implementation.

9.1.1 Diagnostics and Sample Transportation

One of the most promising applications of technological interventions in healthcare is the delivery of medical supplies to remote and hard-to-reach areas. In India, where a significant portion of the population lives in rural regions with limited access to healthcare facilities, drones can play a crucial role in bridging the gap.

In addition to delivering medical supplies, drones can also be used to transport diagnostic samples from remote locations to laboratories for testing. This can significantly reduce the turnaround time for test results, enabling faster diagnosis and treatment of patients.

This section will explore the use of drones for diagnostics and sample transportation in India. It will cover the types of samples that can be transported, the benefits of drone-based transportation, the challenges and limitations, and the potential impact on the healthcare system.

For example, drones can be used to transport blood samples from rural health centres to laboratories in urban areas, ensuring timely analysis and diagnosis. This can be particularly beneficial in cases where timely diagnosis is critical, such as infectious diseases or time-sensitive medical conditions.

9.1.2 Emergency Medical Services

Technological interventions can also play a vital role in emergency medical services, particularly in situations where traditional means of transportation are not feasible or efficient.

For instance, drones can be used to deliver emergency medical supplies, such as blood, vaccines, or antivenom, to the site of an accident or natural disaster. They can also be equipped with defibrillators or other life-saving equipment, enabling first responders to provide immediate care to patients in critical situations.

This section will explore the challenges and limitations of the current emergency medical services (EMS) system in India, the potential impact of technology such as drones and telemedicine, and the future of EMS in India. It discusses investment in infrastructure and technology, training and capacity building, collaboration and coordination, and regulatory compliance.

DOI: 10.1201/9781003451846-9

9.1.3 Telemedicine and Remote Patient Monitoring

In rural areas with limited access to healthcare professionals, drones can be equipped with cameras and communication equipment, enabling remote consultations between patients and doctors. This can help bridge the gap in healthcare access and ensure that patients in remote locations receive timely and appropriate care.

This section will explore the benefits and challenges of telemedicine and remote patient monitoring in India, the role of technology, and the future of these technologies in the Indian healthcare system. It will cover the need for investment in infrastructure, the development of affordable and user-friendly technologies, regulatory and legal reforms, training and capacity building, and public–private partnerships.

9.1.4 Challenges and Regulatory Considerations

The implementation of innovative healthcare solutions and public–private partnerships in the Indian healthcare system presents various challenges and regulatory considerations. Challenges include infrastructure limitations, shortage of trained healthcare personnel, financial constraints, a fragmented healthcare system, and cultural and social barriers. Regulatory considerations encompass data privacy and security, licensure and accreditation, reimbursement policies, telemedicine guidelines, medical devices and equipment regulations, and regulations pertaining to building, manufacturing, and operating drones in India.

To address these challenges and regulatory considerations, measures such as investment in infrastructure, capacity building and training, strengthening regulatory frameworks, fostering collaboration and coordination, and raising awareness and addressing cultural and social barriers are crucial.

This section will explore the challenges and regulatory considerations associated with the implementation of innovative healthcare solutions and public–private partnerships in the Indian healthcare system. It will cover the need for investment in infrastructure, capacity building and training, strengthening regulatory and legal frameworks, fostering collaboration and coordination, and raising awareness.

9.2 DIAGNOSTICS AND SAMPLE TRANSPORTATION

Timely and accurate diagnosis is a critical aspect of healthcare, enabling healthcare providers to make informed decisions about patient care and treatment. In countries like India, where access to diagnostic facilities is often limited in rural and remote areas, the transportation of diagnostic samples to laboratories in urban centres can be a significant challenge. Drones have emerged as a promising solution to address this issue, offering a faster, more efficient, and cost-effective alternative to traditional transportation methods.

This section will explore the various aspects of diagnostics and sample transportation using drones, including the types of samples that can be transported, the benefits of drone-based transportation, the challenges and limitations, and the potential impact on the Indian healthcare system.

9.2.1 Types of Diagnostic Samples Transported by Drones

Drones can be used to transport a wide range of diagnostic samples, including:

- **Blood samples:** Drones can transport blood samples from rural health centres to laboratories in urban areas for analysis, enabling timely diagnosis and treatment of various conditions, such as anaemia, diabetes, and infectious diseases.
- **Pathology samples:** Tissue and biopsy samples can be transported by drones for histopathological examination, facilitating the diagnosis of conditions such as cancer and other diseases.

- **Microbiological samples:** Drones can transport samples for microbiological testing, such as swabs, urine, and stool samples, enabling the identification of bacterial, viral, and parasitic infections.
- **Molecular diagnostics:** Drones can transport samples for molecular diagnostic testing, such as polymerase chain reaction (PCR) and gene sequencing, facilitating the detection of genetic disorders and infectious diseases.
- **Environmental samples:** Drones can transport environmental samples, such as air, water, and soil samples, for analysis, enabling the monitoring of public health and environmental conditions.

9.2.2 Benefits of Drone-Based Diagnostics and Sample Transportation

The use of drones for diagnostics and sample transportation offers several advantages over traditional transportation methods, including:

- **Speed:** Drones can travel at high speeds, enabling faster transportation of diagnostic samples, particularly in emergency situations where time is of the essence.
- **Accessibility:** Drones can navigate difficult terrain and bypass traffic congestion, ensuring that diagnostic samples reach their destination even in remote and hard-to-reach areas.
- **Cost-effectiveness:** Drone-based transportation can be more cost-effective than traditional transportation methods, particularly in rural and remote areas where the cost of transportation infrastructure is high.
- **Reduced sample degradation:** The timely transportation of diagnostic samples by drones can help reduce sample degradation due to delays in transportation, ensuring the accuracy and reliability of test results.
- **Enhanced supply chain management:** The use of drones for diagnostics and sample transportation can improve supply chain management by providing real-time tracking and monitoring of shipments, enabling healthcare providers to better plan and manage their diagnostic services.

9.2.3 Challenges and Limitations of Drone-Based Diagnostics and Sample Transportation

Despite the numerous benefits of using drones for diagnostics and sample transportation, there are several challenges and limitations that must be addressed to ensure the successful implementation of this technology:

- **Payload capacity:** Drones currently have limited carrying capacities, which may restrict the number of diagnostic samples they can transport. However, ongoing research and development efforts are focused on increasing the payload capacity of drones, which will enhance their utility in diagnostics and sample transportation.
- **Sample handling and preservation:** Ensuring the proper handling and preservation of diagnostic samples during transportation is critical to maintaining their integrity and ensuring the accuracy of test results. This requires the development of specialised containers and temperature-controlled systems for drone-based transportation.
- **Safety concerns:** Ensuring the safe operation of drones, particularly in densely populated areas and near sensitive installations such as airports, is a critical concern that must be addressed. This requires the development of robust safety protocols, as well as the integration of advanced collision avoidance and navigation systems.
- **Regulatory compliance:** Drone operators must adhere to the regulations set forth by the DGCA and other relevant authorities. This includes obtaining the necessary permits and certifications and ensuring that drones meet the required safety and performance standards.

- **Infrastructure and capacity building:** The successful implementation of drone-supported diagnostics and sample transportation systems will require investment in infrastructure, such as drone ports and charging stations, as well as training and capacity building for drone operators and healthcare providers.

9.2.4 Impact on the Indian Healthcare System

The integration of drones into the diagnostics and sample transportation system in India has the potential to significantly improve healthcare access and outcomes, particularly in rural and remote areas. Some of the potential impacts include:

- **Improved diagnostic services:** By enabling the timely transportation of diagnostic samples to laboratories in urban centres, drones can help bridge the gap between urban and rural healthcare systems, ensuring that patients across the country receive accurate and timely diagnoses.
- **Enhanced disease surveillance:** The efficient transportation of diagnostic samples by drones can facilitate the monitoring of infectious diseases and public health conditions, enabling healthcare providers and policymakers to make informed decisions about disease prevention and control measures.
- **Cost savings:** The cost-effectiveness of drone-based diagnostics and sample transportation can result in significant cost savings for the healthcare system, freeing up resources that can be invested in other areas, such as infrastructure development and capacity building.
- **Strengthened laboratory networks:** The use of drones for diagnostics and sample transportation can help strengthen laboratory networks, enabling the efficient sharing of resources and expertise between urban and rural healthcare facilities.

9.3 EMERGENCY MEDICAL SERVICES

Emergency medical services play a critical role in providing timely and effective care to patients in emergency situations. In India, the EMS system faces several challenges, including limited resources, inadequate infrastructure, and a shortage of trained personnel. However, the integration of technology, such as drones and telemedicine, has the potential to transform the EMS landscape, enabling faster response times, improved patient outcomes, and enhanced access to care.

This section will explore the various aspects of EMS in India, including the challenges and limitations of the current system, the potential impact of technology on EMS, and the future of EMS in India.

9.3.1 Challenges and Limitations of the Current EMS System

The current EMS system in India faces several challenges and limitations, including:

- **Limited resources:** The EMS system in India is severely underfunded, with limited resources allocated for equipment, vehicles, and personnel. This has resulted in a shortage of ambulances and trained personnel, particularly in rural and remote areas.
- **Inadequate infrastructure:** The lack of adequate infrastructure, such as roads and communication networks, can hinder the timely delivery of emergency medical care, particularly in hard-to-reach areas.
- **Limited access to care:** The limited availability of emergency medical services in India can result in delayed or inadequate care for patients, particularly in rural and remote areas.

- **Lack of trained personnel:** The shortage of trained personnel, including paramedics and emergency medical technicians (EMTs), can limit the quality of care provided to patients in emergency situations.
- **Limited use of technology:** The limited use of technology, such as telemedicine and drones, can hinder the delivery of timely and effective emergency medical care, particularly in hard-to-reach areas.

9.3.2 Potential Impact of Technology on EMS

The integration of technology, such as drones and telemedicine, has the potential to transform the EMS landscape in India, enabling faster response times, improved patient outcomes, and enhanced access to care. Some of the potential impacts of technology on EMS include:

- **Faster response times:** The use of drones for emergency medical transport can significantly reduce response times, particularly in hard-to-reach areas where traditional transportation methods are limited.
- **Improved patient outcomes:** The use of telemedicine can enable remote consultations between healthcare providers and patients, facilitating the timely delivery of care and improving patient outcomes.
- **Enhanced access to care:** The use of technology, such as telemedicine and drones, can improve access to emergency medical care, particularly in rural and remote areas where traditional healthcare services are limited.
- **Improved supply chain management:** The use of technology, such as real-time tracking and monitoring systems, can improve supply chain management for emergency medical supplies and equipment, ensuring that they reach their destination in a timely and efficient manner.
- **Enhanced training and capacity building:** The use of technology, such as simulation training and virtual reality, can enhance the training and capacity building of EMS personnel, enabling them to provide high-quality care to patients in emergency situations.

9.3.3 Future of EMS in India

The future of EMS in India is closely tied to the integration of technology, such as drones and telemedicine, into the existing system. Some of the key areas of focus for the future of EMS in India include:

- **Investment in infrastructure:** The development of adequate infrastructure, such as roads and communication networks, is critical to ensuring the timely delivery of emergency medical care, particularly in hard-to-reach areas.
- **Investment in technology:** The integration of technology, such as drones and telemedicine, into the EMS system, can significantly improve response times, patient outcomes, and access to care.
- **Training and capacity building:** The training and capacity building of EMS personnel, including paramedics and EMTs, is critical to ensuring the delivery of high-quality emergency medical care.
- **Collaboration and coordination:** The collaboration and coordination between healthcare providers, emergency responders, and other stakeholders is critical to ensuring the effective delivery of emergency medical care.
- **Regulatory compliance:** The adherence to regulations and standards set forth by the government and other relevant authorities is critical to ensuring the safety and effectiveness of the EMS system.

9.4 TELEMEDICINE AND REMOTE PATIENT MONITORING

Telemedicine and remote patient monitoring are revolutionising the way healthcare is delivered, particularly in countries like India, where access to healthcare services is often limited in rural and remote areas. By leveraging technology to connect patients with healthcare providers, telemedicine and remote patient monitoring can help bridge the gap between urban and rural healthcare systems, improve patient outcomes, and reduce healthcare costs.

This section will explore the various aspects of telemedicine and remote patient monitoring in India, including the benefits and challenges, the role of technology, and the future of telemedicine and remote patient monitoring in the Indian healthcare system.

9.4.1 Benefits of Telemedicine and Remote Patient Monitoring

Telemedicine and remote patient monitoring offer several benefits for patients, healthcare providers, and the healthcare system as a whole, including:

- **Improved access to care:** Telemedicine can help bridge the gap between urban and rural healthcare systems by connecting patients in remote areas with healthcare providers in urban centres, ensuring that they receive timely and appropriate care.
- **Enhanced patient outcomes:** Remote patient monitoring can enable healthcare providers to track patients' vital signs and health indicators in real time, facilitating early intervention and improving patient outcomes.
- **Reduced healthcare costs:** Telemedicine and remote patient monitoring can help reduce healthcare costs by minimising the need for in-person consultations, hospitalisations, and transportation expenses.
- **Increased patient engagement:** Telemedicine and remote patient monitoring can empower patients to take a more active role in their healthcare, promoting self-management and adherence to treatment plans.
- **Improved healthcare provider collaboration:** Telemedicine can facilitate collaboration between healthcare providers, enabling them to share knowledge, expertise, and resources, ultimately improving patient care.

9.4.2 Challenges of Telemedicine and Remote Patient Monitoring

Despite the numerous benefits of telemedicine and remote patient monitoring, there are several challenges that must be addressed to ensure the successful implementation of these technologies in the Indian healthcare system:

- **Infrastructure limitations:** The lack of adequate infrastructure, such as reliable internet connectivity and power supply, can hinder the effective implementation of telemedicine and remote patient monitoring, particularly in rural and remote areas.
- **Technological barriers:** The limited availability of affordable and user-friendly telemedicine and remote patient monitoring technologies can restrict their adoption, particularly among low-income populations and healthcare providers with limited resources.
- **Regulatory and legal issues:** The implementation of telemedicine and remote patient monitoring requires adherence to various regulations and legal frameworks, such as data privacy and security, licensure, and reimbursement policies.
- **Resistance to change:** The adoption of telemedicine and remote patient monitoring may be met with resistance from healthcare providers and patients who are accustomed to traditional healthcare delivery models.

- **Training and capacity building:** The successful implementation of telemedicine and remote patient monitoring requires the training and capacity building of healthcare providers and the development of appropriate guidelines and protocols.

9.4.3 Role of Technology in Telemedicine and Remote Patient Monitoring

Technology plays a crucial role in the implementation of telemedicine and remote patient monitoring, enabling the delivery of healthcare services over long distances and facilitating real-time communication between patients and healthcare providers. Some of the key technologies used in telemedicine and remote patient monitoring include:

- **Video conferencing:** Video conferencing technologies enable real-time, face-to-face consultations between patients and healthcare providers, facilitating the delivery of healthcare services remotely.
- **Remote patient monitoring devices:** Remote patient monitoring devices, such as wearable sensors and home monitoring systems, enable healthcare providers to track patients' vital signs and health indicators in real time, facilitating early intervention and improving patient outcomes.
- **Electronic health records (EHRs):** EHRs enable the secure storage and sharing of patient information, facilitating collaboration between healthcare providers and improving the continuity of care.
- **Mobile health (mHealth) applications:** mHealth applications can help patients manage their health conditions, track their progress, and communicate with healthcare providers, promoting self-management and adherence to treatment plans.
- **Artificial intelligence (AI) and machine learning:** AI and machine learning technologies can help analyse large volumes of patient data, enabling healthcare providers to make more informed decisions about patient care and treatment.

9.4.4 Future of Telemedicine and Remote Patient Monitoring in India

The future of telemedicine and remote patient monitoring in India is closely tied to the continued development and adoption of technology, as well as the addressing of the challenges and limitations associated with these technologies. Some of the key areas of focus for the future of telemedicine and remote patient monitoring in India include:

- **Investment in infrastructure:** The development of adequate infrastructure, such as reliable internet connectivity and power supply, is critical to ensuring the effective implementation of telemedicine and remote patient monitoring, particularly in rural and remote areas.
- **Development of affordable and user-friendly technologies:** The development of affordable and user-friendly telemedicine and remote patient monitoring technologies can help facilitate their adoption, particularly among low-income populations and healthcare providers with limited resources.
- **Regulatory and legal reforms:** The development of appropriate regulatory and legal frameworks, such as data privacy and security, licensure, and reimbursement policies, is critical to ensuring the successful implementation of telemedicine and remote patient monitoring.
- **Training and capacity building:** The training and capacity building of healthcare providers and the development of appropriate guidelines and protocols are critical to ensuring the effective implementation of telemedicine and remote patient monitoring.
- **Public–private partnerships:** The collaboration between public and private sector stakeholders can help facilitate the development and implementation of telemedicine and remote patient monitoring technologies, ultimately improving patient care and outcomes.

9.5 THE ROLE OF PUBLIC–PRIVATE PARTNERSHIPS IN ADVANCING HEALTHCARE IN INDIA

Public–private partnerships (PPPs) have emerged as a promising approach to address the challenges faced by the Indian healthcare system, including limited resources, inadequate infrastructure, and a shortage of trained personnel. By leveraging the strengths of both the public and private sectors, PPPs can help drive innovation, improve access to care, and enhance the overall quality of healthcare services in India.

This section will explore the various aspects of public–private partnerships in the Indian healthcare system, including the benefits and challenges, the role of technology, and the future of PPPs in advancing healthcare in India.

9.5.1 Benefits of Public–Private Partnerships in Healthcare

Public–private partnerships offer several benefits for the Indian healthcare system, including:

- **Resource mobilisation:** PPPs can help mobilise resources from both the public and private sectors, enabling the development of healthcare infrastructure, the procurement of medical equipment, and the training of healthcare personnel.
- **Innovation and technology adoption:** PPPs can facilitate the adoption of innovative technologies and practices, such as telemedicine and remote patient monitoring, ultimately improving patient care and outcomes.
- **Improved access to care:** PPPs can help bridge the gap between urban and rural healthcare systems by leveraging the expertise and resources of the private sector to expand access to healthcare services in underserved areas.
- **Enhanced quality of care:** PPPs can help improve the quality of healthcare services by promoting the adoption of best practices, standardising protocols, and fostering a culture of continuous improvement.
- **Cost-effectiveness:** PPPs can help reduce healthcare costs by leveraging the efficiencies and economies of scale offered by the private sector, ultimately resulting in more affordable healthcare services for patients.

9.5.2 Challenges of Public–Private Partnerships in Healthcare

Despite the numerous benefits of public–private partnerships in healthcare, there are several challenges that must be addressed to ensure their successful implementation:

- **Aligning interests:** Ensuring that the interests of both the public and private sectors are aligned can be challenging, particularly when it comes to balancing the need for profit with the provision of affordable and accessible healthcare services.
- **Regulatory and legal issues:** The implementation of PPPs in healthcare requires adherence to various regulations and legal frameworks, such as data privacy and security, licensure, and reimbursement policies.
- **Ensuring transparency and accountability:** Ensuring transparency and accountability in the management and operation of PPPs is critical to maintaining public trust and ensuring the successful implementation of these partnerships.
- **Capacity building and training:** The successful implementation of PPPs in healthcare requires the training and capacity building of healthcare providers and the development of appropriate guidelines and protocols.

9.5.3 Role of Technology in Public–Private Partnerships

Technology plays a crucial role in the implementation of public–private partnerships in healthcare, enabling the delivery of healthcare services over long distances, facilitating real-time communication between patients and healthcare providers, and driving innovation in healthcare delivery. Some of the key technologies used in PPPs include:

- **Telemedicine and remote patient monitoring:** These technologies can help expand access to healthcare services in rural and remote areas, ultimately improving patient outcomes and reducing healthcare costs.
- **Electronic health records:** EHRs are a critical component of modern healthcare delivery, enabling healthcare providers to access and share patient information in real time.
- **Mobile health applications:** mHealth applications have the potential to revolutionise healthcare delivery by enabling patients to access healthcare services and information remotely.
- **Artificial intelligence and machine learning:** Drones equipped with AI and ML algorithms can swiftly transport medical supplies, deliver medications, and provide emergency services to remote areas. These technologies improve healthcare accessibility, disease surveillance, and personalised care.

9.5.4 Future of Public–Private Partnerships in Advancing Healthcare in India

The future of public–private partnerships in advancing healthcare in India is closely tied to the continued development and adoption of technology, as well as the addressing of the challenges and limitations associated with these partnerships. Some of the key areas of focus for the future of PPPs in healthcare include:

- **Strengthening regulatory and legal frameworks:** The development of appropriate regulatory and legal frameworks, such as data privacy and security, licensure, and reimbursement policies, is critical to ensuring the successful implementation of PPPs in healthcare.
- **Fostering innovation and technology adoption:** Encouraging the adoption of innovative technologies and practices, such as telemedicine and remote patient monitoring, can help drive improvements in patient care and outcomes.
- **Ensuring transparency and accountability:** Implementing measures to ensure transparency and accountability in the management and operation of PPPs is critical to maintaining public trust and ensuring the successful implementation of these partnerships.
- **Capacity building and training:** The training and capacity building of healthcare providers and the development of appropriate guidelines and protocols are critical to ensuring the effective implementation of PPPs in healthcare.

9.6 CHALLENGES AND REGULATORY CONSIDERATIONS

The rapid advancement of technology and the increasing adoption of public–private partnerships in the Indian healthcare system have brought forth numerous challenges and regulatory considerations. This section will delve into the various challenges faced by the healthcare sector and the regulatory considerations that must be addressed to ensure the successful implementation of innovative healthcare solutions and public–private partnerships in India.

9.6.1 Challenges in the Indian Healthcare System

The Indian healthcare system faces several challenges that must be addressed to ensure the successful implementation of innovative healthcare solutions and public–private partnerships. Some of the key challenges include:

- **Infrastructure limitations:** The lack of adequate infrastructure, such as reliable internet connectivity, power supply, and healthcare facilities, can hinder the effective implementation of innovative healthcare solutions, particularly in rural and remote areas.
- **Shortage of trained healthcare personnel:** The Indian healthcare system faces a significant shortage of trained healthcare personnel, including doctors, nurses, and allied health professionals. This shortage can limit the effectiveness of innovative healthcare solutions and public–private partnerships.
- **Financial constraints:** Limited financial resources can restrict the adoption of innovative healthcare solutions and the implementation of public–private partnerships, particularly among low-income populations and healthcare providers with limited resources.
- **Fragmented healthcare system:** The Indian healthcare system is characterised by a fragmented mix of public and private providers, which can make it challenging to implement innovative healthcare solutions and public–private partnerships on a large scale.
- **Cultural and social barriers:** Cultural and social barriers, such as resistance to change, lack of awareness, and stigma associated with certain health conditions, can hinder the adoption of innovative healthcare solutions and the implementation of public–private partnerships.

9.6.2 Regulatory Considerations in the Indian Healthcare System

The implementation of innovative healthcare solutions and public–private partnerships in the Indian healthcare system requires adherence to various regulations and legal frameworks. Some of the key regulatory considerations include:

- **Data privacy and security:** The implementation of innovative healthcare solutions, such as telemedicine and remote patient monitoring, requires adherence to data privacy and security regulations, such as the Information Technology (Reasonable Security Practices and Procedures and Sensitive Personal Data or Information) Rules, 2011 [1], and the Digital Personal Data Protection Bill 2022 [2]. These regulations aim to protect patients' personal and sensitive health information from unauthorised access, use, and disclosure.
- **Licensure and accreditation:** Healthcare providers involved in the delivery of innovative healthcare solutions and public–private partnerships must adhere to licensure and accreditation requirements, such as the Indian Medical Council Act, 1956 [3], and the Clinical Establishments (Registration and Regulation) Act, 2010 [4]. These regulations aim to ensure that healthcare providers meet the necessary standards of quality and safety.
- **Reimbursement policies:** The implementation of innovative healthcare solutions and public–private partnerships requires the development of appropriate reimbursement policies, such as the Ayushman Bharat Pradhan Mantri Jan Arogya Yojana (AB-PMJAY) [5], which aims to provide financial protection to low-income populations for secondary and tertiary care hospitalisation.
- **Telemedicine guidelines:** The implementation of telemedicine solutions requires adherence to the Telemedicine Practice Guidelines issued by the Ministry of Health and Family Welfare in 2020 [6]. These guidelines aim to provide a framework for the practice of telemedicine in India, including the types of services that can be provided, the responsibilities of healthcare providers, and the ethical considerations involved in the delivery of telemedicine services.

- **Medical devices and equipment regulations:** The implementation of innovative healthcare solutions, such as remote patient monitoring devices, requires adherence to medical device and equipment regulations, such as the Medical Device Rules, 2017 [7], and the Drugs and Cosmetics Act, 1940 [8]. These regulations aim to ensure the safety, quality, and efficacy of medical devices and equipment used in the delivery of healthcare services.
- **Building, manufacturing, and operating drones in India:** The Drone (Amendment) Rules, 2022, governs the requirement for various approvals, including import clearance, remote pilot instructor authorisation, and drone port authorisation [9]. Drones are now classified based on their maximum all-up weight, including payload, and specific components and features are mandated for each category. Operators are required to ensure their drones are NPNT (no permission, no takeoff) compliant and must register on the Digital Sky Platform. The Drone (Amendment) Rules, 2022, streamlined regulations regarding building, manufacturing, and operating drones in India.

9.6.3 Addressing Challenges and Regulatory Considerations

Several measures can be taken to address the challenges and regulatory considerations associated with the implementation of innovative healthcare solutions in the Indian healthcare system:

- **Investment in infrastructure:** The development of adequate infrastructure, such as reliable internet connectivity, power supply, and healthcare facilities, is critical to ensuring the effective implementation of innovative healthcare solutions and public–private partnerships, particularly in rural and remote areas.
- **Capacity building and training:** The training and capacity building of healthcare providers and the development of appropriate guidelines and protocols are critical to ensuring the effective implementation of innovative healthcare solutions and public–private partnerships.
- **Strengthening regulatory and legal frameworks:** The development of appropriate regulatory and legal frameworks, such as data privacy and security, licensure, and reimbursement policies, is critical to ensuring the successful implementation of innovative healthcare solutions and public–private partnerships.
- **Fostering collaboration and coordination:** Encouraging collaboration and coordination between public and private sector stakeholders and between different levels of government can help facilitate the development and implementation of innovative healthcare solutions and public–private partnerships.
- **Raising awareness and addressing cultural and social barriers:** Raising awareness about the benefits of innovative healthcare solutions and public–private partnerships and addressing cultural and social barriers can help facilitate their adoption and implementation.

9.7 CONCLUSION

The integration of technological interventions into the healthcare system in India holds immense promise. The Indian healthcare system is on the brink of a significant transformation, driven by technological advancements, increased collaboration between public and private sector stakeholders, and supportive policy initiatives. Key developments such as the expansion of telemedicine and remote patient monitoring, integration of artificial intelligence and machine learning, development of personalised medicine, and adoption of digital health solutions will reshape the future of healthcare in India.

These technologies will enable the delivery of healthcare services over long distances, facilitate real-time communication between patients and healthcare providers, and drive innovation in healthcare delivery. They will play a critical role in expanding access to healthcare services in rural and remote areas, improving patient outcomes, and reducing healthcare costs.

The integration of technology, such as drones and telemedicine, has the potential to transform the EMS landscape in India, enabling faster response times, improved patient outcomes, and enhanced access to care. Addressing the challenges and limitations of the current system, such as limited resources and inadequate infrastructure, is critical to ensuring the successful implementation of technology-enabled EMS solutions.

Collaboration between public and private sector stakeholders, as well as supportive policy initiatives, will be crucial in shaping the future of healthcare in India. Strengthening regulatory and legal frameworks, fostering innovation and technology adoption, capacity building and training, and raising awareness and addressing cultural and social barriers are key areas of focus for collaboration and policy development.

The development of appropriate regulatory and legal frameworks, such as data privacy and security, licensure, and reimbursement policies, is critical to ensuring the successful implementation of innovative healthcare solutions and public–private partnerships. By investing in infrastructure, building capacity, strengthening regulatory and legal frameworks, fostering collaboration and coordination, and raising awareness, the Indian healthcare system can overcome these challenges and harness the potential of innovative healthcare solutions and public–private partnerships to improve access to care, enhance patient outcomes, and reduce healthcare costs.

As technology advances and the healthcare system in India evolves, the future of innovative healthcare solutions and public–private partnerships is poised for innovation and progress.

REFERENCES

[1] Department of Information Technology, 11 April 2011. [Online]. Available: www.meity.gov.in/writereaddata/files/GSR313E_10511%281%29_0.pdf. [Accessed 23 June 2023].

[2] PRS Legislative Research, "The Personal Data Protection Bill," 2019. [Online]. Available: https://prsindia.org/billtrack/the-personal-data-protection-bill-2019. [Accessed 23 June 2023].

[3] "The Indian Medical Council Act, 1956," 30 December 1956. [Online]. Available: https://lddashboard.legislative.gov.in/sites/default/files/A1956-102_0.pdf. [Accessed 23 June 2023].

[4] Ministry of Health and Family Welfare, "Clinical Establishments (Registration and Regulation) Act," 18 August 2010. [Online]. Available: www.clinicalestablishments.gov.in/WriteReadData/969.pdf. [Accessed 23 June 2023].

[5] National Health Authority, "Ayushman Bharat Pradhan Mantri Jan Arogya Yojana (AB-PMJAY)," 6 May 2022. [Online]. Available: https://setu.pmjay.gov.in/setu/. [Accessed 23 June 2023].

[6] Medical Council of India, "Telemedicine Practice Guidelines," 25 March 2020. [Online]. Available: www.mohfw.gov.in/pdf/Telemedicine.pdf. [Accessed 23 June 2023].

[7] Ministry of Health and Family Welfare, "Medical Devices Rules, 2017," 31 January 2017. [Online]. Available: https://cdsco.gov.in/opencms/resources/UploadCDSCOWeb/2022/m_device/Medical%20Devices%20Rules,%202017.pdf. [Accessed 23 June 2023].

[8] Ministry of Health and Family Welfare, "Drugs and Cosmetics Act, 1940," [Online]. Available: https://cdsco.gov.in/opencms/opencms/system/modules/CDSCO.WEB/elements/download_file_division.jsp?num_id=OTIyNw==. [Accessed 23 June 2023].

[9] Ministry of Civil Aviation, "Drone (Amendment) Rules, 2022," 8 December 2022. [Online]. Available: www.pib.gov.in/PressReleasePage.aspx?PRID=1881767#:~:text=(vii)%20Drone%20(Amendment),notified%20on%2029th%20November%202022. [Accessed 23 June 2023].

10 Disaster and Emergency Healthcare

Haobam Derit Singh, Yaman Hooda, and Jimmy Mehta

10.1 DISASTER

A serious perturbation of the operational dynamics within a community or society, regardless of scale, resulting from the convergence of hazardous occurrences with factors of exposure, vulnerability, and capacity is termed as "disaster". This convergence leads to the occurrence of one or more of the ensuing consequences: human, material, economic, and environmental losses and impacts. Annotations can be defined as impact of a disaster that may manifest as an instantaneous and confined event or a pervasive and enduring phenomenon. Its magnitude may even challenge or surpass the ability of a community or society to manage and address it solely through internal resources. Consequently, external support becomes essential, potentially involving neighboring regions, national entities, or international aid mechanisms. "Emergency" is employed interchangeably with "disaster", particularly when discussing biological and technological hazards or health crises. However, it is crucial to acknowledge that emergencies may encompass hazardous events that do not lead to a severe disturbance in the operations of a community or society. In such cases, the impact might be limited, without reaching the level of serious disruption. Disaster damage pertains to the period encompassing the disaster and its immediate aftermath. This is typically evaluated in tangible measurements like the area of housing affected or length of damaged roads. It involves the complete or partial destruction of physical assets, disruption of essential services, and harm to livelihoods in the affected area. Disaster impact refers to the overall consequences resulting from a hazardous event or disaster, encompassing both negative effects (such as economic losses) and positive effects (such as economic gains). The term comprises the impacts on economic, human, and environmental aspects, encompassing aspects like fatalities, injuries, diseases, and other adverse effects on human physical, mental, and social well-being (Figure 10.1).

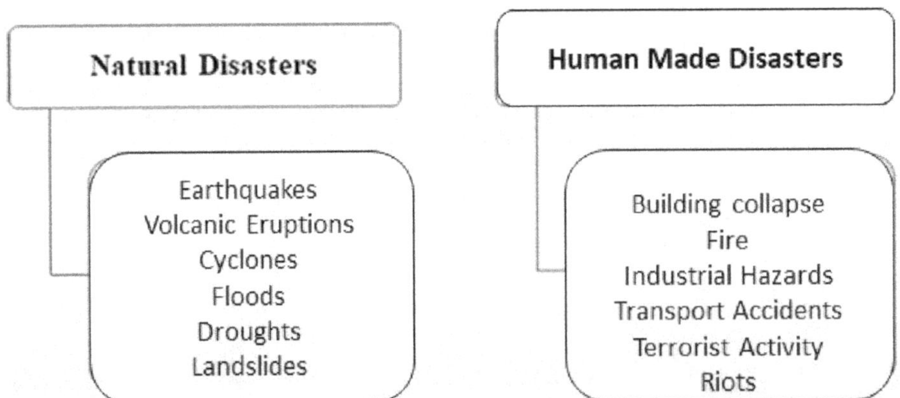

FIGURE 10.1 Types of disasters.

DOI: 10.1201/9781003451846-10

For the purpose of the scope of the Sendai Framework for Disaster Risk Reduction 2015–2030 (para. 15), the following terms are also considered:

- Localized Disaster: This type of disaster affects only specific communities, necessitating assistance from sources beyond the impacted community.
- Widespread Disaster: This type of disaster impacts an entire society, requiring assistance at the national or international level.
- Recurring and Rare Disasters: These are determined by the probability of occurrence and the return period of a particular hazard and its impacts. The effects of recurring disasters can accumulate and become chronic for a community or society.
- Gradual-Onset Disaster: This type of disaster develops gradually over time. Examples include events like drought, desertification, sea-level rise, and epidemic diseases.
- Sudden-Onset Disaster: This type of disaster arises swiftly and unexpectedly due to a hazardous event. Examples include events like earthquakes, volcanic eruptions, flash floods, chemical explosions, critical infrastructure failures, and transport accidents.

10.2 HEALTHCARE

Healthcare refers to efforts aimed at improving people's health through various means, such as disease prevention, diagnosis, treatment, recovery, or alleviation of physical and mental impairments. Health professionals and allied health fields are responsible for delivering healthcare services, which encompass disciplines.

A well-functioning healthcare system plays a vital role in driving a country's economy, fostering development, and promoting industrialization. Across the globe, healthcare is widely recognized as a crucial factor in enhancing the overall physical and mental health and well-being of individuals. An illustrative instance of this impact is the global eradication of smallpox in 1980, a historic achievement recognized by the WHO, as it marked the first successful elimination of a disease through deliberate healthcare interventions.

10.3 EMERGENCY HEALTHCARE

Emergency care in healthcare involves the immediate provision of medical treatment following the onset of a medical condition or injury. Typically, this care is delivered by emergency medical services (EMS) like ambulance services, paramedics, or police.

This type of care often includes life-saving measures such as CPR or the administration of intravenous drugs. Its purpose may also encompass stabilizing patients for transportation to a hospital for further treatment. In some instances, emergency care alone may be sufficient for a patient's recovery. Emergency care plays a vital role within the broader healthcare system, and it is essential for everyone to comprehend its nature and significance.

The term "emergency care" can have varying interpretations across different healthcare settings. Generally, it refers to the medical treatment provided to patients experiencing a medical emergency. This can range from basic life support and oxygen administration to performing surgical procedures or other invasive interventions. A team of healthcare professionals, including doctors, nurses, and paramedics, collaborates to stabilize the patient and achieve the best possible outcome.

In the healthcare context, emergency care refers to the medical attention received for a sudden and unexpected illness or injury. It can be life-saving and is often administered in an emergency room (ER) or designated urgent care center. It is distinct from primary care, which constitutes ongoing healthcare from family doctors or general practitioners, as well as secondary care, which involves specialized treatment for specific illnesses or injuries.

Emergency care in healthcare focuses on promptly treating patients with acute illnesses or injuries that necessitate immediate medical attention. Typically, this care takes place in an emergency room or urgent care facility. Emergency care providers must quickly assess a patient's condition and provide appropriate treatment. They may also need to stabilize the patient for transfer to another facility for more definitive care.

10.4 DISASTER MANAGEMENT CYCLE

Disaster management is typically divided into four stages: prevention, preparedness, response, and recovery. Effectively managing and responding to disasters involves careful consideration of each stage. Although they are distinct stages with specific objectives, the cycle is designed to be comprehensive, with each stage relying on the previous one to achieve better outcomes. During the recovery phase, professionals can gather and analyze performance data to enhance their plans and potentially prevent the disaster or mitigate its effects from recurring. Consequently, with each disaster, outcomes should improve, leading to reduced costs and lessening future hardships for individuals, families, and communities. According to the Federal Emergency Management Agency (FEMA), all communities are involved in at least one stage of emergency management at any given time. The first stage of the disaster management cycle is prevention, which focuses on averting or minimizing the potential impact of a disaster before it occurs. This stage involves identifying potential risks and hazards that could lead to a disaster, conducting environmental analysis, assessing vulnerabilities and risks, and devising measures to prevent or mitigate potential threats. While prevention necessitates preparation before a crisis arises, implementing permanent measures to reduce hazard risk can be advantageous for all stages of disaster management (Figure 10.2).

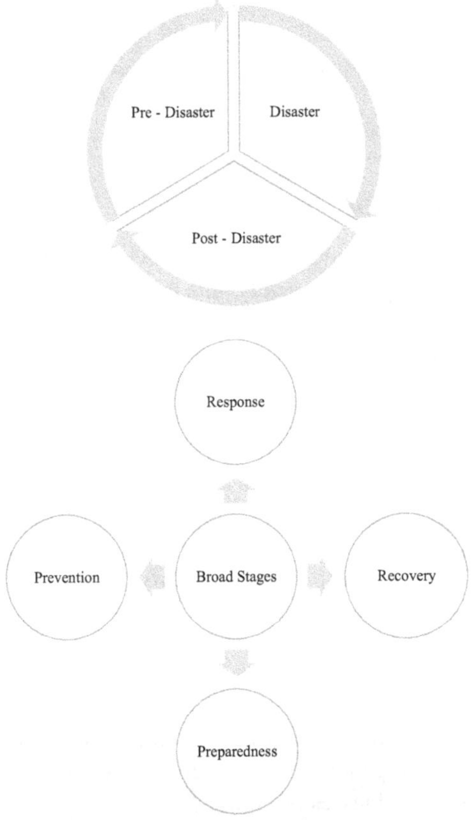

FIGURE 10.2 Stages of disaster management cycle.

1. *Prevention:*

   The only possible way to address any type of disaster is to be proactive, meaning the identification of probable effects and planning precautions for mitigating its impacts. This stage of the disaster management cycle focuses on establishing permanent measures for reducing disaster risk, but it is significant to recognize that disasters and their effects cannot always be prevented.
2. *Preparedness:*

   Preparedness pertains to the development of strategies, plans, and procedures to effectively address potential disasters. It involves creating emergency plans, conducting training, and organizing exercises to ensure that individuals, equipment, and systems are adequately equipped to respond to a disaster. Examples of preparedness measures include safety drills in schools and other community areas, such as active shooter drills, which educate staff and students on how to respond to such events safely and enhance their chances of survival. Fire drills are another instance of preparedness measures, as they familiarize students or employees with proper procedures to follow during a fire, including identifying exits and gathering points away from the building.
3. *Response:*

   The response stage entails the immediate reaction to a disaster. Response measures encompass activities like search and rescue operations, delivering emergency medical assistance, and establishing emergency shelters. Response teams work to stabilize the situation and minimize the potential for further harm. Illustrative examples of emergency response include deploying emergency workers to guide residents towards evacuation routes or relocating emergency supplies to a pre-designated safety area where community members can gather in the event of a displacing flood.
4. *Recovery:*

   The recovery stage is centered on returning the impacted community to a state of normality. Recovery efforts encompass activities like reconstructing infrastructure, delivering medical aid and social services, and assisting individuals and families in recovering financially. A recovery plan may encompass ongoing medical assistance, such as physical therapy, for individuals who sustained injuries during the disaster. Additionally, it may involve establishing support groups for those who experienced emotional trauma due to the event.

10.5 IMPLEMENTING HEALTH EMERGENCY AND DISASTER RISK MANAGEMENT

Health systems play a central role in managing risks and mitigating the consequences of emergencies and disasters across various hazards. The health sector is particularly adept at handling infectious risks and responding to outbreaks. However, it also has a critical responsibility in preventing and minimizing the health impacts of emergencies caused by natural, technological, and societal hazards.

The first stage of the disaster management cycle is prevention, which focuses on averting or minimizing the potential impact of a disaster before it occurs. This stage involves identifying potential risks and hazards that could lead to a disaster, conducting environmental analysis, assessing vulnerabilities and risks, and devising measures to prevent or mitigate potential threats. While prevention necessitates preparation before a crisis arises, implementing permanent measures to reduce hazard risk can be advantageous for all stages of disaster management. Ensuring sound risk management is crucial to safeguard the development and implementation of various global, regional, and national frameworks, including the Sustainable Development Goals (SDGs), universal health coverage (UHC), the Sendai Framework for Disaster Risk Reduction 2015–2030, International Health Regulations, and the Paris Agreement on Climate Change.

The field of health emergency and disaster preparedness pertains to the knowledge and capabilities required to effectively anticipate, respond to, and recover from the impacts of potential, imminent, or existing hazardous events or conditions. Governments, response and recovery organizations, communities, and individuals can take preparatory actions to build the necessary capacities for handling all types of emergencies and achieving a systematic transition from response to sustained recovery. These actions, founded on a thorough analysis of disaster risks and well connected with early warning systems, involve contingency planning, stockpiling essential equipment and supplies, establishing and testing coordination mechanisms, raising risk awareness, disseminating public information about protective behaviors, and conducting relevant training and field exercises.

10.6 LATEST TECHNOLOGICAL ADVANCEMENTS IN EMERGENCY HEALTHCARE

With the emerging technological advancements in every sector of society, healthcare systems are also adapting to ongoing trends so as to provide the best services to patients in times of need. When a place is hit by a disaster, that area becomes more remote for providing healthcare facilities and services. In such difficult scenarios, where normal emergency healthcare operations and services cannot be performed, applications of some advanced technological sectors play a vital role in serving the purpose. The various technological advancements being applied in emergency healthcare systems are as follows (Figure 10.3):

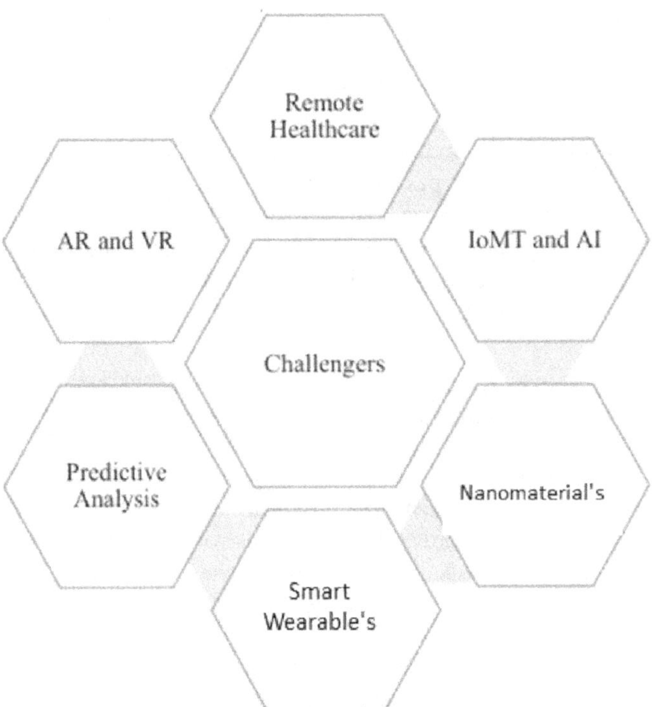

FIGURE 10.3 Latest technological advancements in emergency healthcare.

1. *Remote Healthcare:*

   Telehealth, or remote healthcare, is a term used to describe one of the latest technological advancements used worldwide. With the help of this technological boon, consultation with a doctor is possible without meeting them personally by getting out of the house. This technological advancement is specifically beneficial for wide clusters of patients, including elderly people, people living in remote or rural areas, and many more. It can be performed by using device applications. With applications installed on devices (mobile phones or laptops), one can get the benefits of the following services:

- Booking an appointment
- Consultation with a doctor in a specialized domain
- Records of medicine intake
- Overall medical record
- Services available at a particular location
- Visit history
- Communication between patient and doctor
- Emergency care

With the records maintained on the application, the doctor analyses them on a monthly or yearly basis and recommends medication accordingly.

During post-disaster scenarios, with the help of telehealth, a doctor can easily visualize and predict medication post first aid so that the life of the patient can be saved or enough time is available to the patient for transfer from the site of emergency to nearby healthcare services like hospitals, medical centers, medical institutions, and clinics. Some healthcare facilities assessed ways the application of technology could help remote parties assist in post-disaster conditions.

A well-distributed communication platform enables healthcare professionals to support emergency services. Mobile telehealth units and services tends to improve victim care without any major hurdles in situations where all hospital facilities are damaged immensely after the occurrence of a natural disaster. If the line of communication is open during challenging circumstances, teams on the ground can discuss specifics when it comes to injury and illness. Remote professionals can guide rescue workers on how to treat and aid those affected.

2. *Internet of Medical Things:*

The Internet of Medical Things (IoMT) refers to a collection of network-connected medical services and devices and software or hardware technologies through the internet. The most basic advantage of the IoMT is that since a large number of the devices are interconnected with each other, transmission and storage of data are done easily. Furthermore, this stored big data is used in determining and providing medication to patients at a much faster rate. The most important application of the IoMT is found in diagnosing chronic diseases and in emergency scenarios [1–3].

IoMT devices are already available in limited areas of the world and find applications as smart robot nurses for monitoring the blood pressure of the patients and SpO_2 levels in patients during COVID-19 emergencies.

Per the literature review, around 600,000 IoMT devices are in practical use in the following systems:

- Smart wearables
- Smart pills
- Smart beds
- Automated temperature readers
- Ingestible cameras/sensors
- Inhaler delivery systems

3. *Nanomedicine:*

The application of nanoparticles, nano-objects, or nanoscale materials in the healthcare–medicine sector is termed "nanomedicine". The technological advancement of nanomedicine finds its application in targeted cancer treatment and drug injection. In scenarios of emergency healthcare disasters, the application of nanomedicine plays a vital role in providing medical treatment for victims suffering from medical conditions. Also, some medical instruments have been converted into smaller dimensions by the application of nanomedicine, proving beneficial to patients of remote or disaster-affected areas.

4. *Smart Wearables:*

   Smart wearables is and will be one of the most important innovations among all the sectors of demographics, considering the part of notable technological advancements in the medical sector. Focusing on medical-related approaches, these smart watches and trackers finds their application as:

   - Recording heartbeat
   - Recording blood oxygen levels
   - Tracking daily activities
   - Recording ECG reports

   With such applications, smart watches give an indication when any health parameter they measure is critical, thus saving the life of the wearer. During post-disaster scenarios, such instruments can be used in measuring heart rate and blood oxygen level (as stated), helping first-aid medical teams focus on critical patients for lifesaving.

   Besides these smart watches and fitness trackers, one of the most popular smart wearables is smart bio patches. Smart bio patches find applications in monitoring blood vitals without being connected to a smart watch or any other related device.

5. *Artificial Intelligence in Healthcare Systems:*

   One of the most prominent technological advancements that finds application in disaster-related healthcare facilities is artificial intelligence (AI) and machine learning (ML). Various medical operations have been operated with the help of robots, and it has been noted that such applications of AI and ML proved effective and efficient even in micro areas of the healthcare sector. Following are some of the applications of AI in the healthcare sector:

   - With the help of AI, the healthcare services are able to reach most inaccessible and underdeveloped regions.
   - Effective diagnosis with a negligible rate of errors has been noticed after implementing AI techniques during different diagnoses.
   - Gathering, storing, and managing data effectively.
   - With recent advancement, it has been reported that AI is playing a crucial role in the development of next-generation automated–predictive radiology equipment.
   - Detection of cancer in early stages.

   With the application of AI in healthcare systems, installation and gathering information from early warning systems and risk assessment become more effective. Also, it finds application in epidemiological surveillance and outbreak management during disaster risk reduction measures [4, 5].

6. *Augmented Reality (AR) and Virtual Reality (VR):*

   Augmented reality and virtual reality have been considered useful tools for professionals in the healthcare industry for giving assistance and training to young professionals to performing critical treatments. With technologies like the Microsoft Hololens, surgeons are able to perform operations with more accuracy.

   In post-disaster scenarios, the applications of AR and VR in healthcare systems are a boon, as this technology can be accessed for faraway places from the point of the source of disaster, where healthcare professionals need to wear VR lenses and guide the people available on-site for medical treatment and surgeries. Also, they find applications in targeting veins correctly for taking blood samples. AR also allows healthcare professionals to treat patients through voice commands, where the surgeon in charge can also give suggestions/recommendations to other patients without disturbing the ongoing surgery with the help of voice commands.

7. *Predictive Analysis:*

   A technique of providing improved healthcare is known as predictive analysis. It includes the usage of the medical data and records of past patients and formation of an algorithm based on the concept of machine learning for showing insights for the treatment of upcoming patients.

The collection of data through the IoMT and implementation of AI and ML in the analysis of the data will predict and provide outcomes beforehand in terms of a pattern that was created based on the large amount of stored data of similar types. The advantages of implementing predictive analysis in healthcare services for disaster-affected areas include:

- Faster diagnosis
- Improved patient care
- Enriched decision making in emergency situations
- Faster availability of medicine

Healthcare management around the world is always attentive towards the occurrence of disasters and strategies during pre- and post-disaster scenarios. Predictive analysis software determines and examines the medical records of all the victims from past disaster-related situations and makes a prediction about the percentage of population being prone to any type of medical illness, depending upon the type, magnitude, and location of the source and effects of the disaster. Medical services and aids are being prepared on the basis of predictive analysis so that many more people will be treated in less time, aiming to save the life of every person.

Satellite mapping plays a vital role in determination of disaster-hit areas. During flood conditions, healthcare systems may come to a halt. It takes days for floodwater to recede, and it is not possible to perform an assessment of flood damage until the level of water comes to its natural point. In such a situation, satellite mapping comes into action.

The local authorities can address mass causality incidents (MCIs) skillfully when they have all the necessary information regarding actual and potential damage. An MCI can be understood as an emergency situation dealing with loss of multiple lives, depending upon which they have been categorized into different domains: terrorist activities, active shooting conditions, and natural disasters.

Another technological advancement that is gaining much attention worldwide is the application of chatbots in the treatment of patient symptoms at their own locations. Various health organizations around the world are using chatbots, which is decreasing emergency room visits. In post-disaster conditions, these chatbots can be treat as a helping aid to the doctors or healthcare personnel present over the affected location. The main function of a chatbot is to recognize the symptoms of a disease, so they are helpful in cases where patients require immediate treatment. Healthcare personnel also used the application as a part of suggesting the treatments for the disease of said symptoms. The advantage of this exercise was making patients calmer about their suffering, helping with the psychological aspects of the disaster-victimized population. This application can be used by hospital staff for the purpose of interaction with victims, and they can hire additional staff if the existing ones are unable to handle patients effectively and efficiently.

REFERENCES

1. Yongwan Chun, Mei-Po Kwan, Daniel A. Griffith (2019) Uncertainty and Context in GIScience and Geography: Challenges in the Era of Geospatial Big Data, International Journal of Geographical Information Science, 33:6, 1131–1134, DOI: 10.1080/13658816.2019.1566552.
2. Alan T. Murray, Tony H. Grubesic, Ran Wei, Elizabeth A. Mack (2015) A Hybrid Geocoding Methodology for Spatio-Temporal Data, https://doi.org/10.1111/j.1467-9671.2011.01289.x.
3. Y. Hooda (2022) "IoT and Remote Sensing," in Computer Vision and Internet of Things. Chapman and Hall/CRC, pp. 111–140.
4. Yaman Hooda, Haobam Derit Singh (2023) "Digital Reforms in Public Services and Infrastructure Development & Management," in Technological Prospects and Social Applications of Society 5.0, Chapman and Hall/CRC, pp. 219–237.
5. Haobam Derit Singh, Yaman Hooda (2023) "Resilience of Digital Society to Natural Disasters," in Technological Prospects and Social Applications of Society 5.0, Chapman and Hall/CRC, pp. 185–199.

11 Deep Learning and IoT in Healthcare

Mrinalika Durairaju, Mrinalini Durairaju, Vallidevi Krishnamurthy, Sakthivel V, and Surendiran Balasubramanian

11.1 INTRODUCTION

Deep learning, a subset of machine learning, has shown great potential in revolutionising the field of healthcare. One key factor that contributes to the success of deep learning algorithms is the availability of large amounts of data. With the advent of big data, healthcare organisations now have access to vast amounts of information that can be used for training and validating deep learning models. In the healthcare industry, machine learning algorithms have a lot of potential because there is a lot of data generated for each patient [1]. This data includes medical records, imaging data, genomics data, wearable sensor data from IoT devices, and more.

The wealth of healthcare data allows deep learning algorithms to learn and extract meaningful patterns that can be used for various healthcare applications. For example, deep learning has been used for image analysis in radiology, where algorithms are trained on large datasets of medical images to accurately detect and classify abnormalities or diseases. Furthermore, deep learning has also shown promise in natural language processing and text mining tasks, allowing for more efficient analysis of medical literature and patient records. In addition to the availability of large amounts of data, another factor that contributes to the success of deep learning in healthcare is advancements in technology.

Big data is a methodology for data analysis made possible by a new generation of technological and architectural advancements that facilitate high-velocity data capture, storage, and analysis. Data sources go beyond the typical company database to include email, mobile device output, sensor-generated data, and social media output [2]. Rather than being limited to organised database records, data now also includes unstructured data, or data with no set structuring.

Big data necessitates enormous amounts of storage. Network-attached storage (NAS) clusters will often serve as the foundation of a big data storage and analysis infrastructure. Clustered NAS infrastructure necessitates the setup of many NAS "pods," each of which is made up of a number of storage devices connected to a NAS device. In order to enable extensive data sharing and querying, the sequence of NAS devices is then connected [3].

Cloud computing has completely changed how computing infrastructure is used and is one of the most successful service-oriented computing paradigms. Infrastructure as a Service (IaaS), Platform as a Service (PaaS), and Software as a Service (SaaS) are the top three cloud models. Features of cloud computing include flexibility, pay to use each time, low investment, quick time to market, and risk transfer. Cloud infrastructure facilitates management of a large volume of databases by updating important workload applications and maintaining support systems. This has been the vision of the research community. Designing scalable systems for these workloads has received a lot of research attention. Distributed databases for workloads that require frequent updates and analytical task-based database systems are examples of early architectures. Parallel databases went from prototype systems to big commercial systems.

The creation of new systems like key-value stores stemmed from shifts in application data access patterns and the need to expand to numerous commodity machines for scalability. The MapReduce model [4] and its open-source implementation Hadoop [5] have also been widely used in both

DOI: 10.1201/9781003451846-11

industry and academics in the field of data analysis. Traditional data warehouses find it difficult to handle and analyse data because of the Vs of big data, as shown in Figure 11.1. Big data is characterised as data that is processed more quickly than by traditional database systems. It suggests that the data count is excessive, the data values change too quickly, or the data does not abide by the conventions of traditional database management systems (such as consistency). In order to execute analytics, one needs new skills in the fields of data management and systems management. This deals with analysing and designing large volume of data. This requires more CPU and memory resources, which are provided by distributed processors and storage in cloud environments [6].

When considering the usage of big data analytical approaches, small- to medium-sized organisations should consider data storage via cloud computing. On-demand network access to computing resources is known as cloud computing.

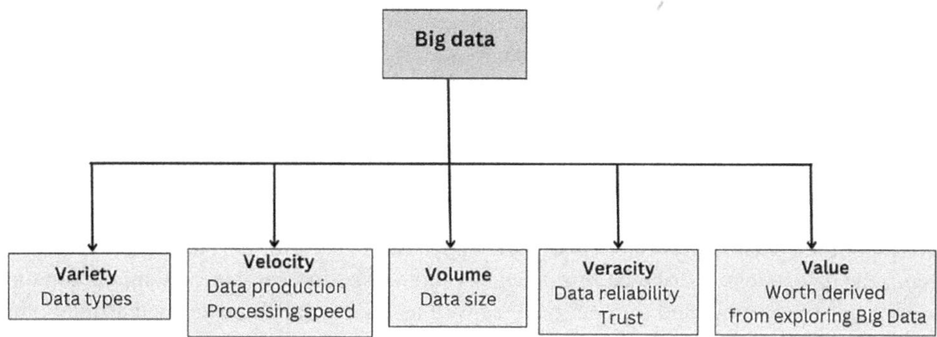

FIGURE 11.1 Some Vs of big data.

11.2 BIG DATA: CONCEPT AND DEFINITION

Big data is a term used to describe how conventional data architectures cannot effectively handle the new data sets. Data set-at-rest characteristics like volume and variety of data from various domains or types, as well as data-in-motion characteristics like velocity, or rate of flow, and variety (most often referring to a change in velocity), force a new architectural design to achieve efficiencies [7]. To achieve the requisite efficiency, each of these elements leads to a unique design or sequencing of the data lifecycle process. This is represented by Figure 11.1.

The size of the data (latest big data), whether in motion or at rest, makes data management a key factor in the design of the architecture. The big data paradigm makes a shift in the data system topologies from vertically (faster discs or processors) to horizontally scaled systems. Since the advent of massively parallel processing (MPP) computers for scientific simulations over two decades ago, the simulation industry has undergone a transformation. Computational scientists were able to significantly expand their modelling capabilities by varying the ways in which code and data were distributed between independent processors. As a result, there were a number of problems that inevitably arose, including message forwarding and data migration.

Large volumes of data are stored and retrieved with the intention of performing analysis that leads to the discovery of new data. In the past, analysis was frequently performed on a sample of data that was selected at random.

11.2.1 Big Data Engineering

Big data engineering describes the data manipulation and storage methods that make use of a set of horizontally coupled resources to achieve performance that is almost linear. New engineering techniques have been developed at the data layer as a result of the growing popularity of data types that cannot be efficiently handled in a conventional design. The creation of software based on name/key-value pairs, big tables, document-based data, and graph paradigms was prompted by the requirements for scalable access to data.

11.2.2 Non-Relational Model

Non-relational models are logical data models that are used to store and access non-tabular data sets more efficiently. Examples of these models include document, graph, key value, and others.

11.2.3 NoSQL

NoSQL refers to a type of database management system that is not based on the traditional relational database model. Instead, it provides a flexible and scalable way of storing and retrieving data that is not restricted by the constraints of relational databases. The term "NoSQL" is sometimes interpreted as "not only SQL," as these systems often incorporate other data models, such as key-value or document-oriented models, in addition to traditional SQL-based models.

11.2.4 Big Data Models

The concept of big data models refers to different approaches used for the storing and manipulation of large-scale data across distributed resources. It encompasses processing or computation models, including batch, streaming, and transactional, as well as logical data models such as relational and non-relational models. These models leverage widely scaled resources to be efficient in handling the big data difficulties of enormous volume, high velocity, and high diversity.

11.2.5 Schema-on-Read

The schema required for organising (and frequently cleaning) the data is discovered and modified as the data are queried in schema-on-read big data, which is often stored in a raw form dependent on its generation. This is significant because the data needs to be organised to allow the many algorithms or processing frameworks used for many analytics to run effectively.

11.2.6 Big Data Analytics

Both the functionality and underlying programming model of big data analytics are evolving quickly. Such analytical functions facilitate the integration of findings from parallel analyses of dispersed data from one or more data sources.

11.2.7 Big Data Paradigm

The big data model involves distributing data systems across horizontally coupled independent resources to achieve the scalability needed for effective handling of enormous information collections.

Using the new big data paradigm, analytical operations can be performed throughout the full data set or even in real time across a continuous stream of data. Analysis may even combine several data sources from various organisations. Consider the following case: "The relationship exists between insect-borne diseases, temperature, precipitation, and changes in foliage". Aerial photography, weather information, and statistics on illness incidence would all need to be included in the research in order to provide a definitive response.

Until a new paradigm shift occurs, the current trend of leveraging multiple horizontally coupled resources for data processing and storage is likely to continue. This approach represents a one-time shift, analogous to the transition that occurred in the simulation community. However, we can expect ongoing evolution in the techniques used to achieve scalability across distributed resources in a cost-effective manner.

These technology innovations have other effects on the big data paradigm. Along with logical data storage, direct queries against this storage as well as the parallel distribution of data and code in the physical file system have undergone changes.

The conventional data lifecycle alters as a result of the mental shift. The four categories of the end-to-end data lifecycle steps are collection, preparation, analysis, and implementation. The features of the data sets that are at rest or in motion as well as the length of the end-to-end data lifecycle can be used to categorise various big data use cases. Data lifecycle procedures are affected by data set features in a variety of ways, such as the point in the lifetime when the data is placed in persistent storage. The data is stored after preparation in a conventional relational model. Persistent storage is only supplied to the data in a high velocity use case after it has been prepared and examined for alerting. Before applying the preparation processes to organise the data, the existing data in a volume is frequently stored in the raw state in which it was produced. Due to the permanence of data in its unprocessed state, data models or schemas are only applied when the data is retrieved, a practise known as schema on read.

The third effect of big data engineering, which involves the decentralisation of processing resources and the execution of processing tasks on the data nodes themselves, reduces the need to transfer large amounts of data across the network. As a result, the analysis programme is split up across the data storage resources, and only the findings are gathered on a different resource, as the data is too big to query and move to another resource for analysis. To optimise data transfer and avoid issues with I/O bandwidth, an alternative approach is to embed query and filtering software directly within the storage media itself. This would allow for more efficient processing of data directly where it is stored, minimising the need for large-scale data transfer across multiple resources.

Fundamentally, big data is about extending data stores and processing over large scaled resources, much like the computer-intensive simulation community did when it adopted huge parallel computing. Historically, a wide range of communication and synchronisation constructs were used by classical parallel computing applications to generate a number of communications mechanisms. On the other hand, contemporary distributed processing frameworks that allow map-reduce patterns offer a trustworthy, high-level, commercially viable computing model based on cost-effective computing resources, dynamic resource scheduling, and synchronisation algorithms. This is because data sets are now growing to petabyte and exabyte scales [7].

Big data refers to datasets with properties like large volume, rapid growth, high diversity, significant variation, and significant veracity that can't be processed efficiently using conventional technologies and approaches to extract insights and value in a particular problem domain at a given moment.

Although the term "big data" covers a wide range of applications, it varies from standard transactional processing and business intelligence in that it refers to datasets that have properties that cannot be processed effectively using present technology and approaches. In order to produce consistent and distinctive value, big data processing is the primary goal. Regardless of the volume of data, powerful analytics are used to the full corpus to achieve this. The value debate for big data use cases is better framed by parsing the objective data.

1. Ability to operate and process data at any scale: using the complete body of relevant data rather than just a few samples or subsets. Furthermore, it seeks to integrate past, present, and future decision-support time horizons by utilising statistically produced insights into large data sets that span all of those dimensions.
2. Ensuring data trustworthiness: Obtaining reliable insights either through the consolidation and cleaning of deep data into a single version of the truth or by statistical models that sift through huge piles of unorganised data to uncover the right insights.
3. Advanced analytics: More rapid findings from data patterns employing a variety of analytical and mining approaches, such as "long tail" studies, micro-segmentations, and others

that are unworkable if you are restricted to less data, slower speeds, narrower alternatives, and inaccurate veracities.

Big data primarily relies on the self-referential notion that data is massive because it needs scalable systems to handle it and that the requirements to handle big data have resulted in the creation of solutions with greater scalability [7].

11.3 USING THE CLOUD FOR DATA MANAGEMENT

In a data management system, data can be ingested, extracted, transformed, loaded, processed, archived, and destroyed. When moving one or more phases of the data lifecycle to the cloud, it is important to take the following things into account:

1. Security: It's crucial to check that the right security protocols are in place to safeguard sensitive and private data when migrating data management to the cloud. This includes implementing authentication and access controls, encrypting data at rest and in transit, and adhering to industry-specific compliance requirements such as HIPAA or the General Data Protection Regulation (GDPR).
2. Availability of Reliable Cloud Services: It is essential to confirm that the cloud services can deliver the required level of data service reliability before migrating data management to the cloud. One way to achieve this is by replicating application components across multiple cloud instances, ensuring that if any one instance fails, another instance can take over without causing downtime. Furthermore, cloud service providers could establish service-level contracts that ensure uptime and other performance indicators.
3. Cloud Service Availability: Specific levels of availability assurances are provided by cloud service providers. While data warehousing uses lengthy searches to produce reports, transactional data processing demands instantaneous results. While one may be comfortable placing analytical infrastructure in the cloud, they may be hesitant to place their transactional data there. It is important to consider the availability guarantees offered by the cloud provider before moving any stage of the data lifecycle to the cloud.
4. Maintainability: The maintenance aspect of data management requires a high level of expertise, which involves decisions on how to organise data, maintain indices and views, and so on. This should be considered when shifting data management to the cloud.

Thanks to the cloud, organisations now have the opportunity to completely transform the way data is created, processed, and shared. This approach has been shown to be superior at upholding the performance and expansion needs of analytical applications, and when combined with cloud computing, it provides significant advantages.

11.4 MANAGING BIG DATA IN ENVIRONMENTS OF CLOUD COMPUTING

Cloud computing is a setting where people use and offer services. Service-oriented systems can be grouped into a number of different areas. One of the most common criteria used to categorise these systems is the abstraction level offered to the system user. As seen in Figure 11.2, these are the three tiers of service [8].

The benefits of cloud computing include scalability in terms of resource usage, reduced administrative effort, flexibility in cost structure, and portability for software users.

Figure 11.3 shows an example of a typical big data analytics framework. A management organisation architecture based on a four-layer structure with the following components [9] may be found to be the most appropriate management organisation architecture when focusing on the structure of the data management industry.

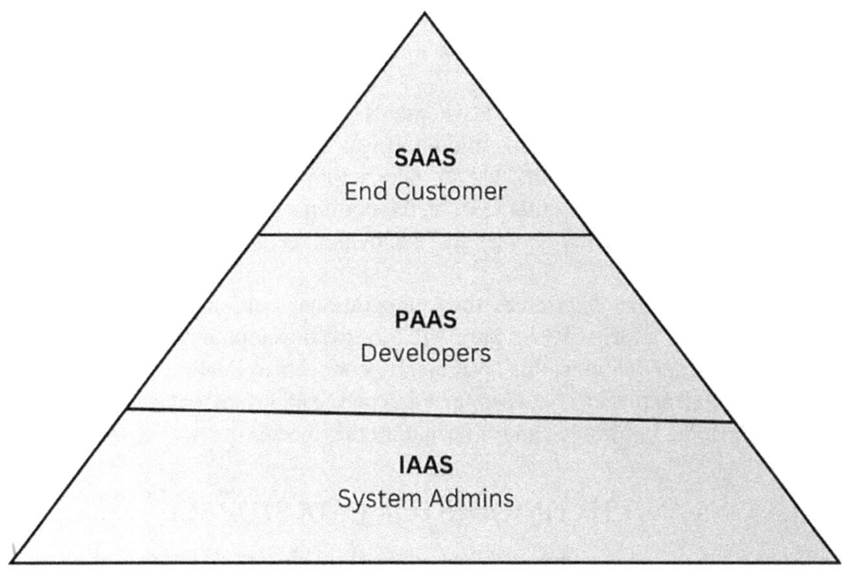

FIGURE 11.2 Illustration of the layers for service-oriented computing.

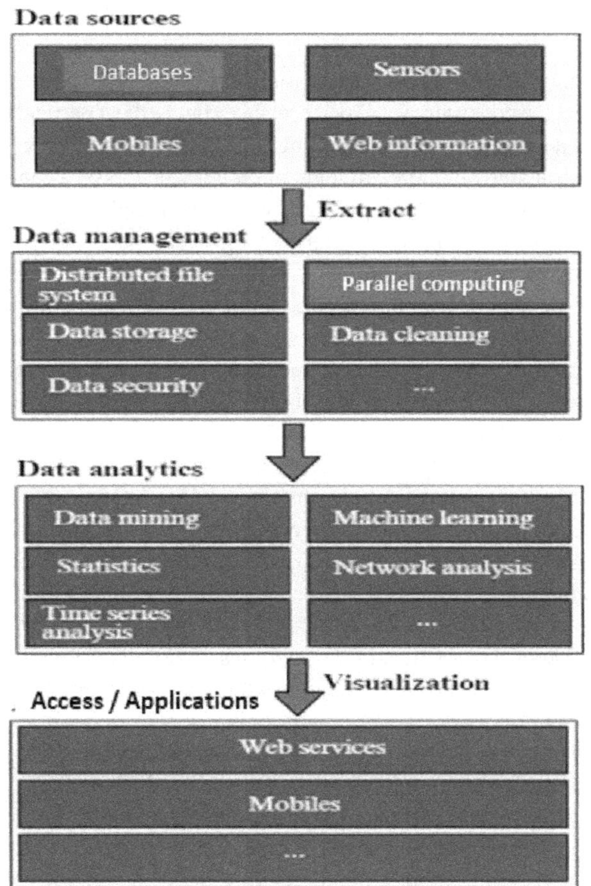

FIGURE 11.3 Big data framework [8].

1. A file system for the preservation of big data or a huge number of records. The implementation of this layer falls under the IaaS level since it provides the organisational structure for the consecutive tiers.
2. DBMS for organising data; since it has elements of both the IaaS and PaaS models, it can be seen as falling somewhere in the middle. It was used by developers to access data, but hardware dictates how it is put into use. A PaaS actually serves as an interface, containing the implementation for a particular IaaS on the bottom side and providing its functionality on the top. This functionality enables the deployment of applications across several IaaS without rewriting them.
3. An application tool that distributes the computational burden among cloud computers. Because it serves as a form of "software API" for the development of business intelligence (BI) and big data applications, this layer clearly connects to PaaS.
4. A search mechanism that sits between the PaaS and SaaS layers and is used by the system's users to retrieve the knowledge and information they need.

11.5 SOLUTIONS AND TECHNIQUES FOR DATA STORAGE

To store and access the massive volumes of data required by big data, a number of methods were put forth, some of which are already implemented in clouds. The resilience, scalability, and dependability that some Internet applications require are attempted by Internet-scale file systems. To increase redundancy, scalability, and data availability, some technologies offer object-store features where files can be reproduced over various geo-graphical sites. Examples include Windows Azure Binary Large Object (Blob) storage, OpenStack Swift, Nirvanix Cloud Storage, and Amazon Simple Storage Service (S3). Although these solutions give many cloud applications the scalability and redundancy they need, they occasionally fail to meet the consistency and performance standards of particular analytics applications.

Data localisation is a crucial factor in achieving high performance for big data analytics applications. This is because transferring large amounts of data for processing can be prohibitively expensive. In traditional high-performance computing systems, data could be transferred to the computing units because the ratio of time required to transfer is low compared to time need to process. This approach would, however, produce an unfavourable high ratio of data transfer time to processing time in the setting of big data. Thus, a new approach that brings the computing closer to the data source is preferred. This approach involves deploying computational resources closer to the data source to minimise data movement, reduce latency, and increase performance. By doing so, the computational resources can process the data more efficiently without incurring the high cost of transferring large amounts of data.

MapReduce is a useful tool in the field of big data analytics for enhancing the functionality of applications by localising data. The Hadoop Distributed File System (HDFS) is a distributed file system that makes it simpler for mappers to access and process the data in a distributed fashion by storing and managing massive datasets by partitioning and duplicating them across several nodes. Hadoop is an open-source version of MapReduce and it is possible to replicate data to a configurable number of nodes using HDFS, which reduces the effects of failures by taking advantage of the concurrency of many nodes. In practice, many analytics tasks are performed on Hive-Hadoop clusters, where the platform uses replication, compression, and columnar Hive7 compression to store massive volumes of data.

While relational databases have been widely used to store structured data, they are not the most suitable option for storing unstructured data. A traditional DBMS requires data to be transferred to data warehouses for analysis and retrieval, which can be infrequent. For relational data analysis, models like MapReduce are generally not the optimal choice.

The architecture for parallel database analytics described in reference [10] allows combining various data sources using MapReduce and MYSQL on top of a DBMS. Analytics and data mining solution providers are experimenting with models like MapReduce by shifting some of the processing processes closer to the area where the data is stored in order to lower the expenses related to data preparation, storage, and processing. In order to enable reuse across different datasets, data processing and analytics capabilities are being implemented in data hubs or are progressing towards enterprise data warehouses.

NoSQL databases have gained popularity due to their ability to handle unorganised data and their compatibility with remote systems. The use of non-relational models to store data is a key feature of NoSQL databases, which includes object-oriented, hierarchical, and graph databases that have been available for over 50 years. Newer models have recently grown in acceptance, including key-value stores, column-oriented stores, and document-based stores. According to Leavitt [11], the growing interest in NoSQL databases is driven by various factors, including better performance and the ability to handle unstructured data.

The summary of NoSQL databases in reference [12] focuses on the advantages and disadvantages of these databases when used with cloud computing. The survey categorises NoSQL systems into clusters according to their capabilities in managing different combinations of the CAP (consistency, availability, partitioning) principles. It also delves into the data models that these surveyed NoSQL systems support.

11.6 BIG DATA FRAMEWORKS

The current big data technology landscape provides a broad array of options, ranging from popular ones like Hadoop, Spark, Hive, and Strom to emerging ones like Flink and Heron and practical ones like Presto and MapReduce. Extensive research has identified these popular technologies and functionality in processing and analysing large-scale data. While other frameworks such as Samza and Kudu are less recognised, they can also be valuable in certain contexts. These top big data frameworks were identified through comprehensive research that assessed their popularity and functionality.

11.6.1 Hadoop

The Apache Hadoop project is an open-source tool from the Apache Software Foundation that has transformed the way large datasets are processed and stored. Many big data software tools either utilise Hadoop or follow its standards. Hadoop is designed for distributed, scalable computations and functions as a general-purpose file storage system. Its three essential components are the Hadoop Distributed File System, which stores data in the Hadoop cluster; the MapReduce system, which is designed for processing massive amounts of data in a cluster; and the YARN (Yet Another Resource Negotiator) resource management core.

To overcome the memory limitations of modern DBMS, Hadoop employs an intermediate layer between a query engine and data storage. Its performance improves as the amount of data stored increases, and it can be further expanded by adding more nodes to the data store. Hadoop has the capability to store and handle several petabytes of data, and its quickest operations only take a few seconds to complete. It prohibits making changes to data that has already been processed and saved in the HDFS system.

Hadoop is particularly useful for business initiatives, data lakes, and customer analytics. It is suitable for significant batch processing operations that do not require immediate access to data or atomicity, consistency, isolation, and durability (ACID)-compliant storage.

Although Hadoop is popular, new objectives and demands are emerging due to technological advances. As more innovative alternatives enter the market, they are likely to gradually replace it.

11.6.2 MapReduce

MapReduce is a programming model used in Hadoop for processing and analysing large datasets. It was initially developed by Google and later adopted by Hadoop. The model divides the input data into multiple chunks and processes them in parallel across many nodes in a Hadoop cluster. The results of the processing are then combined to generate the final output. This approach enables scalable processing of large volumes of data.

The three stages of processing data in the MapReduce engine are as follows:

1. Map: This stage involves pre-processing and data filtration. The input data is divided into smaller chunks and processed in parallel across multiple nodes in the cluster. The map function is applied to each chunk of data, transforming it into intermediate key-value pairs.
2. Shuffle: In this stage, the intermediate key-value pairs produced by the map function are sorted and grouped based on their keys. Each unique key is sent to a specific reducer node, which will process all the intermediate values associated with that key.
3. Reduce: The reduce function is applied to each group of intermediate values with the same key. The output of the reduce function is typically a smaller set of key-value pairs that represent the final result of the MapReduce job. The reduce function is controlled by the user and determines the outcome for various output data categories.

Reduce is the final step in the MapReduce operation, and it returns the majority of all values. Data may be automatically parallelised with MapReduce, and it offers effective balancing and fail-safe performance.

It has been a standard in the sector and is employed alongside other well-known big data technologies. The Apache Tez alternative to MapReduce is one of these solutions. It is a lot quicker and highly customisable. It manages resources considerably more effectively.

11.6.3 Spark

Apache Spark is a very powerful big data framework that was developed as an open-source alternative to Apache Hadoop. Although it was initially designed as a more sophisticated alternative, it has since become one of the most widely used big data frameworks. A key difference between these two solutions is the data processing model used.

Each stage of the MapReduce algorithm is recorded by Hadoop in a data file that is stored on the hard disc. In contrast, Spark uses random-access memory to implement all operations. As a result, Spark performs quickly and enables processing of large amounts of data. High performance and fail-safety are the key components and functional pillars of Spark.

The Apache Spark framework supports multiple programming languages such as Scala, Java, Python, and R, among others. It consists of a core and four libraries that enhance big data processing capabilities. One of the specific framework libraries that support structured data processing is Spark SQL. Using Data Frames, Hadoop Hive requests can be answered up to 100 times faster.

Sparkling Water 2.3.0 is a product of Spark and is known for its excellent AI capabilities. Additionally, Spark Streaming is another tool that supports real-time processing of data streams. However, it should be noted that in practice, Spark Streaming operates more like a micro-batch processor than a true stream processor, as demonstrated by benchmarks.

Instead of functioning as a true stream processor like Flink, Heron, or Samza, Spark behaves more like a micro-batch processor. Spark is often referred to as a real-time alternative to Hadoop. It can be used in conjunction with Hadoop and other well-known big data Frameworks, but like all parts of the Hadoop ecosystem, it may also be utilised independently of them.

11.6.4 Hive

Hive is a big data analytics tool that was developed by Facebook to leverage the scalability of one of the most popular big data frameworks. It is an engine that converts a series of SQL queries into MapReduce tasks.

The engine is composed of the following components:

1. Parser (organises incoming SQL requests),
2. Optimizer (increases efficiency of the requests), and
3. Executor (starts MapReduce framework activities).

For the study of massive data volumes, Hadoop can be connected with Hive (as a server component). Hortonworks released Hive 3. Tez replaced MapReduce as the default search engine. It integrates with other well-known big data frameworks and features machine learning capabilities.

11.6.5 Storm

Apache Storm is Twitter's first big data framework; it focuses on handling a significant real-time data flow. Scalability and swift downtime recovery are two of Storm's primary characteristics. Along with Python, Ruby, and Fancy, Java can be used to work with this solution.

Storm stands out from its counterparts in several ways, one of which is the Tuple, a crucial data representation component that facilitates serialisation. Another distinctive feature is the Stream, which also adopts the Tuple's field naming approach. Spout is responsible for ingesting data from external sources, transforming it into a Tuple, and feeding it to the Stream for processing.

Topology, a collection of elements with information on how they interact, and Bolt, a data processor, are present. When all of these components are used together, they can help developers control massive flows of unstructured data.

The performances of both Flink and Spark have a higher latency than Storm. Its throughput is worse. Twitter, the main supporter of Storm, switched to a new framework called Heron. The Storm project, which is an open-source real-time computation system, is still widely used by many companies, including Yelp, Yahoo!, and Alibaba. Despite the emergence of newer alternatives such as Apache Flink and Apache Samza, Storm remains a popular choice for real-time data processing and analysis.

11.6.6 Flink

Apache Flink is a popular open-source framework for big data processing that supports both batch and stream processing. It was originally developed as a research project and has gained popularity due to its powerful features and high performance.

Flink offers many advanced features, including stateful stream processing, batch processing, and extract, transform, and load (ETL) capabilities. It is well-suited for a Lambda architecture and can be used to combine batch and stream processing. Flink is also able to extract timestamps from streamed data, enabling more accurate time-based analysis. Another advantage is its built-in support for machine learning, making it a powerful tool for advanced data analysis. As a component of the Hadoop ecosystem, it can be easily integrated into existing architectures and has a history of integration with MapReduce and Storm. Its scalability is also good for big data applications.

Flink is ideal for event-driven application design and supports checkpoints to maintain progress in the event of processing failure. In addition, it is compatible with Zeppelin, a popular data visualisation tool.

Alibaba has successfully leveraged Flink's advanced features, including its machine learning capabilities, to monitor consumer behaviour and search engine rankings during Singles' Day. This has resulted in a significant boost in sales, with an increase of 30%.

11.6.7 Heron

Apache Heron is a modern big data processing engine developed by Twitter to replace its older software, Storm. Designed for trend analysis, ETL jobs, and real-time spam detection, Heron represents the next generation of data processing engines.

The transition to Apache Heron from Storm is simple and entirely backward compatible. Low latency, good and predictable scalability, and simple management are among its design objectives. Process isolation is highly valued by developers for simple debugging and consistent resource consumption. Twitter benchmarks reveal a considerable upgrade over Storm.

This framework is currently under development, so if you're looking for a piece of tech to implement quickly, this might be it. Heron is probably going to become the next big thing shortly because it works so well with Storm and has Twitter's strong support. And some, like Stanford University and Microsoft, have already caught up.

11.6.8 NoSQL Databases

NoSQL databases are different from traditional relational databases in that they do not require data to follow a predetermined schema or structure. This makes them better suited to handling vast amounts of semi-structured and unstructured data, as they can accommodate various data models. NoSQL databases are more adaptable than relational databases and have been shown to be faster and more scalable. Some well-known examples of NoSQL databases include MongoDB, Apache CouchDB, and Azure Cosmos DB.

Business intelligence and big data analysis applications can collect data in structured, unstructured, or hybrid forms. Traditional database systems were not sufficient to handle the diversity of data, but the emergence of NoSQL databases such as MongoDB has provided a solution. NoSQL databases offer flexible schemas that can accommodate unstructured and semi-structured data, while their scale-out architecture enables load distribution by adding new nodes.

To make sense of large amounts of data, data visualisation tools such as charts, graphs, and infographics are often used. Initially, business intelligence tools were designed to work with tabular data sourced from relational databases. However, the rise of non-relational databases has spurred the development of new data visualisation tools. These tools can access data from both relational and non-relational sources. MongoDB, which is currently the most popular NoSQL database according to DB-Engines, is frequently used in these tools.

11.6.8.1 MongoDB Charts

MongoDB Charts is a cloud-based tool that enables users to visualise data from MongoDB. The tool was designed to take advantage of the document-based architecture of MongoDB and is capable of handling complex data structures such as embedded objects and arrays, making it possible to create comprehensive data visualisations.

The charts are arranged using dashboards. In order to securely collaborate with others, dashboards can be shared with various permissions. Individual charts can also be embedded using an iframe or SDK.

MongoDB Charts is integrated with MongoDB Atlas, a database-as-a-service offering, as well as MongoDB Atlas Data Lake. With these integrations, real-time analytics can be performed without the need for data copying or migration.

11.6.8.2 MongoDB Compass

MongoDB Compass is a graphical user interface that enables users to explore the structure of their MongoDB database and run ad-hoc queries.

Compass employs a variety of field visualisation techniques. A field can be represented using one of the following depending on the type of data it contains and the level of cardinality:

1. a histogram
2. graded bars
3. a world map
4. sample data

11.6.8.3 Studio 3T

Studio 3T is a graphical user interface application for MongoDB that allows users to view and manage data collections. One of the features of Studio 3T is the Schema Explorer, which provides a visual representation of data distribution and can help identify missing fields, duplicate records, and other data irregularities. This feature can be useful for data analysis and quality control purposes, enabling users to more easily identify and resolve issues with their data.

11.6.8.4 Business Intelligence Tools

Business intelligence tools are software applications that collect, analyse, and transform large datasets from multiple sources. The purpose of these tools is to generate artifacts that can be used to derive business insights. By analysing data from various sources, business intelligence tools can provide a more comprehensive view of an organisation's operations, enabling better decision-making.

11.6.8.5 Knowi

Knowi is a business intelligence platform that offers native integrations with several NoSQL databases, including MongoDB, MongoDB Atlas, Apache Cassandra, and Couchbase. It also supports unstructured data and cloud APIs, enabling integration with various data sources without requiring data relocation or alteration.

Knowi provides three separate real-time data analysis products, Knowi HUB, Knowi ELEVATE, and Knowi EMBED. Knowi HUB is a tool for combining and visualising data. With Knowi ELEVATE, questions can be asked and prompt responses can be received via Slack and Microsoft Teams. Using an iframe or a JavaScript API, Knowi EMBED enables integration of dashboards and charts into applications.

11.6.8.6 Pentaho Data Integration

Pentaho Data Integration (PDI) is a data integration platform that provides access to, transforms, analyses, and generates value from both traditional and big data sources. A no-code graphical user interface can be used to create transformations, which are data pipelines. Using the Adaption Execution Layer (AEL), data can be imported from some NoSQL databases, including MongoDB. The Pentaho transformations are converted by AEL into operators specific to the source engine, such as MongoDB query operators.

11.6.8.7 Tableau

Tableau is popular data visualisation and business intelligence software that allows users to connect, visualise, and share data in an interactive and meaningful way. Interactive dashboards can be built with the Tableau Desktop application's straightforward drag-and-drop interface. Tableau provides a diverse set of capabilities, such as the ability to conduct advanced statistical analysis, build interactive maps, and connect with popular data analysis languages like R or Python.

Tableau is built on SQL. The MongoDB Connector for BI, on the other hand, allows linking MongoDB data in Tableau.

11.6.8.8 SAP Lumira

SAP Lumira is a data visualisation and analytics tool that can be used by business users. The software has a drag-and-drop interface that enables users to collect data from various sources and create visualisations such as charts, crosstabs, and geo maps. SAP Lumira also provides default UI elements to facilitate the visualisation process. Additionally, users can create infographics by combining text, images, and other graphical components. SAP Lumira has the ability to connect to SAP enterprise data models and external data sources such as MongoDB via a Java Database Connectivity (JDBC) driver, allowing for queries to be performed on the data.

SAP Lumira is data visualisation software that allows users to connect to various data sources, including SAP enterprise data models and external sources like MongoDB. To connect to these databases, SAP Lumira utilises a Java Database Connectivity driver. By establishing a connection with these databases through JDBC, the software can perform queries on the data and visualise the results in various formats.

Applications for data visualisation are essential resources for acquiring business intelligence in contemporary organisations. The top data analysis tools today support MongoDB and other NoSQL data sources, despite having historically been designed to work with the relational database model.

11.6.9 Challenges in the Visualisation of NoSQL Databases

Traditional BI solutions like Tableau were built to work with tabular data from relational databases, which use SQL as their query language. NoSQL databases, on the other hand, have a different architecture and do not rely on SQL. As a result, integrating NoSQL databases as a data source can be more challenging compared to traditional relational databases. However, modern BI tools have evolved to support a wide range of data sources, including NoSQL databases like MongoDB, making it easier to incorporate them into data analytics and reporting workflows. Contemporary business intelligence tools have advanced to encompass a diverse array of data origins, like MongoDB and other NoSQL databases, in order to deliver a broader adaptable solution for data analytics.

The earliest strategy used by data analysis tools involves converting NoSQL data to a relational representation before visualising it. The analysis process is slowed down as a result of having to move the data between sources or alter it. The MongoDB Business Intelligence Connector offers a different approach.

The Connector is responsible for translating the SQL commands generated by the data analysis software into MongoDB commands, which are then executed against the database. This allows for seamless integration of NoSQL databases, such as MongoDB, with BI solutions originally designed for SQL databases. For visualisation, the results are supplied back to the data analysis tool in tabular format. The MongoDB BI Connector, for instance, enables the integration of many tools with MongoDB. Similar methods are used by other data analysis tools, however they each have their unique connectors. These tools include SAP Lumira and Pentaho Data Integration.

The best course of action might be to never modify or translate requests. We also looked at Knowi, Studio 3T, MongoDB Charts, and MongoDB Compass, which are all native NoSQL database visualisation tools.

11.7 ADVANTAGES OF BIG DATA APPLICATIONS

Big data applications are designed to handle large-scale distributed systems that typically involve massive amounts of data. The need for these applications arises from the challenges of traditional data processing methods when dealing with complex and voluminous data. Google's MapReduce framework and Apache Hadoop are the leading software systems used for big data applications, as they can handle large amounts of intermediate data. Two primary fields where big data applications are used are manufacturing and bioinformatics.

The use of big data can bring transparency to the manufacturing industry by helping to identify and analyse relationships among variables such as component performance and availability. The process typically begins with data collection, which can include various types of sensory data such as pressure, vibration, acoustics, voltage, current, and controller data. This data is then processed and analysed using big data tools and techniques to extract insights and patterns that can help improve processes, reduce waste, and optimise performance. This is the foundation of the conceptual framework of predictive manufacturing. The manufacturing industry's big data is built using a combination of historical data and sensory data. This combination produces big data, which is used as an input by prognostic and health management systems [13, 14].

The field of bioinformatics, which includes next-generation sequencing and other biological domains, is another significant application for Hadoop. Hadoop is used in bioinformatics, which calls for extensive data analysis. Along with computer clusters and online interfaces, cloud computing introduces the parallel distributed computing framework [15].

Software packages for big data offer a wide range of tools and possibilities, including the ability to map the entirety of a company's data landscape. This can allow organisations to assess internal risks and identify any potentially sensitive information that is not being properly protected, ensuring that it is stored in accordance with regulatory standards. Protecting data is one of the key benefits of big data, and big data solutions can provide advanced security measures to safeguard against cyber threats and data breaches. Additionally, big data can enable organisations to identify and respond to security threats more quickly by analysing large amounts of data in real time.

Big data is characterised by the following features:

1. Big data integrates both structured and unstructured data sources.
2. Big data solutions address scalability and speed, mobility and security, flexibility and stability.
3. The time taken to obtain insights from multiple data sources, including mobile devices, RFID, the web, and a growing range of automated sensing technologies, is crucial in big data.

While cloud storage offers benefits such as speed, capacity, and scalability, it is not specific to big data. Additionally, the abilities to visualise data and discover new business opportunities are not unique to cloud storage or big data. However, data analytics does allow for real-time customisation of website content or design based on the needs of individual visitors, which is a benefit of big data. Predictive analytics in combination with big data creates a difficulty for many industries. Exploration of these four domains emerges from the combination:

1. Identify potential risks that come with significant investments.
2. Detect, prevent, and investigate cases of financial fraud.
3. Improve collection of late payments.
4. Deploy effective marketing strategies to enhance business value.

11.8 FACTORS OF BIG DATA FRAMEWORKS

Many companies, research teams, and IT sectors are experiencing the impact of various transformational and disruptive big data solutions and technologies that are emerging to support innovation and data-driven operational decisions. Cloud computing services for big data now offer infrastructures, technologies, and analytics that speed up and reduce the cost of analysing large data sets.

Although there are numerous possibilities, the key is choosing the framework that is most appropriate for a certain organisation. This decision usually comes down to the application needs and balancing the benefits and drawbacks of each situation. A lot of these are dependent on the usage scenarios for the applications, and they probably include some trade-offs. There are a few important things that need to be defined before a big data app is deployed on the cloud. The advantages and disadvantages of choosing each major management framework type will now be covered.

11.8.1 Processing Speed

Processing speed, which is dependent on the speed of data transmission reads and writes (I/O) to memory or disc, is a crucial performance assessment tool for assessing the effectiveness of various resource management mechanisms. Additionally, it calculates the speed at which data is transferred during a specific time period between two communication components. Naturally, certain resource management frameworks will function better than others. It has been discovered via study, nevertheless, that although some frameworks performed better for simpler tasks, others handled larger data source sets far more quickly. However, when the dataset input increased, all frameworks noticed a decrease in their "speed-up" ratio.

11.8.2 Fault Tolerance

Fault tolerance is the process of evaluating how well the system as a whole continues to operate when a single component fails. When a certain activity is carried out in a high-performance computing system, hundreds of intricately coupled nodes are examined. Failure in one should have little to no impact on the calculation as a whole. Certain frameworks perform better than others when there is a lot of data transmission going on. Some frameworks are substantially more fault tolerant than others. The performance of various frameworks has been studied using the PageRank method, and it has been discovered that performance measures well for smaller data sets, but the "speed-up" decreases as data sets get larger. Certain systems may just be unable to handle dealing with some datasets without crashing as they grow in size.

11.8.3 Scalability

Timely processing of data is essential in order to address high-value business issues. Multiple computations on a large scale can be performed simultaneously, which can reduce the time taken, effort put in, and complexity of the computations. Scalability refers to the storage and changes in workload by allocating extra resources at runtime. Increasing or reducing them can help achieve scalability. Many different criteria are integrated to form a single algorithm through scalability.

11.8.4 Security

The majority of big data applications are abandoning internal data storage in favour of a cloud environment, which enables several users to quickly access and record the same information that requires privacy. Although data security and integrity have always been top priorities, big data platforms' extensive use of cloud computing services has made this issue much more important. Because the data is accessible to several users, each of whom is looking for the information for different purposes, there is a correspondingly greater danger to the data's security and privacy.

Big data frameworks and tools offer different levels of security measures that can be categorised into authentication and authorisation. These categories have varying access requirements and use different levels of encryption for security. Some frameworks provide password-controlled access and encryption measures, while others have encryption integrated into their access scheme. However, there are also frameworks that do not include any built-in system security measures.

11.9 ADVANTAGES OF BIG DATA AND CLOUD COMPUTING FRAMEWORKS

The integration of cloud computing into large-scale projects offers several benefits. Big data requires several servers due to the vast amount of data it uses, its scale, and the high velocity and variety it demands. Multiple servers must operate simultaneously to meet the high demand of big data. Cloud computing is an ideal solution for storing and analysing big data due to the availability of multiple servers and resource allocation. Using cloud environments can result in improved efficiency and performance for big data analysis. Cloud systems utilise remote multi-servers, which enable the management of large amounts of data simultaneously. This makes it possible for big data to handle vast amounts of data using advanced analytics methods. By integrating cloud computing with big data, costs can be minimised, as there is no need to build new servers and storage volumes. Instead, cloud computing systems can serve as the foundation for all the servers and volumes required for big data processing. This approach offers greater flexibility and scalability and eliminates the need for substantial investments in big data computers and servers.

The simplicity and practicality of cloud server provisioning also contribute to faster processing of big data. The cloud environment can be easily scaled up or down according to the processing requirements of the big data. This is particularly important since the value of big data diminishes over time, and quick provisioning can help to ensure that data is processed in a timely and efficient manner. Big data and cloud computing are often integrated to provide a flexible and shared computing environment that requires low overhead and administration work. This integration enables multi-tenancy, increases automation, and strengthens the environment. Moreover, it makes it easier to manage, monitor, and report on large data resources. Additionally, this connectivity streamlines processes and boosts efficiency. Therefore, cloud-based approaches are considered the best models for delivering big data due to all these benefits.

11.10 CHALLENGES AND RISKS OF BIG DATA AND CLOUD COMPUTING FRAMEWORKS

Integrating big data and cloud computing can be beneficial, but there are potential challenges and risks to consider. Security is a significant concern in the big data cloud environment, with platform heterogeneity being a well-known vulnerability. When deploying big data on a cloud system, it is essential to develop new security tools that are compatible with these platforms, such as authentication measures, access control protocols, encryption methods, intrusion detection systems, event logging tools, and event monitoring solutions. Additionally, goals for consolidating the data and relevant security standards should be considered to minimise risks and ensure data remains protected. Despite the challenges, leveraging the capabilities of the cloud is often more cost effective than building an infrastructure to handle the processing and storage requirements of big data.

Integrating big data and cloud computing poses several challenges, including managing the type and location of the data, optimising the big data cloud topology, and deciding whether to process the data in a processing environment or in situ. The data may be stored in various locations, some of which may not be available in the cloud environment. Furthermore, the manner in which data is processed, including parallel processing and location of processing, adds further complexity. To overcome these challenges, it is necessary to optimise the topology of the big data cloud by defining the ideal configuration and size of clouds, clusters, and nodes to achieve the best big data cloud model. In addition, new security tools must be developed, including authentication measures, access control protocols, encryption methods, intrusion detection systems, event logging tools, and event monitoring solutions, to ensure the security of big data in a cloud environment. It is also essential to consider the goals for consolidating the data and relevant security standards when integrating big data with cloud computing.

While integrating big data and cloud computing poses various challenges, these obstacles can be surmountable through different means. Thus, it is often more practical and cost effective to utilise the capabilities of the cloud rather than investing large amounts of money to create an infrastructure that can manage the immense storage and processing demands of big data.

11.11 REVOLUTIONISING HEALTHCARE

The integration of deep learning, facilitated by expansive datasets known as big data, has brought about transformative changes in various sectors, with healthcare being a prominent beneficiary. Deep learning algorithms, a subset of artificial intelligence (AI), have demonstrated remarkable capabilities in discerning complex patterns and making precise predictions. The efficacy of deep learning in the healthcare domain, however, relies heavily on the availability of extensive datasets, which is made feasible through big data frameworks. Furthermore, the incorporation of the Internet of Things (IoT) devices has significantly amplified the potential of deep learning in healthcare, enabling real-time data collection, analysis, and tailored patient care. This chapter examines the intricate interplay between deep learning, big data, and the IoT in revolutionising healthcare and reshaping medical practices.

11.11.1 The Role of Big Data in Empowering Deep Learning

Central to the proficiency of deep learning algorithms is their data-centric nature. Exposure to copious data enhances their ability to recognise intricate patterns and render accurate predictions. In healthcare, these algorithms exhibit promise across various applications, such as the analysis of medical images, disease diagnosis, drug discovery, and personalised treatment recommendations. However, the success of these algorithms hinges on access to a diverse and comprehensive dataset, a role fulfilled by big data.

Within the healthcare context, big data encompasses an extensive repository of patient records, medical images, genomic sequences, electronic health records (EHRs), clinical trial data, and more. The availability of such data empowers deep learning models to glean intricate patterns, contributing to refined disease detection and enhanced prediction accuracy. For instance, in medical imaging, deep learning models trained on vast datasets can discern subtle anomalies in X-rays, MRIs, and CT scans that might elude human observers. This capability has significantly elevated early detection and diagnosis rates for a range of diseases, including various forms of cancer.

11.11.2 Harnessing Cloud Computing for Data Storage and Processing

Meeting the storage and processing demands of big data often surpasses the capacities of conventional computing infrastructure. Cloud computing offers a scalable remedy through on-demand access to substantial computational resources. In healthcare, cloud platforms facilitate the secure and efficient storage of extensive volumes of medical data. Furthermore, they simplify the deployment of intricate deep learning models without necessitating substantial upfront investments in hardware.

Healthcare providers and research institutions can exploit cloud-based solutions to collaborate, exchange, and analyse patient data while upholding stringent privacy and security mandates. Cloud-based data storage also encourages interoperability, facilitating the seamless exchange of information among disparate healthcare systems and fostering a comprehensive and patient-centric approach to healthcare.

11.11.3 IoT Devices: Augmenting Healthcare Data Collection

The emergence of the Internet of Things has introduced a novel dimension to healthcare by enabling real-time collection of patient data through interconnected devices. Wearables, remote monitoring sensors, and intelligent medical equipment continuously amass data like heart rate, blood pressure, glucose levels, and physical activity metrics. This continuous data stream provides a holistic view of an individual's health status, enabling early identification of irregularities and proactive interventions.

The integration of deep learning algorithms with IoT-generated data permits real-time analysis of these dynamic data streams, supplying actionable insights to both healthcare providers and patients. As an example, an IoT-enabled wearable can monitor an individual's vital signs and transmit alerts to medical professionals upon detecting anomalies. These insights grounded in data empower healthcare providers to make informed decisions and offer customised treatment strategies.

11.11.4 Personalised Medicine and Customised Treatment Strategies

The amalgamation of deep learning, big data, and IoT in the healthcare sector has paved the way for the concept of personalised medicine. In contrast to traditional healthcare models that often employed generalised treatment methods, the rich availability of expansive datasets empowers healthcare providers to curate interventions according to individual patient needs. By delving into a patient's medical history, genetic composition, lifestyle choices, and real-time data gleaned from IoT devices, deep learning models can forecast susceptibilities to various diseases and recommend interventions tailored to the specific individual.

This approach represents a departure from the one-size-fits-all methodology that has been predominant in medical practice. Through the synthesis of diverse data streams, deep learning algorithms can uncover unique patterns and correlations that provide a comprehensive understanding of a patient's health profile. This information then forms the basis for crafting personalised treatment strategies that are more effective, efficient, and aligned with the patient's distinct requirements.

11.11.4.1 Conclusion

The advent of big data has introduced a significant challenge in managing and analysing large volumes of data that may have varying degrees of reliability, high velocity, and diverse formats. These factors present difficulties for traditional data warehouses, making it challenging to process big data. Therefore, hosting big data workloads on the cloud has emerged as a viable option due to its scalability, flexibility, and affordability. However, deploying big data on the cloud comes with its own unique challenges. It requires reconciling two different design philosophies, which can be incompatible. On one hand, big data systems such as Hadoop are built on the shared-nothing principle, where each node is independent and self-sufficient. On the other hand, cloud computing emphasises consolidation and resource sharing. Balancing these two approaches is necessary to deploy big data effectively on the cloud. Integrating big data and cloud computing may present certain challenges, but it also has immense potential for businesses and educational institutions alike. One major benefit of combining big data and cloud computing is the availability of massive storage capacity and processing power. Cloud computing provides access to a vast array of resources and infrastructure that can accommodate this integration in the most efficient and effective manner possible. While the integration of big data and cloud computing has many advantages, there are also some challenges that need to be addressed. One of the major concerns is security. When deploying big data on the cloud, the user may not have complete physical control over the data, which increases the risk of security breaches. Therefore, new security tools and standards must be developed to ensure the safe and secure storage and processing of data in the cloud. Authentication, access control, encryption, intrusion detection, event logging, and monitoring of events are some examples of security tools that can be used to protect data in the cloud. Additionally, the type and location of the data, as well as the kind of processing required, may pose difficulties when deploying big data on a cloud system. The optimisation of the cloud topology, which describes the configuration, size, and nodes that should be included in the ideal big data cloud model, is another challenge that must be addressed. Despite these challenges, the integration of big data and cloud computing provides vast potential for businesses and educational institutions by providing access to vast data storage and processing power.

However, big data security is based on an automated framework for security evaluation and analysis, which reduces security design time and increases knowledge of security parameters. Thus, it facilitates the adoption of cloud architectures, which is essential for managing big data sets. The integration of deep learning, big data, and the IoT fosters a paradigm shift from reactive healthcare to proactive and pre-emptive care. As the synergy between these technologies continues to evolve, the healthcare field is poised to witness a revolution where treatments are not just informed by general guidelines but are finely tailored to each individual, resulting in more precise, impactful, and patient-centric medical interventions.

REFERENCES

[1] Al-Maliki, D. S. Q. A., Kuppuswamy, P., John, R. K., and Sivakumar, N. R. COVID-19: An efficient big data analytics for SARS-CoV-2 mutations prediction: A machine learning approach. Indian Journal of Science and Technology. 1:20–33.

[2] Villars, R. L., Olofson, C. W., and Eastwood, M (2011). Big data: What it is and why you should care. IDC White Paper. Framingham, MA: IDC.
[3] White, C. (2011). Data communications and computer networks: A business user's approach (6th ed.). Boston, MA: Cengage Learning.
[4] Sharma, L. (Ed.). (2020). Towards smart world: Homes to cities using internet of things (1st ed.). USA: Chapman and Hall/CRC. doi:10.1201/9781003056751
[5] Apache Hadoop Project (2009). http://hadoop.apache.org/core/
[6] Gupta, R., Gupta, H., and Mohania, M. (2012) Cloud computing and Big data analytics: What is new from databases perspective?. In S. Srinivasa and V. Bhatnagar (Eds.) BDA 2012, LNCS 7678. Berlin; Heidelberg: Springer-Verlag, pp. 42–61.
[7] ISO/IEC JTC 1 (2015). Information technology Big Data, Preliminary Report 2014. ISO/IEC.
[8] Ferandez, A., Sara del, R., Opez, V., Bawakid, A., del Jesus, M. J., Benitez, J. M., and Herrera, F. (2014). Big Data with cloud computing: An insight on the computing environment, MapReduce, and programming frameworks. WIREs Data Mining Knowl Discov, 4:380–409. doi:10.1002/widm.1134
[9] Kambatla, K., Kollias, G., Kumar, V., and Grama, A. (2014). Trends in big data analytics. J Parallel Distrib, 74:2561–2573. doi:10.1016/j.jpdc.2014.01.003
[10] Cohen, J., Dolan, B., Dunlap, M., Hellerstein, J.M., Welton, C. (2009). MAD skills: New analysis practices for big data. Proc. VLDB Endow, 2(2):1481–1492. doi:10.14778/1687553.1687576
[11] Leavitt, N. (2010). Will NoSQL databases live up to their promise? Computer, 43(2):12–14. doi:10.1109/MC.2010.58
[12] Han, J., Le, G., and Du, J. (2011). Survey on NoSQL database, in: 6th International Conference on Pervasive Computing and Applications (ICPCA 2011), IEEE, Port Elizabeth, pp. 363–366.
[13] Muhtaroglu, F. C. P., Demir, S., Obali, M., and Girgin, C. (2013). Business model canvas perspective on big data applications, in: Big Data, 2013 IEEE International Conference, Silicon Valley, CA, October 6–9, pp. 32–37.
[14] Zhao, Y., and Wu, J. (2013). Dache: A data aware caching for big-data applications using the MapReduce framework, in INFOCOM, 2013 Proceedings IEEE, Turin, April 14–19, pp. 35–39. doi:10.1109/infcom.2013.6566730
[15] Li, X.-B., Jiang, W.-R., Jiang, Y., and Zou, Q. (2012). Hadoop applications in bioinformatics, in Open Cirrus Summit (OCS), 2012 Seventh, Beijing, June 19–20, pp. 48–52.

12 Improved Patient Care Using Robotics in the Healthcare Industry
Benefits, Real-Time Applications, and Challenges

Mukesh Carpenter, Lavanya Sharma, and Sudhriti Sengupta

12.1 INTRODUCTION

With technological advancements in the healthcare industry, robotics has become more and more established and also provides various benefits to both healthcare workers and patients. It enables high-end patient care, efficient medical processes, and a safe environment for both patients and medical practitioners. In the 1980s, the first medical robots which appeared provided surgical assistance via robotic arm technologies. Automation and robotics are widely used in research laboratories to automate manual, monotonous, and tedious job so that specialists can focus their attention on more strategic tasks, which can lead to faster innovations [1–9]. Medical robots result in streamlined workflows, risk reduction, and less time used to complete a particular task as compared to manual work. With the advancement of artificial intelligence and robotics technologies in the medical domain, the scope is expanding day by day by replacing human workers and delivering effective outcomes [7, 10, 11].

In today's world, robots are changing the way surgeries are performed in the medical domain by streamlining supply delivery, antisepsis, and time duration for healthcare providers to interact with patients. In operating theatres (OTs), robots are also used to assist medical practitioners and improve patient care. During the COVID-19 pandemic, robots are used in various hospitals and clinics for several tedious tasks to help in less exposure to pathogens. Overall, the operational competences and risk reduction provided by medical robotics add more value in the healthcare industry [11–22]. Furthermore, the global use of robots in healthcare makes it clear that robotics will become more common in the future. It has the potential to revolutionize the domain due to its various real-time applications and advantages as a benefit to both patients and healthcare workers [23–29].

Medical robotics, which uses robots in the healthcare or medical field, has grown in popularity in recent years. With the advancement in technologies, robots in the healthcare sector have become more established these days and provide various advantages to both healthcare providers and patients, as shown in Figure 12.1. For example, the da Vinci surgical system gives surgeons more exact control for a range of procedures and interventions in the operating room. With the help of magnified 3D high-definition vision and controls that strap to a surgeon's wrists and hands, this robot makes small, accurate incisions that human hands might not. This provides improved control to surgeons, and surgery becomes less invasive compared to conventional surgery, resulting in less healing time for admitted patients [21, 22, 24, 30, 31].

DOI: 10.1201/9781003451846-12

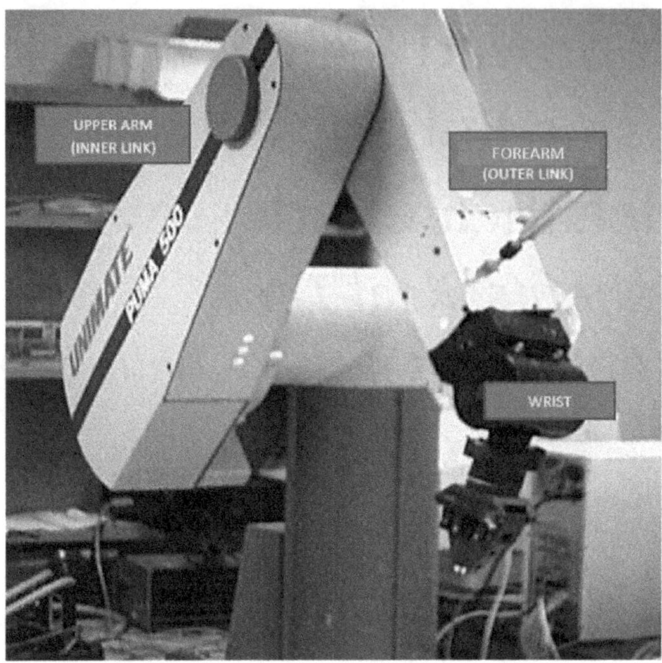

FIGURE 12.1 The first surgical robot, PUMA 560.

12.2 MAJOR BENEFITS OF ROBOTICS IN THE HEALTHCARE INDUSTRY

Robotics has various advantages in today's world. Some of them are listed as follows.

12.2.1 High-End Healthcare

Medical robots are very useful in minimally invasive surgery (MIS), personalized and continuous monitoring for patients with prolonged illnesses, smart therapies, and social engagement for older patients. Nursing robots can perform jobs similar to human nursing staff without being tired out. While nursing robots can also handle less important workloads, nurses and other staff can focus on more significant tasks such as promoting the patient's long term well-being [20, 29–42].

12.2.2 Safer Work Environment

Heavy lifting tasks by nursing robots, such as changing the position of beds or lifting patients in hospitals, eliminates some workplace hazards for staff workers. They can be used for transportation of goods and linens in hospitals and clinics where microbe and virus exposure is a risk for healthcare workers [4, 9, 12, 15, 30, 39, 42–49]. Using robots for cleaning and disinfection also help reduce infections while limiting virus exposure.

12.2.3 Simplified Hospital Workflows

Autonomous mobile robots (AMRs) help in reducing physical demands on human power while ensuring more reliable procedures. These kind of robots can help in addressing human power shortages and issues by checking inventory and placing it accurately to ensure medication, equipment, and other supply materials can be easily available per requirements [36–38, 46]. These robots also allow hospital rooms to be speedily sanitized and prepared for new inpatients.

12.2.4 Surgical Robots in Operating Theatres

Robots are now not only assisting surgeons in setting up surgery tables in OTs, but they also contribute to interventions or procedures. These robots play an important role in the process as they allow surgeons to perform surgery with high accuracy. Furthermore, these robots also enable surgeons to perform complex operations or surgical interventions with better flexibility, precision, vision, and control. Because of smaller incisions, robotic surgery, in particular, has reduced the risk of infection and resulted in shorter hospitalization times. Furthermore, because it is less invasive, robotics in healthcare reduces blood loss and transfusions and improves patient recovery time. As a result, surgery will be more successful with fewer incisions or scars, less pain, and a lower risk of infection. Patients have shorter hospital stays as compared to those with traditional surgery [45–60].

With the adoption of robots in sectors like healthcare and its allied fields, the applications and capabilities of robots are improving day by day [41, 45, 61–66]. Today robots are used for complicated surgeries, clinical training, medicine dispensing, personal care, and many other applications.

12.3 EXAMPLES OF ROBOTICS

There are various robots used in the medical domain. The top advancements in medical robotics that will change your life are listed here.

12.3.1 da Vinci Surgical Robots

This is one of the oldest and most commonly used robots in the medical world. This device blurs the gap between robots and surgical tools, as it is always under the control of a surgeon. With the help of this robot, various operations can be performed with fewer minor incisions with maximum precision, less bleeding, rapid post-op healing, and lower chances of infection [34–36, 66, 67]. da Vinci robotic surgery at St. Paul hospital is presented in Figure 12.2.

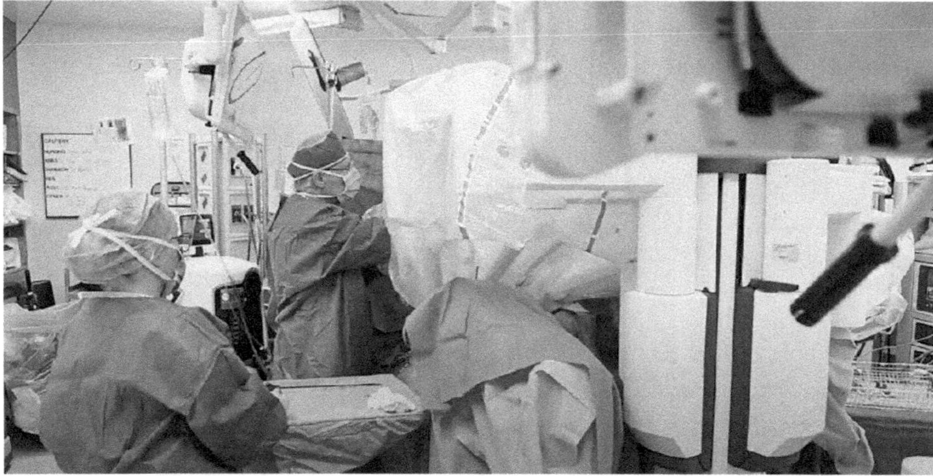

FIGURE 12.2 da Vinci robotic surgery.

12.3.2 Capsule Endoscope Robots

An endoscopy is a procedure to look onto the body of a patient where a wire with small camera is inserted into the patient's body through a natural opening such as the mouth to examine for any kind of damage, foreign particles, or signs of disease. It is a very uncomfortable procedure, but with the advancement of technology, companies such as medineering are using flexible robots which be used like an RC car to a particular place as per the requirement. They can then attach there without the movement of human hands, as shown in Figure 12.3 [50, 52, 54, 55].

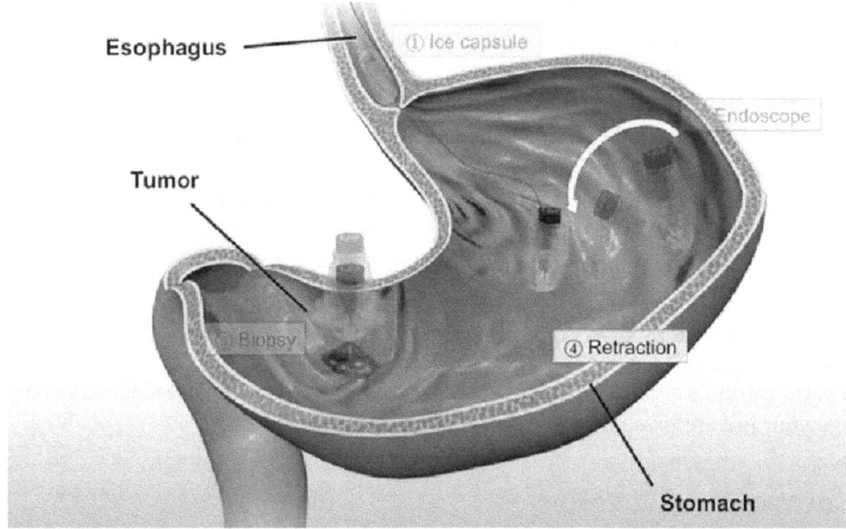

FIGURE 12.3 Endoscopy using capsule robots.

12.3.3 Orthoses (a.k.a. Exoskeletons)

Exoskeletons are used to help with walking in the case of paralyzed patients and to correct abnormality or provide rehabilitation after a brain or spinal injury by providing fragile muscles with the help they need to perform activities and begin to heal. These orthoses work on the basis of pre-set movements and user input, as shown in Figure 12.4. These exoskeletons make walking more comfortable and less tiring [20, 23–28, 30, 45–57].

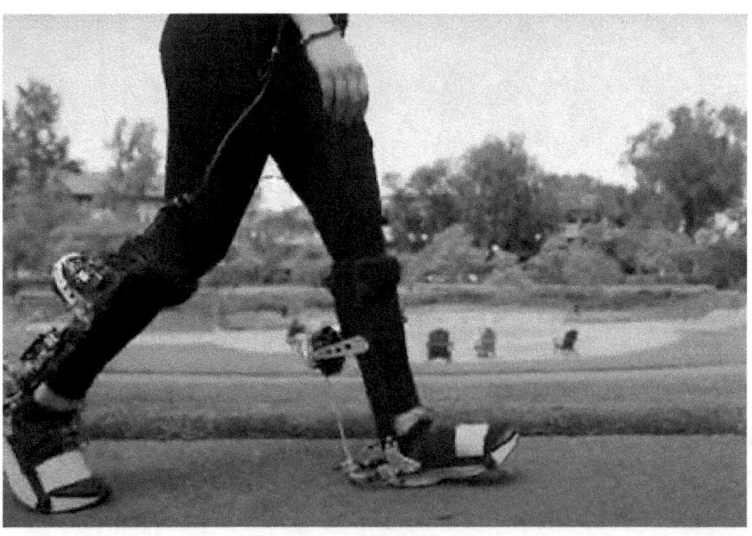

FIGURE 12.4 Exoskeletons help in performing activities.

12.3.4 Disinfectant Robots

These robots are widely used in hospitals and clinics. Since hospitals routinely administer huge amounts of antibiotics, they become a major source of the most virulent antibiotic-resistant bacteria. In order to make them clean and free from pathogens and infections, disinfectant robots are commonly used worldwide. These robots move autonomously to each hospital room where a patient is being discharged, and all the microorganisms can be killed using high-powered ultraviolet (UV) radiation for a few minutes, as shown in Figure 12.5. A DeKonBot is used for cleaning and disinfection purposes [60–63].

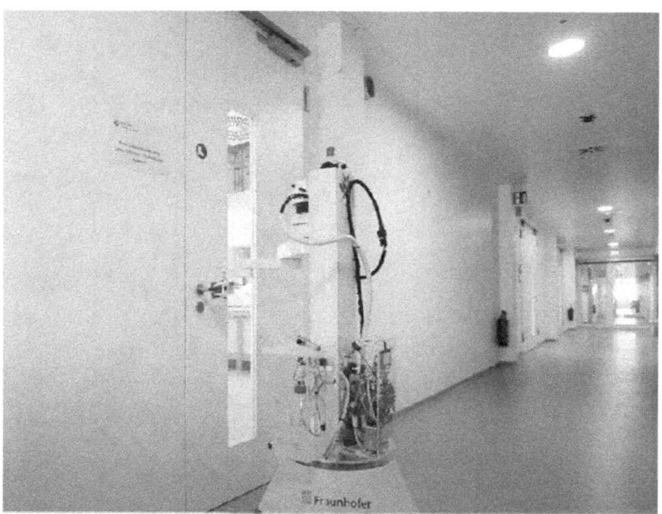

FIGURE 12.5 Cleaning and disinfection work done using DeKonBot robots.

12.3.5 Companion Robots

There are billions of elderly or mentally disabled persons worldwide who are suffering from prolonged loneliness and lack stimulation. These kind of patients need regular follow-ups from caretakers, which can be a significant problem if there is a shortage of human power. In such cases, these robots can make patients' lives comfortable and better. For example, BUDDY can interacts with its owners at an ever-changing emotional level. It won the Best of Innovation Award in 2018 for its advancements [2, 7, 28, 40–49]. Robin is a friendly robot that can express emotions and have interactive discussions with children, as shown in Figure 12.6.

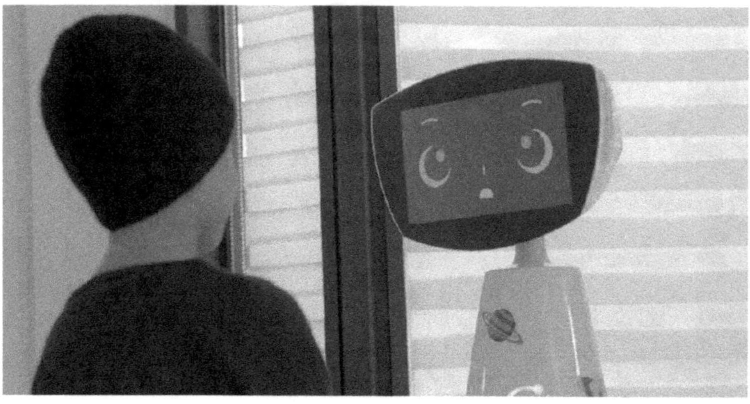

FIGURE 12.6 Companion robots interacting with children at hospital.

12.3.6 Robotic Nurses

In healthcare systems, nurses and other staff are miracle workers and the true lifeblood of any medical setting. But in the case of shortage of manpower or high workload, robotic nurses can be used. These robots can work like humans, such as filling forms at the hospital at a patient billing counter, and can monitor patient vitals and also help in taking care of patients [55–66], as shown in Figure 12.7. Moxi robots assist the nursing staff by performing time-consuming jobs such as delivering laboratory samples from one place to another and medicine collection from pharmacy stores. They can also travel to shops to pick up items for patients.

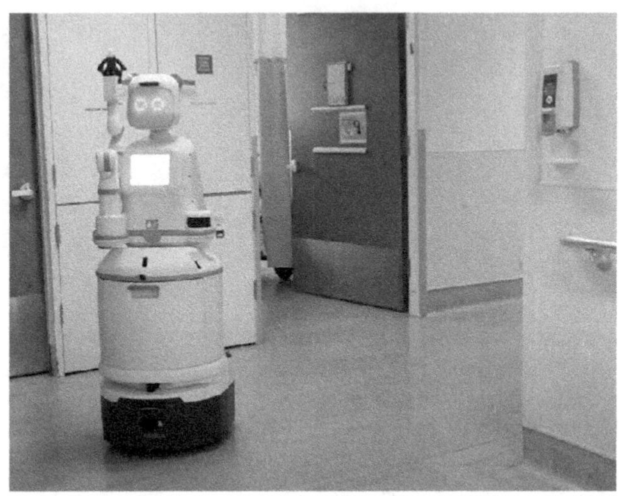

FIGURE 12.7 Nursing robot performing various delivery of samples in a hospital.

12.3.7 Robotic-Assisted Biopsy

With the advancement of technology, a new potentially life-saving technology has come from a project known as MRI and ultrasound robotic-assisted biopsy (MURAB). Basically, it is a minimally invasive technique (magnetic resonance tomography, MRT) for early detection of cancer where a robotically steered transducer is guided to a biopsy site using an innovative technique known as the MRI/ultrasound combination technique. It allows surgeons to precisely place a biopsy needle into various domains of the nodule in real time, as shown in Figure 12.8 [20, 30, 34, 47, 48–57].

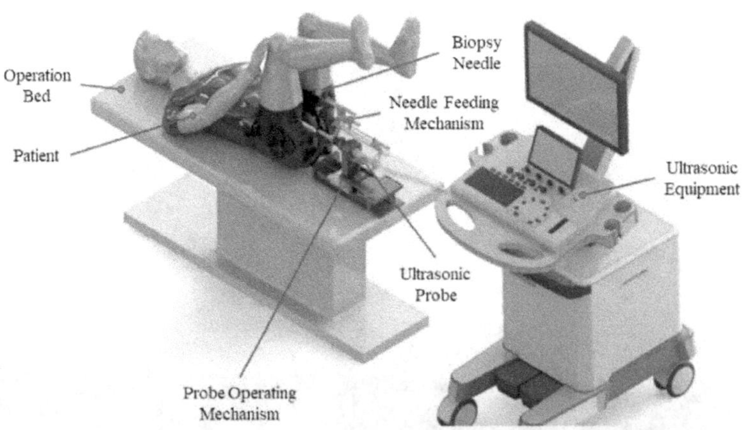

FIGURE 12.8 Robotic guided transperineal prostate biopsy.

12.3.8 Antibacterial Nanorobots

These are active structures capable of sensing, handling, actuating, signaling, and processing data at the microscopic level. In heath care systems, basically, these are small machines built of gold nanowire-coated platelets and red blood cells (RBCs) capable of clearing pathogens or bacterial infections directly from a patient's blood using a bacterium and its toxin's target when the bacteria is collected in nanomesh, as shown in Figure 12.9. They can also be directed using ultrasound sonography (USG) for fast clearance procedures and to treat local infections. Instead of using broad-spectrum antibiotics, these can be used, and they have a great impact on the fight against various antibiotic-resistant diseases [58–64].

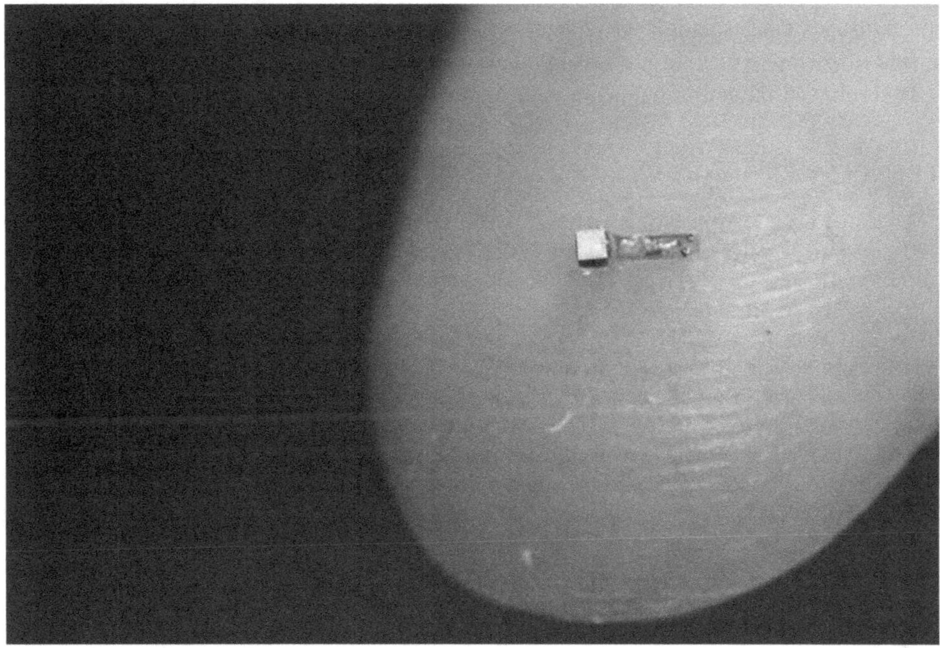

FIGURE 12.9 Antibacterial nanorobots.

12.4 CHALLENGING ISSUES IN ADOPTING ROBOTICS

Apart from various benefits of using robots in healthcare, there are several open challenges also present in deployment of these systems. There is a high possibility of error and chances of failure [67]. As there is a scope of human error or machine failure with medical robots, a minute mistake or error can cost patient lives [34, 39, 47–66, 68]. Some of the major disadvantages of these systems are:

1. In the case of surgical robots, a small amount of bleeding during a surgical intervention or procedure or any kind of infection cannot be neglected, as it costs patient lives.
2. The use of surgical robots in developing countries or advanced clinics is limited due to the high cost of employment of robots in healthcare. A normal person cannot afford robotic surgeries.
3. Robots can replace nursing staff employed in hospitals, which can lead to unemployment.

12.5 FUTURE OF ROBOTICS

With advancements in AI technology, medical robots can increase accuracy, quality, and safety in delivery services. Medical robots can perform surgeries more accurately. With the improvement in hardware and software systems, there is a large scope of robotics in other healthcare domains also. The collaboration of robotic manufacturers and healthcare providers will further boost the healthcare robot market [60, 61, 63–66]. However, the cost of robots and affordability for normal people will remain challenging issues to address.

12.6 CONCLUSION

With the advancement of AI and robotics, robotics are widely used in hospitals and can perform various tasks efficiently and with high precision. This chapter presents a detailed description of medical robots, major advantages and disadvantages, and their future, along with open key challenges that could lead to unemployment of humans in the near future. In this chapter, various current examples of medical robots used in the healthcare industry are also given.

REFERENCES

1. Medical Robots. Available at: https://interestingengineering.com/lists/15-medical-robots-that-are-changing-the-world [accessed on 20 July 2023].
2. Medical Robots. Available at: https://theappsolutions.com/blog/machine-learning/medical-imaging/ [accessed on 20 July 2023].
3. Medical Robots. Available at: www.analyticsinsight.net/what-are-the-benefits-of-robotics-in-the-healthcare-industry/ [accessed on 20 July 2023].
4. Intuitive Surgical Incorporation. "Webpage on da Vinci clinical evidence," March 2012. Available at: www.intuitivesurgical.com/company/clinical-evidence.
5. Intuitive Surgical Incorporation. "Webpage on da Vinci regulatory approval," March 2012. Available at: www.intuitivesurgical.com/company/regulatory-clearance.html.
6. H. Lavery, D. Samadi, and A. Levinson, "Not a zero-sum game: The adoption of robotics has increased overall prostatectomy utilization in the united states," in *Proceedings of the American Urological Association Annual Meeting, Poster Session*, Washington, DC, 2011.
7. R. D. Howe and Y. Matsuoka, "Robotics for surgery," *Annual Review of Biomedical Engineering*, vol. 1, pp. 211–240, 1999.
8. R. H. Taylor and D. Stoianovici, "Medical robotics in computer-integrated surgery," *IEEE Transactions on Robotics and Automation*, vol. 19, no. 5, pp. 765–781, 2003.
9. A. R. Lanfranco, A. E. Castellanos, J. P. Desai, and W. C. Meyers, "Robotic surgery: A current perspective," *Annals of Surgery*, vol. 239, no. 1, pp. 14–21, 2004.
10. B. Davies, "A review of robotics in surgery," *Proceedings of the Institution of Mechanical Engineers H*, vol. 214, no. 1, pp. 129–140, 2000.
11. P. Berkelman, J. Troccaz, and P. Cinquin, "Body-supported medical robots: A survey," *Journal of Robotics and Mechatronics*, vol. 16, pp. 513–519, 2004.
12. L. Guo, X. Pan, Q. Li, F. Zheng, and Z. Bao, "A survey on the gastrointestinal capsule micro-robot based on wireless and optoelectronic technology," *Journal of Nanoelectronics and Optoelectronics*, vol. 7, no. 2, pp. 123–127, 2012.
13. C. Stüer, F. Ringel, M. Stoffel, A. Reinke, M. Behr, and B. Meyer, "Robotic technology in spine surgery: Current applications and future developments," *Intraoperative Imaging*, vol. 109, pp. 241–245, 2011.
14. S. Badaan and D. Stoianovici, "Robotic systems: Past, present, and future," in *Robotics in Genitourinary Surgery*, pp. 655–665, Springer, New York, NY, 2011.
15. I. Singh, "Robotics in urological surgery: Review of current status and maneuverability, and comparison of robot-assisted and traditional laparoscopy," *Computer Aided Surgery*, vol. 16, no. 1, pp. 38–45, 2011.
16. G. P. Moustris, S. C. Hiridis, K. M. Deliparaschos, and K. M. Konstantinidis, "Evolution of autonomous and semi-autonomous robotic surgical systems: A review of the literature," *International Journal of Medical Robotics and Computer Assisted Surgery*, vol. 7, no. 4, pp. 375–392, 2011.

17. B. Challacombe and D. Stoianovici, "The basic science of robotic surgery," *Urologic Robotic Surgery in Clinical Practice*, pp. 1–23, 2009.
18. H. Kenngott, L. Fischer, F. Nickel, J. Rom, J. Rassweiler, and B. Muller-Stich, "Status of robotic assistance: A less traumatic and more accurate minimally invasive surgery?" *Langenbeck's Archives of Surgery*, vol. 397, no. 3, pp. 1–9, 2012.
19. P. Gomes, "Surgical robotics: Reviewing the past, analysing the present, imagining the future," *Robotics and Computer-Integrated Manufacturing*, vol. 27, no. 2, pp. 261–266, 2011.
20. A. M. Okamura, M. J. Matarić, and H. I. Christensen, "Medical and health-care robotics," *IEEE Robotics and Automation Magazine*, vol. 17, no. 3, pp. 26–37, 2010.
21. S. Najarian, M. Fallahnezhad, and E. Afshari, "Advances in medical robotic systems with specific applications in surgery—a review," *Journal of Medical Engineering and Technology*, vol. 35, no. 1, pp. 19–33, 2011.
22. J. Rosen, B. Hannaford, and R. Satava, Eds., *Surgical Robotics: Systems Applications and Visions*, Springer, New York, NY, 2011.
23. T. Haidegger, L. Kovacs, G. Fordos, Z. Benyo, and P. Kazanzides, "Future trends in robotic neurosurgery," in *Proceedings of the 14th Nordic-Baltic Conference on Biomedical Engineering and Medical Physics (NBC '08)*, pp. 229–233, Springer, June 2008.
24. Y. S. Kwoh, J. Hou, E. A. Jonckheere, and S. Hayati, "A robot with improved absolute positioning accuracy for CT guided stereotactic brain surgery," *IEEE Transactions on Biomedical Engineering*, vol. 35, no. 2, pp. 153–160, 1988.
25. D. Glauser, H. Fankhauser, M. Epitaux, J. L. Hefti, and A. Jaccottet, "Neurosurgical robot Minerva: First results and current developments," *Journal of Image Guided Surgery*, vol. 1, no. 5, pp. 266–272, 1995.
26. T. R. K. Varma and P. Eldridge, "Use of the NeuroMate stereotactic robot in a frameless mode for functional neurosurgery," *International Journal of Medical Robotics and Computer Assisted Surgery*, vol. 2, no. 2, pp. 107–113, 2006.
27. Q. H. Li, L. Zamorano, A. Pandya, R. Perez, J. Gong, and F. Diaz, "The application accuracy of the NeuroMate robot—a quantitative comparison with frameless and frame-based surgical localization systems," *Computer Aided Surgery*, vol. 7, no. 2, pp. 90–98, 2002.
28. P. Morgan, T. Carter, S. Davis, et al., "The application accuracy of the pathfinder neurosurgical robot," *International Congress Series*, vol. 1256, pp. 561–567, 2003.
29. G. Deacon, A. Harwood, J. Holdback, et al., "The pathfinder image-guided surgical robot," *Proceedings of the Institution of Mechanical Engineers H*, vol. 224, no. 5, pp. 691–713, 2010.
30. N. Nathoo, M. C. Çavuşoğlu, M. A. Vogelbaum, and G. H. Barnett, "In touch with robotics: neurosurgery for the future," *Neurosurgery*, vol. 56, no. 3, pp. 421–431, 2005.
31. L. Sharma and N. Lohan, "Internet of Things with object detection," in *Handbook of Research on Big Data and the IoT*, pp. 89–100, IGI Global, 2019. doi:10.4018/978-1-5225-7432-3.ch006.
32. J. Brodie and S. Eljamel, "Evaluation of a neurosurgical robotic system to make accurate burr holes," *International Journal of Medical Robotics and Computer Assisted Surgery*, vol. 7, no. 1, pp. 101–106, 2011.
33. L. Joskowicz, R. Shamir, Z. Israel, Y. Shoshan, and M. Shoham, "Renaissance robotic system for keyhole cranial neurosurgery: in-vitro accuracy study," in *Proceedings of the Simposio Mexicano en Ciruga Asistida por Computadora y Procesamiento de Imgenes Mdicas (MexCAS '11)*, 2011.
34. L. Sharma and P. Garg, Eds., *From Visual Surveillance to Internet of Things*, Chapman and Hall/CRC, New York, 2020. https://doi.org/10.1201/9780429297922
35. L. Sharma and N. Lohan, "Performance analysis of moving object detection using BGS techniques in visual surveillance", *International Journal of Spatiotemporal Data Science, Inderscience*, vol.1, pp. 22–53, January 2019.
36. A. Anand, V. Jha, and L. Sharma, "An improved local binary patterns histograms techniques for face recognition for real time application", *International Journal of Recent Technology and Engineering*, vol. 8, no. 2S7, pp. 524–529, July 2019.
37. L. Sharma and D. K. Yadav, "Histogram based adaptive learning rate for background modelling and moving object detection in video surveillance", *International Journal of Telemedicine and Clinical Practices,* 2016. doi:10.1504/IJTMCP.2017.082107.
38. L. Sharma and N. Lohan, "Performance analysis of moving object detection using BGS techniques", *International Journal of Spatio-Temporal Data Science*, vol. 1, no. 1, pp. 22–53, 2019.
39. L. Sharma, "Introduction: From visual surveillance to Internet of Things," in *From Visual Surveillance to Internet of Things*, vol. 1, p. 14, USA: Taylor & Francis, CRC Press , 2019.

40. L. Sharma and P. K. Garg, "Block based adaptive learning rate for moving person detection in video surveillance," in *From Visual Surveillance to Internet of Things*, vol.1, p. 201, USA: Taylor & Francis, CRC Press, 2019.
41. S. Makkar and L. Sharma, A face detection using support vector machine: Challenging issues, recent trend, solutions and proposed framework. In: M. Singh, P. Gupta, V. Tyagi, J. Flusser, T. Ören, and R. Kashyap (eds) *Advances in Computing and Data Sciences. ICACDS 2019. Communications in Computer and Information Science*, vol. 1046. Springer, Singapore. https://doi.org/10.1007/978-981-13-9942-8_1
42. L. Sharma and P. K. Garg, "IoT and its applications," in *From Visual Surveillance to Internet of Things*, vol. 1, p. 29, USA: Taylor & Francis, CRC Press.
43. L. Sharma, D. K. Yadav, and S. K. Bharti, "An improved method for visual surveillance using background subtraction technique," in *2015 2nd International Conference on Signal Processing and Integrated Networks (SPIN)*, 2015, pp. 421–426, doi:10.1109/SPIN.2015.7095253.
44. D. K. Yadav, L. Sharma, and S. K. Bharti, "Moving object detection in real-time visual surveillance using background subtraction technique," in *2014 14th International Conference on Hybrid Intelligent Systems*, 2014, pp. 79–84, doi: 10.1109/HIS.2014.7086176.
45. L. Sharma, A. Singh, and D. K. Yadav, "Fisher's linear discriminant ratio based threshold for moving human detection in thermal video," in *Infrared Physics and Technology*, USA: Elsevier, March 2016.
46. L. Sharma, Ed., *Towards Smart World*, Chapman and Hall/CRC, New York, NY, 2021. https://doi.org/10.1201/9781003056751
47. L. Sharma, "Human detection and tracking using background subtraction in visual surveillance", in *Towards Smart World*, pp. 317–328, Chapman and Hall/CRC, New York, 2020. https://doi.org/10.1201/9781003056751
48. L. Sharma, D. K. Yadav, and S. K. Bharti, "An improved method for visual surveillance using background subtraction technique," in *IEEE, 2nd International Conference on Signal Processing and Integrated Networks (SPIN-2015)*, Amity University, Noida, February 19–20, 2015.
49. D. K. Yadav, L. Sharma, and S. K. Bharti, "Moving object detection in real-time visual surveillance using background subtraction technique," in *IEEE, 14th International Conference in Hybrid Intelligent Computing (HIS-2014)*, Gulf University for Science and Technology, Kuwait, December 14–16, 2014.
50. L. Sharma, D. K. Yadav, and M. Kumar, "A morphological approach for human skin detection in color images", in *2nd national conference on "Emerging Trends in Intelligent Computing & Communication"*, GCET, Noida, April 26–27, 2013.
51. L. Sharma, S. Sengupta, and B. Kumar, "An improved technique for enhancement of satellite images," *Journal of Physics: Conference Series*, vol. 1, pp. 1–8, January 2021.
52. S. Singh, L. Sharma, and B. Kumar, "A machine learning based predictive model for coronavirus pandemic scenario," *Journal of Physics: Conference Series*, vol. 1, pp. 20–29, January 2021.
53. G. Jha, L. Sharma, and S. Gupta, "Future of augmented reality in healthcare department," in P. K. Singh, S. T. Wierzchoń, S. Tanwar, M. Ganzha, and J. J. P. C. Rodrigues (eds) *Proceedings of Second International Conference on Computing, Communications, and Cyber-Security. Lecture Notes in Networks and Systems*, vol 203, Springer, Singapore, 2021. https://doi.org/10.1007/978-981-16-0733-2_47.
54. G. Jha, L. Sharma, and S. Gupta, "E-health in Internet of Things (IoT) in real-time scenario," in P. K. Singh, S. T. Wierzchoń, S. Tanwar, M. Ganzha, and J. J. P. C. Rodrigues (eds) *Proceedings of Second International Conference on Computing, Communications, and Cyber-Security. Lecture Notes in Networks and Systems*, vol. 203. Springer, Singapore, 2021. https://doi.org/10.1007/978-981-16-0733-2_48
55. S. Kumar, P. Gupta, S. Lakra, L. Sharma, and R. Chatterjee, "The Zeitgeist Juncture of "Big Data" and Its Future Trends," in *2019 International Conference on Machine Learning, Big Data, Cloud and Parallel Computing (COMITCon)*, 2019, pp. 465–469, doi: 10.1109/COMITCon.2019.8862433.
56. S. Sharma, S. Verma, M. Kumar, and L. Sharma, "Use of motion capture in 3D animation: Motion capture systems, challenges, and recent trends," in *2019 International Conference on Machine Learning, Big Data, Cloud and Parallel Computing (COMITCon)*, 2019, pp. 289–294, doi: 10.1109/COMITCon.2019.8862448.
57. M. Carpenter, "An accidentally detected diaphragmatic hernia with acute appendicitis," *Asian Journal of Case Reports in Surgery*, vol. 9, no. 2, pp. 19–24, 2021. www.journalajcrs.com/index.php/AJCRS/article/view/30260
58. Artificial Intelligence Technologies, Applications, and Challenges. Available at: www.routledge.com/Artificial-Intelligence-Technologies-Applications-and-Challenges/Sharma-Garg/p/book/9780367690809 [accessed on 20 July 2021].

59. L. Sharma, "Computer-aided lung cancer detection and classification of CT images using convolutional neural network," in *Computer Vision and Internet of Things: Technologies and Applications*, pp. 247–262, USA: Taylor & Francis, CRC Press, May 2022.
60. L. Sharma, "Analysis of machine learning techniques for airfare prediction," in *Computer Vision and Internet of Things: Technologies and Applications*, pp. 211–231, USA: Taylor & Francis, CRC Press, May 2022.
61. L. Sharma, "Innovation and emerging computer vision and artificial intelligence technologies in coronavirus control," in *Computer Vision and Internet of Things: Technologies and Applications*, pp. 177–192, USA: Taylor & Francis, CRC Press, May 2022.
62. L. Sharma, "Self-driving cars: Tools and technologies," in *Computer Vision and Internet of Things: Technologies and Applications*, pp. 99–110, USA: Taylor & Francis, CRC Press, May 2022.
63. L. Sharma, "Computer vision in surgical operating theatre and medical imaging," in *Computer Vision and Internet of Things: Technologies and Applications*, pp. 75–96, USA: Taylor & Francis, CRC Press, May 2022.
64. L. Sharma, "Preventing security breach in social media: Threats and prevention techniques," *Computer Vision and Internet of Things: Technologies and Applications*, pp. 53–62, USA: Taylor & Francis, CRC Press, May 2022.
65. L. Sharma and M. Carpenter, "Use of robotics in real-time applications," in *Computer Vision and Internet of Things: Technologies and Applications*, pp. 41–50, USA: Taylor & Francis, CRC Press, May 2022.
66. L. Sharma et al., "An overview of security issues of Internet of Things," in *Computer Vision and Internet of Things: Technologies and Applications*, pp. 29–40, USA: Taylor & Francis, CRC Press, May 2022.
67. L. Sharma, "Rise of computer vision and Internet of Things," in *Computer Vision and Internet of Things: Technologies and Applications*, pp. 5–17, USA: Taylor & Francis, CRC Press, May 2022.
68. L. Sharma, and M. Carpenter, Eds. *Computer Vision and Internet of Things: Technologies and Applications* (1st ed.). USA: Chapman and Hall/CRC, 2022. doi: 10.1201/9781003244165

13 Deep Learning Processes in MRI Images

Sudhriti Sengupta, Lavanya Sharma, and Mukesh Carpenter

13.1 INTRODUCTION

In the digital world, image processing is used to enhance the quality of the information included in an image. The development of an automated diagnosis system for numerous types of diseases depends on effective and efficient processing of medical images. Medical resonance imaging (MRI) is an important medical imaging technique that uses radio waves to scan the body. It is a type of tomographic imaging that is mostly employed in the radiology industry. MRI has the benefit of being a non-invasive diagnostic technology, which enables medical professionals to clearly depict images of the anatomy and physiological processes taking place in the body, enabling early disease identification and treatment. These images, when utilized in conjunction with image processing methods, may be used to detect tumors or other ailments that are difficult to spot with the unaided eye [1, 2]. Detection of diseases can be done manually by doctors and specialists for identification of various diseases. This is a very challenging task due to the subjective diagnosis and understanding by human experts and also the wide variety of pathologies and physiologies of the human body. It is difficult to detect diseases quickly and accurately on human expertise alone, and this leads to the need for computerized diagnostic systems using MRI as the chief mode. The creation of an automated diagnostic system requires certain precise and essential steps of image processing, commonly image pre-processing, feature extraction, segmentation, classification, and any post-processing steps. Both classical and artificial intelligence–based techniques are developed and utilized in the detection and processing of MRI images. Wavelet transformation, filtering, extraction of the gray-level co-occurrence matrix (GLCM) for texture features, and object labelling are often used in preprocessing of MRI images. Fuzzy c-means, Otsu thresholding, edge detection operators, and others are popular techniques used in segmentation and feature extraction of MRI images. Section 13.2 describes the processing of MRI images. MRI image processing using deep learning techniques and applications in MRI images is described in Sections 13.3 and 13.4, respectively. Sections 13.5 and 13.6 present the application of deep learning in MRI image pre-processing and a conclusion, respectively.

13.2 PROCESSING OF MRI IMAGES

A medical image is composed of different types of images of body parts, and its main objective is to promote health and treat diseases. The vast expansion of medical data is utilized by applications of machine learning and deep learning techniques. In recent years, medical images have better perception quality with the application of artificial intelligence techniques. The main aims of processing medical images are detecting various diseases, recuperating corrupted images, identifying individual elements, and improving image quality. There are various categories of medical images obtained by applying different techniques, each serving a specific clinical purpose. Some common examples of medical images are x-rays (radiography), computed tomography (CT), magnetic resonance imaging, ultrasounds, nuclear medicine, positron emission tomography (PET), mammograms, endoscopies, electrocardiograms (ECG or EKG), and many more [3, 4]. These various

DOI: 10.1201/9781003451846-13

kinds of medical images are extremely important for diagnosing, monitoring, and treating medical disorders in a variety of healthcare specializations. Every type of image offers distinct insights into the bodily structures and processes, assisting healthcare professionals in giving patients accurate and effective medication. One important and popular type of medical image is the MRI. Magnetic resonance imaging is a effective medical imaging technique that uses strong magnetic fields and radio waves to produce intricate images of the internal structures of the body. MRI is widely used by healthcare providers for diagnosis, monitoring disease progression, and guiding treatment plans [5]. Magnetic resonance imaging is increasing in popularity due to its non-invasive nature and successful soft tissue contrast. A physician may examine the organs, tissues, and skeletal system utilizing MRI, which is a non-intrusive technique. It generates comprehensive images of the internal structure of the human body to help in the diagnosis of many ailments. Spine and brain imaging most frequently employ MRI. It is frequently utilized to help in determining the cause of the following conditions: cerebral ruptures, eye and inner ear diseases, multiple sclerosis (MS), spinal cord disorders, strokes, tumors, and traumatic brain injuries. MRI of the bones and joints may be helpful in finding osteoarthritis, torn ligaments or cartilage, bone infections, or bone tumors. Mammography and MRI of the breasts can be used to detect breast cancer, particularly in those with heavy breast tissue or those who may be at high risk for the illness. The scope and potential uses of MRI technology are steadily expanding. In order to enhance the quality and extract valuable data from MRI images, image processing techniques are required. These methods can help in reducing noise, image clarity, medical research, and diagnosis. One of the challenges faced by researchers in MRI image analysis is to improve tumor detection while discovering more about the nature of disorders [6–8]. The steps in a general image processing method are image acquisition, preprocessing, segmentation, feature extraction, classification, and any other post-processing steps.

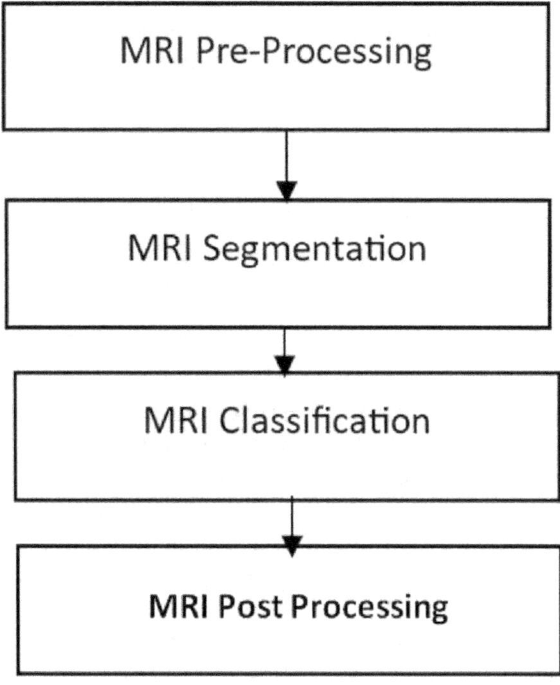

FIGURE 13.1 Processing of MRI images.

In the subsequent sections, the different stages of image processing applied to MRI images are discussed in brief.

13.2.1 Preprocessing

Preprocessing MRI images is a crucial step in analyzing MRI images, as it helps improve image quality, eliminate artifacts, and make the images ready for subsequent tasks like segmentation, feature extraction, and classification. The first step in image processing is typically pre-processing, where MRI images are processed for contrast enhancement, noise removal, image resizing, and removal of artifacts. The pre-processed images are improved images, which promises to give better-quality output in the next steps of MRI image processing. Some common tasks performed in pre-processing are:

- Increasing image brightness in a dark MRI image.
- Filtering images to remove noise and other artifacts.
- Image scaling to resize the image based on dimensions or pixels.
- Grayscale conversion for eliminating unwanted background.
- Color correction for adjusting the color balance and accuracy of the MRI image.

13.2.2 Segmentation

The process of partitioning an MRI image into segments depending on the underlying anatomical or pathological components is known as segmentation. MRI images require segmentation for simpler and more reliable data perception from the image. Segmentation plays a important part in tasks like tumor detection, organ analysis, quantitative analysis, and treatment management. MRI image segmentation helps in the identification of particular structures or regions of interest (ROIs) within MRI images. Some of the common MRI segmentation techniques are threshold techniques, edge-based segmentation techniques, active contour models, watershed segmentation techniques, and machine learning based segmentation techniques. The three categories of image segmentation are pixel-based, edge-based, and region-based, used for the purpose of collecting information about the MRI image being processed. The threshold technique is a pixel-based technique where a threshold value is specified for conversion of a grayscale image to a binary image. The Otsu threshold method is popular in MRI image segmentation. Clustering is also a type of pixel-based segmentation where data with similar properties is put together to form clusters. Active contour, gradient mode, and edge detection operators are examples of edge-based detection. This technique uses the pixel values at the edges or borders to partition objects. Region-based detection categorizes the image into groups by the pixel value. Region growing, split and merge, and graph cut are some types of region-based detection.

13.2.3 Classification

Image classification is the method of categorizing and labeling a number of pixels within an image according to specific guidelines. In MRI image analysis, image segmentation is crucial for activities like accurate and timely disease detection and providing correct treatment. Classifying MRI imaging is challenging because of its complexity and variances. One of the effective techniques used in the classification of MRI images is support vector machine (SVM). Large data sets can be used to train the SVM and examine the data model. Naïve Bayes, fuzzy C means, principal component analysis, and machine learning techniques are also used in classification of MRI images [9]. With the advances in deep learning, numerous methods for deep learning have been developed to enhance the performance of MRI image processing and analysis. Deep learning can uncover new characteristics that have never been discovered previously by researchers. Traditional feature extraction techniques frequently require certain a priori knowledge and can only extract some features related to a specific application. Hence application of deep learning techniques is a popular emerging field to process and analyze MRI images. The aim of the following section is to give a comprehensive overview of MRI image processing and analysis using deep learning.

13.3 MRI IMAGE PROCESSING USING DEEP LEARNING TECHNIQUES

Deep learning is an approach used in artificial intelligence (AI) that trains computers to interpret data in a manner modeled after the human brain. Deep learning models can identify complex patterns in images, text, audio, and other types of data to generate accurate analyses and predictions. Deep learning is a type of machine learning in which the algorithms are modeled like the architecture and function of the brain, called artificial neural networks. The human brain has millions of connected neurons that collaborate to process and learn new information. Similar to this, deep learning neural networks are constructed inside computers from numerous layers of synthetic neurons. Artificial neurons are software components (nodes) that process data using mathematical operations. These nodes are used by artificial neural networks to resolve complex problems. Large sets of labeled data and neural network architectures that automatically extract features from the data are used to train deep learning models. The following are the main components of a deep neural network.

13.3.1 Input Layer

A number of nodes provide data in an artificial neural network, forming the input layer.

13.3.2 Hidden Layer

The input layer of the neural network processes and sends the data to the next level, called the hidden layer. These hidden layers employ several levels of data processing, modifying their behavior in response to new data. Deep learning networks examine a problem from multiple viewpoints because they can use numerous hidden layers.

13.3.3 Output Layer

The nodes that output the data constitute the output layer. Deep learning models which produce "yes" or "no" answers consist of two nodes in the output layer. However, those that produce an increased number of outputs have more nodes.

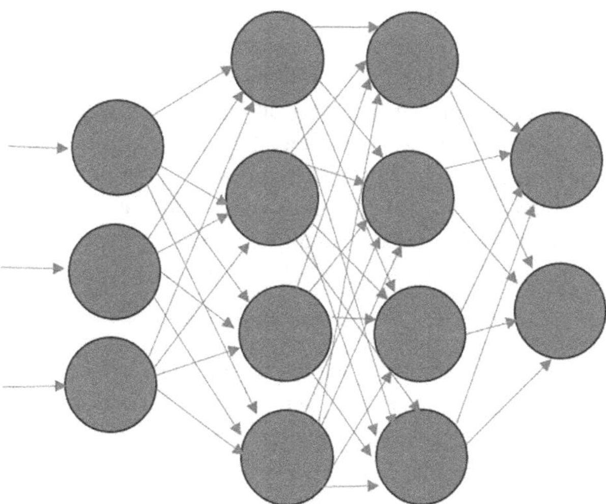

FIGURE 13.2 Neural networks (a set of interconnected nodes).

Convolutional neural networks (CNNs), recurrent neural networks (RNNs), and deep belief networks (DBNs) are some of the popular types of deep learning architectures. Deep learning can be used for reinforcement learning as well as supervised and unsupervised learning. Deep learning algorithms, such as recurrent neural networks and convolutional neural networks, are utilized for a variety of supervised applications like image classification and recognition, sentiment analysis, and language translations. Unsupervised tasks like clustering, dimensionality reduction, and anomaly detection are performed using deep learning techniques like automatic encoders and generative models. Deep reinforcement learning techniques, such as deep Q networks and deep deterministic policy gradients (DDPGs) are utilized to reinforce tasks like robotics and game playing. Deep learning has made substantial progress in a number of areas, including speech recognition, image recognition, natural language processing, and recommendation systems.

13.4 DEEP LEARNING APPLICATIONS IN MRI IMAGES

Many deep learning techniques, including those for image detection, registration, segmentation, and classification, have been presented recently for use in the field of MRI image processing and analysis. All of these issues can be framed as challenges related to feature representation, and consequently, they can be efficiently addressed by employing deep learning techniques to discover an effective set of features. In this part of the chapter, we focus on the progress of deep learning applications in the field of image pre-processing, segmentation, and classification.

13.4.1 Pre-Processing of MRI Images Using Deep Learning

Image pre-processing is an important stage in various applications of image processing for getting meaningful output. Some of the steps in pre-processing of MRI images are:

- The images have all been scaled to the same size.
- Filtering process, like mean filtering, is done.
- Contrast enhancement is done using techniques like histogram equalization.

In their research, Periera et al. [2] proposed brain tumor segmentation using convolutional neural networks in MRIs.

Brain tumor segmentation using deep neural networks was proposed by Devy et al. [10], who additionally examined intensity inhomogeneity correction and data normalization for each input channel. As a preprocessing phase, Zikic et al. [11] proposed segmentation of brain tumor tissues using convolutional neural networks, examining intensity inhomogeneity correction in each MRI channel. Structures with convolutional neural networks for multimodal brain tumor segmentation was proposed by Dvorak et al. [12]. They investigated the bias field correction and intensity normalization of MRI images as a pre-processing step. Preprocessing with a deep learning approach aids in the most accurate and reliable design of computer vision applications. With this goal in mind, we used Resnet preprocessing for the quantitative analysis of MRI images.

13.4.2 MRI Image Segmentation Using Deep Learning

In current clinical procedures and medical research, automatic tissue segmentation in MRI images is crucial. Many deep learning techniques have been presented to perform segmentation of different tissues in MRI images. Gray matter (GM), white matter (WM), and cerebrospinal fluid (CSF) segmentation are some of the most popular image segmentations used in MRI brain scans. Zhang et al. [13] suggested using convolutional networks to segment newborn brain tissue images into GM, WM, and CSF by merging multi-modal MRI data, which include T1, T2, and fractional anisotropy (FA) images.

Additionally, Moeskops et al. [14] segmented pictures of neonatal brain tissue into the following areas: brain stem (BS), cortical GM (cGM), myelinated WM (mWM), basal ganglia and thalami (BGT), unmyelinated WM (uWM), ventricular CSF (vCSF), extracerebral CSF (eCSF), and cerebellum (CB).

Using a convolutional network with tiny convolutional kernels, Pereira et al. [2] were able to segment gliomas, the most prevalent and dangerous brain tumors, in MRI scans.

Avendi et al. [15] suggested a method that used deep learning architectures and deformable object recognition to separate left ventricular (LV) from MRI image models to carry out this task.

For automatic segmentation of LV using MRI images, Ngo et al.'s merged method of deep learning architecture and a level set algorithm was proposed [16].

A fully automatic heterogeneous segmentation using a support vector machine (FAHS-SVM) was proposed for segmenting brain tumors [17] by Jia et al.

Through the use of convolutional neural networks based on U-Net for tumor segmentation and transfer learning based on a pre-trained convolution-base of Vgg16 and a fully connected classifier for tumor grading, tumor segmentation and grading using magnetic resonance imaging are made possible [18].

13.4.3 MRI Image Classification Using Deep Learning

Image classification is crucial for cognitive recognition and automatic disease diagnosis. This includes the classification of various diseases according to severity and the identification such as different brain activities. Many deep learning techniques have been proposed for using MRI images to perform image classification tasks. Suk et al. [19] introduced a deep learning method for locating high-level latent and common features from two imaging modalities, MRI images and positron emission tomography images, in order to diagnose Alzheimer's disease (AD) and its prodromal stage, mild cognitive impairment (MCI). A stacked sparse autoencoder and a softmax regression layer were integrated in a deep learning technique created by Liu et al. [20] to diagnose AD and MCI. MRI and PET imaging modalities were used to train the stacked sparse autoencoder to extract high-level latent features.

In order to identify patients with schizophrenia (SCZ) from healthy controls, Pinaya et al. [21] trained a deep neural network that combined a deep belief network with a softmax layer to extract high-level latent information from MRI images.

A deep neural network with numerous hidden layers and a softmax layer were also introduced by Kim et al. [22] to separate high-level latent information from low-level features retrieved from MRI images. Koyamada et al. [23] trained a feedforward deep neural network from fMRI images to carry out this task, which involved identifying various brain processes such as emotions, social, motor, working memory, gambling, relational, and language activities. Jang et al. [24] used fully connected feedforward deep neural networks with a number of hidden layers to identify a variety of sensorimotor tasks, including left-hand clenching, right-hand clenching, and attentiveness to aural stimuli.

Several deep learning tools have been developed in recent years, such as Caffe, Torch, Theano, Pylearn2, Keras, TensorFlow, Chainer, and MXNet. On the basis of general deep learning tools, certain deep learning methods used with MRI images have also been developed in recent years. Some of them are BrainNet, LiviaNet, DIGITS, mrbrain, and DeepMedic [25].

13.5 APPLICATION OF DEEP LEARNING IN MRI IMAGE PREPROCESSING

In this section, we give real examples of enhancement of MRI images using deep learning methods. We consider ten MRI images for experimentation and simulation. As a preprocessing method, the popular DnCNN model is chosen. DnCNN is an effective deep learning model for estimating the resulting image from an input image with noise. Many low-level vision challenges have been successfully handled by convolutional neural networks. One such persistent issue with computer vision is image denoising. The main aim of image denoising is to obtain a clean image I from a noisy image NI = I + N. It is presumed that N is additive white Gaussian noise (AWGN). Model-based methods and discriminative learning-based methods can generally be used to categorize image denoising techniques. Model-based approaches can handle denoising problems with a variety of noise levels, but their execution takes a long time. To address these issues, discriminative methods have been proposed. Both batch normalization and residual learning are used to accelerate training and improve denoising performance [26]. Discriminative denoising models seek to train a mapping function F(NI) = I in order to forecast the latent clean image. DnCNN is one of the popular techniques of discriminative denoising models. In this chapter, we have applied DnCNN to nine test images, as shown in Figure 13.3.

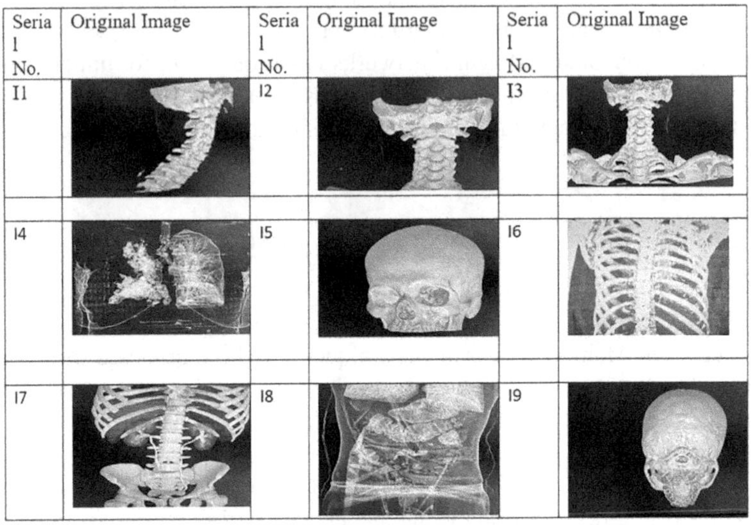

Serial No.	Original Image	Serial No.	Original Image	Serial No.	Original Image
I1		I2		I3	
I4		I5		I6	
I7		I8		I9	

FIGURE 13.3 Original MRI images.

Figure 13.3 depicts the real MRI images which will be used in experimentation and simulation for pre-processing using DnCNN techniques.

It can be observed that the images in Figure 13.4 have clearer features and perception. For quantitative analysis, histograms of the pre-processed images are observed. The tonal distribution and intensity of each pixel are displayed in the image's histogram. The image is scanned in a single pass before the number of pixels at each intensity level is counted in order to create a histogram.

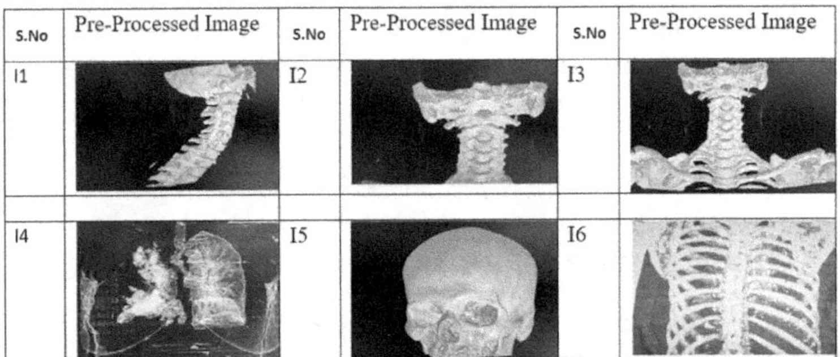

S.No	Pre-Processed Image	S.No	Pre-Processed Image	S.No	Pre-Processed Image
I1		I2		I3	
I4		I5		I6	
I7		I8		I9	

FIGURE 13.4 Pre-processed MRI images.

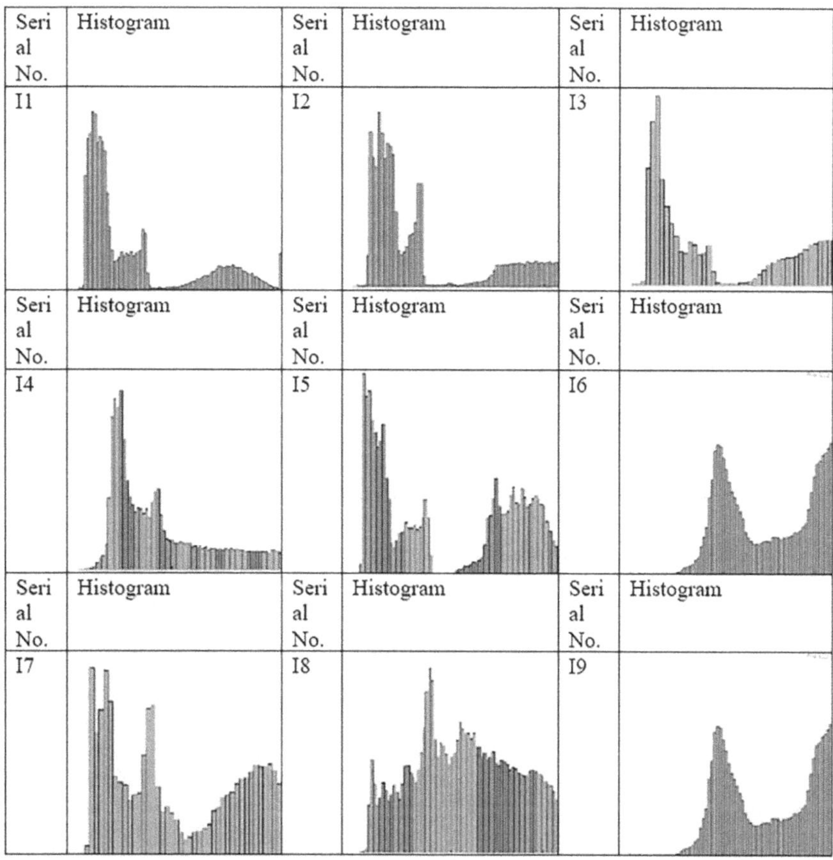

FIGURE 13.5 Histogram of pre-processed images.

It can be seen from the following table that all of the histograms' intensity values are very distributed. This demonstrates that the images are exposed properly. The pre-processed image has strong contrast due to the intensity values' wide distribution and the substantial disparity between their maximum and minimum values. These histograms demonstrate the efficacy of the pre-processing stage.

These simulations and results are a demonstration of the application of the deep learning process in MRI images. As stated, we applied DnCNN techniques on MRI images to achieve better contrast and quality of the image as a pre-processing step. Different methods can also be applied for analysis and processing of MRI images.

13.6 CONCLUSION

MRI is the process in which a magnetic field and radio waves are produced by a computer to generate exact images of a patient body's organs and tissues. It produces intricate images of the inside of the body which help in the diagnosis of numerous ailments. The use of computational techniques to evaluate MRI images is a way similar to that of a radiologist studying the ground truth from the images. MRI image analysis has experienced tremendous growth as a result of the emergence of low-cost, high-performance computing technology and concurrent advancements in computer vision. Of these, deep learning techniques are gaining immense popularity. Using a deep learning technique has several advantages, one of which is its own autonomy in performing feature engineering, leading to better and quicker performance. This chapter presents the various methods of MRI image analysis and processing with an emphasis on deep learning techniques. This chapter also describes simulation and its resultant experiments of applying DnCNN methods of pre-processing in real MRI images.

REFERENCES

[1] G. Wang et al., "Interactive medical image segmentation using deep learning with image-specific fine tuning," IEEE Transactions on Medical Imaging, vol. 37, no. 7, pp. 1562–1573, July 2018, doi: 10.1109/TMI.2018.2791721.

[2] S. Pereira, A. Pinto, V. Alves and C. A. Silva, "Brain tumor segmentation using convolutional neural networks in MRI images," IEEE Transactions on Medical Imaging, vol. 35, no. 5, pp. 1240–1251, May 2016, doi: 10.1109/TMI.2016.2538465.

[3] I. Scholl and A. Til, "Challenges of medical image processing," Computer Science—Research and Development, vol. 26, pp. 5–13, 2011

[4] I. Bankman, ed. Handbook of medical image processing and analysis. Elsevier, 2008.

[5] MRI, www.mayoclinic.org/tests-procedures/mri/about/pac-20384768, Accessed on 30th September 2023.

[6] J. John, "Image processing techniques for identifying tumors in an MRI image," Computer Vision and Pattern Recognition, 2021, arXiv: 2103.15152.

[7] S. Sengupta, A. Negi, "Comparative analysis of contrast enhancement techniques for MRI images," Proceeding of the International Conference on Computer Networks, Big Data and IoT (ICCBI-2019), 2019, pp. 290–296.

[8] S. Sengupta, A. Dubey, N. Mittal, "Analysis of MRI images using image processing technique," Proceeding of the International Conference on Computer Networks, Big Data and IoT (ICCBI-2019), 2019, pp. 267–274.

[9] A. R. Matthew, A. Prasad, P. B. Anto, "A review on feature extraction techniques for tumor detection and classification from brain MRI," 2017 International Conference on Intelligent Computing, Instrumentation and Control Technologies (ICICICT), 2017. doi:10.1109/icicict1.2017.8342838

[10] S. Pereira, A. Pinto, V. Alves, C. A. Silva, Deep Convolutional Neural Networks for the Segmentation of Gliomas in Multi-sequence MRI. Springer International Publishing, 2016, pp. 131–143.

[11] D. Zikic, Y. Ioannou, M. Brown, A. Criminisi, "Segmentation of brain tumor tissues with convolutional neural networks," MICCAI-BRATS Proceedings, 2014.

[12] P. Dvorak, B. Menze, "Structured prediction with convolutional neural networks for multimodal brain tumor segmentation," Proceeding of the Multimodal Brain Tumor Image Segmentation Challenge, 2015, pp. 13–24.

[13] W. L. Zhang, R. J. Li, H. T. Deng, L. Wang, W. L. Lin, S. W. Ji, D. G. Shen, "Deep convolutional neural networks for multi-modality isointense infant brain image segmentation," NeuroImage, vol. 108, pp. 214–224, 2015.

[14] P. Moeskops, M. A. Viergever, A. M. Mendrik, L. S. de Vries, M. J. N. L. Benders, I. Isgum, "Automatic segmentation of MR brain images with a convolutional neural network," IEEE Transactions on Medical Imaging, vol. 35, no. 5, pp. 1252–1261, 2016.

[15] M. R. Avendi, A. Kheradvar, H. Jafarkhani, "A combined deep-learning and deformable-model approach to fully automatic segmentation of the left ventricle in cardiac MRI," Medical Image Analysis, vol. 30, pp. 108–119, 2016.

[16] T. A. Ngo, Z. Lu, G. Carneiro, "Combining deep learning and level set for the automated segmentation of the left ventricle of the heart from cardiac cine magnetic resonance," Medical Image Analysis, vol. 35, pp. 159–171, 2017.

[17] Z. Jia, D. Chen, "Brain tumor identification and classification of MRI images using deep learning techniques," IEEE Access. doi: 10.1109/ACCESS.2020.3016319.

[18] M. A. Naser, M. Jamal Deen, "Brain tumor segmentation and grading of lower-grade glioma using deep learning in MRI image," Computers in Biology and Medicine, vol. 121, 2020.

[19] H. I. Suk, S. W. Lee, D. G. Shen, "Hierarchical feature representation and multimodal fusion with deep learning for AD/MCI diagnosis," NeuroImage, vol. 101, pp. 569–582, 2014.

[20] S. Q. Liu, S. D. Liu, W. D. Cai, S. Pujol, R. Kikinis, D. G. Feng, "Early diagnosis of Alzheimer's disease with deep learning," Proceedings of the 2014 IEEE 11th International Symposium on Biomedica, 2014.

[21] W. H. Pinaya, A. Gadelha, O. M. Doyle, C. Noto, A. Zugman, Q. Cordeiro, A. P. Jackowski, R. A. Bressan, J. R. Sato, "Using deep belief network modelling to characterize differences in brain morphometry in schizophrenia," Scientific Reports, vol. 6, p. 38897, 2016.
[22] J. Kim, V. D. Calhoun, E. Shim, J. H. Lee, "Deep neural network with weight sparsity control and pre-training extracts hierarchical features and enhances classification performance: Evidence from whole brain resting-state functional connectivity patterns of schizophrenia," NeuroImage, vol. 124, pp. 127–146, 2016.
[23] S. Koyamada, Y. Shikauchi, K. Nakae, M. Koyama, S. Ishii, "Deep learning of fMRI Big Data: A novel approach to subject-transfer decoding," 2015, arXiv: 1502.0009.
[24] H. Jang, S. M. Plis, V. D. Calhoun, J. H. Lee, "Task-specific feature extraction and classification of fMRI volumes using a deep neural network initialized with a deep belief network: Evaluation using sensorimotor tasks," NeuroImage, vol. 145, pp. 314–328, 2017.
[25] J. Liu, Y. Pan, M. Li, Z. Chen, L. Tang, C. Lu, C. Lu, J. Wang, "Applications of deep learning to MRI Images: A survey," Big Data Mining and Analytics, vol. 1, no. 1, March 2018.
[26] https://adityarastogi2k12.github.io/Projects/NNLS/

14 Artificial Intelligence and Robotics in Healthcare

Transforming the Indian Landscape

Naman Kumar Agrawal, Rajeev Kumar, and Himanshu Kumar Agrawal

14.1 INTRODUCTION

A diverse and populous country, India has made significant advances in various fields, including technology, education, and economic growth. However, the healthcare industry continues to encounter various obstacles in providing high-quality treatment to its residents. With a population of over 1.4 billion people [1], the demand for healthcare services is enormous, and the present infrastructure is struggling to meet the people's demands. The Indian healthcare system has inadequate infrastructure; a shortage of competent workers; limited access to medical services, particularly in rural regions; and a high burden of communicable and non-communicable diseases.

In recent years, the advent of AI and robotics has shown immense potential in revolutionising the healthcare landscape in India. These technologies can transform healthcare delivery, making it more accessible, affordable, and efficient. By leveraging AI and robotics, India can address the challenges in its healthcare sector and pave the way for a brighter, healthier future for its citizens.

The potential of AI and robotics in healthcare is vast, ranging from diagnostics and telemedicine to drug discovery and precision medicine. These technologies can help bridge the gap between urban and rural healthcare, improve the quality of care, and enable personalised treatments for patients with chronic conditions. Moreover, AI and robotics can drive research and innovation in healthcare, leading to the development of novel treatments and therapies.

This introduction aims to provide an overview of the role of AI and robotics in transforming healthcare in the Indian context. It will discuss the factors that have contributed to the growing interest in these technologies, the key players in the Indian AI and robotics healthcare ecosystem, and the potential impact of these technologies on various aspects of healthcare.

14.1.1 Factors Contributing to the Growing Interest in AI and Robotics in Indian Healthcare

Several factors contribute to the growing interest in AI and robotics in Indian healthcare. Here are some key factors:

- **Rising Healthcare Demands:** With a growing population and increasing healthcare needs, there is a demand for more efficient and effective healthcare services. AI and robotics offer the potential to improve diagnosis, treatment, and patient care, leading to better healthcare outcomes.

DOI: 10.1201/9781003451846-14

- **Shortage of Healthcare Professionals:** India faces a shortage of healthcare professionals, especially in rural and remote areas. AI and robotics can help bridge this gap by providing automated and remote healthcare solutions, enabling access to quality healthcare services where medical professionals are scarce.
- **Data Availability and Digitisation:** The digitisation of healthcare data and the availability of large amounts of healthcare data have created opportunities for AI and robotics applications. These technologies can analyse vast amounts of data, identify patterns, and generate insights supporting clinical decision-making and personalised healthcare.
- **Government Initiatives and Support:** The government of India has recognised the potential of AI and robotics in healthcare and has launched various initiatives to promote their adoption. These initiatives include policy support, funding programs, and collaborations with industry and academia to drive research and innovation in healthcare technologies.
- **Industry Investments and Collaborations:** Both domestic and international companies are investing in AI and robotics for healthcare applications in India. Collaborations between healthcare providers, technology companies, and research institutions are leading to the development of innovative solutions and driving the adoption of these technologies in the healthcare sector.
- **Patient-Centric Care:** The focus on patient-centric care and personalised medicine drives the interest in AI and robotics. These technologies can enable better understanding of patient needs, facilitate precision medicine, and improve patient outcomes by tailoring treatments to individual characteristics.
- **Need for Cost-Effective Solutions:** The high cost of healthcare services is a significant barrier to access for many Indians. AI and robotics have the potential to reduce costs by automating routine tasks, improving efficiency, and enabling more accurate diagnoses and treatments.
- **Increasing Prevalence of Chronic Diseases:** India is witnessing a rise in the prevalence of chronic diseases, such as diabetes, cardiovascular diseases, and cancer. AI and robotics can play a crucial role in the early detection, management, and treatment of these conditions, ultimately reducing the burden on the healthcare system.
- **Technological Advancements:** Rapid advancements in AI and robotics technologies have made them more accessible and affordable, leading to increased interest in their applications in healthcare. This has opened opportunities for innovation and the development of new solutions to address healthcare challenges.
- **Rise of Digital Health:** The increasing adoption of digital technologies in healthcare, such as electronic health records, telemedicine, and mobile health applications, has created a conducive environment for the integration of AI and robotics.

Overall, the growing interest in AI and robotics in Indian healthcare is driven by technological advancements, healthcare demands, shortage of healthcare professionals, data availability, government support, industry investments, and the need for patient-centric care. These factors collectively contribute to the development and adoption of AI and robotics solutions, transforming healthcare delivery and improving patient outcomes in India.

14.1.2 Key Players in the Indian AI and Robotics Healthcare Ecosystem

A wide range of actors, including startups, well-established businesses, research institutions, and government efforts, make up the Indian AI and robotics healthcare ecosystem. Startups, well-established businesses, research facilities, government programmes, non-governmental organisations, and multi-lateral organisations are a few of the ecosystem's major actors. In this chapter, we shall cover the specifics of these important payers in detail with examples.

14.1.3 Potential Impact of AI and Robotics on Indian Healthcare

AI and robotics have the potential to transform various aspects of healthcare in India, such as:

- **Accessibility and affordability:** By automating routine tasks, improving efficiency, and enabling more accurate diagnoses and treatments, AI and robotics can help make healthcare services more accessible and affordable for the masses.
- **Quality of care:** AI and robotics can improve the quality of care by reducing errors, enhancing decision-making, and enabling personalised treatments for patients with chronic conditions.
- **Healthcare workforce:** The integration of AI and robotics in healthcare can create new job opportunities and require upskilling and reskilling of the existing workforce.
- **Research and innovation:** AI and robotics can drive research and innovation in healthcare, leading to the development of novel treatments and therapies.
- **Global collaboration:** India can collaborate with other countries and international organisations in developing and deploying AI and robotics in healthcare, positioning itself as a global leader in this field.

14.2 THE EMERGENCE OF AI AND ROBOTICS IN INDIAN HEALTHCARE

The emergence of AI and robotics in Indian healthcare is a relatively recent phenomenon, but it has already shown immense potential in transforming the sector. The use of AI and robotics in healthcare is not new, but the advancements in technology and the increasing availability of data have made it more accessible and affordable. In India, the adoption of AI and robotics in healthcare has been driven by several factors, including the need for cost-effective solutions, the rise of digital health, the increasing prevalence of chronic diseases, and government initiatives.

14.2.1 Need for Cost-Effective Solutions

The high cost of healthcare services is a significant barrier to access for many Indians. According to the Economic Survey of India 2022–23, the total health expenditure of India stands at only 3.2% of its GDP [2], which is much lower than the global average of 10.89% in 2020 [3]. This low spending has resulted in inadequate infrastructure; a shortage of skilled professionals; and limited access to medical facilities, especially in rural areas. AI and robotics have the potential to reduce costs by automating routine tasks, improving efficiency, and enabling more accurate diagnoses and treatments.

For example, AI algorithms can analyse medical images, such as X-rays, CT scans, and MRIs, for early detection of diseases like cancer, tuberculosis, and diabetic retinopathy. This can reduce the need for expensive and time-consuming manual analysis by radiologists and improve the accuracy of diagnoses. Similarly, robotics-assisted surgery can enhance precision, reduce complications, and improve patient outcomes, ultimately reducing the cost of healthcare services.

14.2.2 Rise of Digital Health

The increasing adoption of digital technologies in healthcare, such as electronic health records, telemedicine, and mobile health applications, has created a conducive environment for the integration of AI and robotics. Digital health has enabled the collection and analysis of vast amounts of data, which can be used to train AI algorithms and develop predictive models for disease diagnosis and treatment.

Telemedicine, in particular, has emerged as a promising application of AI and robotics in Indian healthcare. The deployment of AI-powered chatbots and virtual assistants can provide remote consultations, triage, and follow-up care, bridging the gap between urban and rural healthcare. This can improve access to healthcare services for millions of Indians who live in remote areas and have limited access to medical facilities.

14.2.3 Increasing Prevalence of Chronic Diseases

India is witnessing a rise in the prevalence of chronic diseases, such as diabetes, cardiovascular diseases, and cancer. Non-communicable diseases (NCDs) are a contributor to the overall disease burden in India, and their management requires long-term care and monitoring. Per the Indian Council of Medical Research (ICMR), it is estimated that the proportion of deaths due to non-communicable Diseases in India has increased from 37.9% in 1990 to 61.8% in 2016 [4].

AI and robotics can play a crucial role in the early detection, management, and treatment of these conditions, ultimately reducing the burden on the healthcare system. For example, precision medicine, which involves using AI to analyse genetic, environmental, and lifestyle data to develop personalised treatment plans for patients with chronic conditions, can improve the effectiveness of treatments and reduce the risk of adverse events.

14.2.4 Government Initiatives

The government of India has recognised the transformative potential of artificial intelligence (AI) and robotics in healthcare and has taken several initiatives to promote their adoption. These initiatives aim to leverage AI and robotics technologies to improve healthcare delivery, enhance patient outcomes, and address healthcare challenges. Here are some key government initiatives for AI and robotics in healthcare in India:

- **National Health Policy 2017:** The National Health Policy 2017 by the government of India [5] emphasises the need to leverage technology, including AI and robotics, to improve healthcare delivery. The policy recognises the potential of these technologies to improve diagnosis, treatment, and patient outcomes. It also highlights the need for research and development in this field and encourages collaboration between the government, industry, and academia to promote innovation in healthcare.
- **National Strategy for Artificial Intelligence:** The National Strategy for Artificial Intelligence [6] aims to leverage AI to improve disease diagnosis, drug discovery, and personalised medicine. It also emphasises the need for data privacy and security in healthcare and encourages collaboration between the government, industry, and academia to promote innovation in this field. It also highlights the importance of developing a skilled workforce to support the growth of AI and robotics in healthcare.
- **National Digital Health Mission:** The National Digital Health Mission (NDHM) aims to leverage technology, including AI and robotics, to improve healthcare delivery and access [7]. The mission aims to create a digital health ecosystem that will enable the seamless exchange of health data between patients, healthcare providers, and other stakeholders. The NDHM also emphasises the need for data privacy and security in healthcare and encourages the development of AI-powered tools for disease diagnosis and treatment. The mission aims to improve the quality of care provided and to make healthcare more accessible and affordable for all.
- **Atal Innovation Mission:** The Atal Innovation Mission (AIM) is an initiative of NITI Aayog to promote innovation and entrepreneurship in India [8]. It has established Atal Incubation Centres that support startups working on AI and robotics solutions in healthcare. AIM provides funding, mentorship, and networking opportunities to these startups.

These government initiatives are driving the adoption of AI and robotics in healthcare, fostering innovation, and creating an ecosystem for collaboration between government, academia, and industry. They are transforming the Indian healthcare landscape by leveraging the potential of AI and robotics to improve healthcare access, delivery, and outcomes for the benefit of the population.

14.2.5 Key Players in the Indian AI and Robotics Healthcare Ecosystem

The Indian AI and robotics healthcare ecosystem comprises a diverse range of players, including startups, established companies, research institutions, and government initiatives. Key players in the Indian AI and robotics healthcare ecosystem include:

- **Startups:** Several Indian startups are working on innovative AI and robotics solutions for healthcare. A few examples include:
  - **Niramai Health Analytix:** Niramai Health Analytix uses AI and machine learning to develop automated solutions for critical healthcare problems [9]. Their flagship product, Thermalytix, is a non-invasive, painless, and radiation-free computer-aided diagnostic engine that uses thermal sensing and cloud-hosted analytics to detect breast cancer at an early stage.
  - **SigTuple:** SigTuple uses AI and machine learning to develop automated solutions for medical diagnosis. Their flagship product, AI100, is a cloud-hosted platform that uses computer vision and machine learning to analyse medical images and videos for diagnosis [10]. SigTuple has conducted clinical trials and partnered with several hospitals and diagnostic centres in India to deploy their solutions.
  - **HealthifyMe:** HealthifyMe is an Indian digital health and wellness company that provides an app for calorie tracking, nutrition, and fitness advice [11]. The app offers personalised diet plans and workout routines created by an AI-driven digital nutritionist.
  - **Onco.com:** Onco.com is a Bangalore-based startup that provides an online platform for cancer care advisory services using AI-driven algorithms and expert oncologists [12]. The platform offers personalised treatment plans, remote consultations with oncologists, and access to a network of cancer care providers.
  - **mfine:** mfine is an AI-powered on-demand healthcare startup that provides customers with access to online appointments and hospital-based linked healthcare [13]. Their platform enables rapid and ongoing communication with top doctors in the best hospitals, making use of cutting-edge technology to keep track of health indicators and keep all health data under control and accessible.
- **Established companies:** Major technology companies, such as Wipro, Tata Consultancy Services, and Infosys, are also investing in AI and robotics for healthcare in India. These companies are collaborating with hospitals, research institutions, and government agencies to develop and deploy AI and robotics solutions.
  - **Wipro:** With Wipro's AI- and ML-based platforms, organisations can improve their approaches to drug discoveries, genetics research, and patient diagnoses [14]. With their autonomous robotics solutions, care providers can complete essential patient-monitoring tasks that ensure safety and accuracy, as well as benefit from self-driving bots that handle drug deliveries and Covid-related sanitisation tasks.
  - **Tata Consultancy Services (TCS):** TCS has developed several AI and robotics solutions for the healthcare industry including a cognitive assistant application for personalised healthcare [15], a teleoperated humanoid robot nurse named Asha [16], and a pharmacogenomics and AI-powered future for managed care [17].
  - **Infosys:** Infosys Nia for healthcare is an AI-powered platform that uses machine learning and natural language processing to automate tasks such as claims processing, medical coding, and fraud detection [18]. The platform also provides predictive analytics and insights to help healthcare organisations improve patient outcomes and reduce costs. Nia for healthcare is designed to help healthcare providers streamline their operations and improve the quality of care they provide to patients.
- **Research institutions:** Indian research institutions, such as the Indian Institutes of Technology (IITs) and the Indian Institute of Science (IISc), are conducting cutting-edge

research in AI and robotics for healthcare. These institutions are also collaborating with industry partners and international organisations to advance the development and adoption of these technologies.

- **Indian Institute of Technologies:** IITs have developed AI and robotics applications for healthcare, including an AI-powered diagnostic tool for tuberculosis, a robotic exoskeleton for stroke patient rehabilitation, an AI-powered tool for diabetic retinopathy, and a robotic system for minimally invasive surgery. They are actively involved in research and development in this field and is working on several other projects as well. Some examples are:
- **AI-powered diagnostic tool for tuberculosis:** Researchers at IIT Delhi have developed an AI-powered diagnostic tool for tuberculosis that can analyse chest X-rays and provide accurate results in just a few seconds [19].
- **Robotic exoskeleton for rehabilitation:** Researchers at IIT Hyderabad have developed a robotic exoskeleton that can help stroke patients with their rehabilitation [20]. The exoskeleton provides support to the patient's arm and helps them perform exercises to improve their motor function.
- **Robotic surgery:** Researchers at IIT Madras have developed a robotic system for minimally invasive surgery [21]. The system uses a combination of robotics and AI to provide surgeons with greater precision and control during surgery.
- **Indian Institute of Science:** ARTPARK is a non-profit organisation promoted by the Indian Institute of Science that aims to foster innovations in AI and robotics. One of its key areas of focus is healthcare, where it seeks to develop solutions that can improve the lives of people [22]. ARTPARK is working on creating language data and AI that understands all Indians so that Digital India is inclusive. It has also launched Project Vaani, a pan-India inclusive language data initiative for open-sourcing datasets, which will amplify the Indian government's Digital India efforts by including more diverse regional and local languages [23]. With more than 150,000 hours of curated speech and 100 million phrases of text in Indian scripts, it will expand the size and diversity of India's open-source language data.

- **Government initiatives:** The Indian government has launched various initiatives to promote AI and robotics in healthcare, such as the National Health Policy 2017, the National Digital Health Mission, and the National Artificial Intelligence Mission. These initiatives aim to create a conducive environment for the development and adoption of AI and robotics in healthcare by providing funding, infrastructure, and policy support.

These are just a few examples of the key players in the Indian AI and robotics healthcare ecosystem, with many more startups, companies, research institutions, and organisations contributing to the advancement and adoption of AI and robotics in healthcare.

14.3 AI AND ROBOTICS APPLICATIONS IN INDIAN HEALTHCARE

The integration of AI and robotics in Indian healthcare has led to the development of various applications that have the potential to revolutionise the sector. These applications span different areas of healthcare, such as diagnostics, treatment, patient care, and research. In this section, we will explore some of the most promising AI and robotics applications in Indian healthcare.

14.3.1 Diagnostics

AI-powered diagnostics have emerged as a game-changer in Indian healthcare, enabling faster and more accurate detection of diseases. By analysing medical images and other data, AI algorithms can identify patterns and anomalies that may be indicative of a disease, even at its early stages. Some of the key AI-driven diagnostic applications in Indian healthcare include:

1. **Medical Imaging:** AI algorithms can analyse medical images, such as X-rays, CT scans, and MRIs, to detect diseases like cancer, tuberculosis, and diabetic retinopathy. Synapsica Healthcare is an Indian AI startup that focuses on medical imaging and radiology [24]. They develop solutions to improve the accuracy and efficiency of radiology diagnostics. Their AI-powered platform, Synapsica, uses deep learning algorithms to analyse medical images and provide insights to radiologists. The platform can assist in the diagnosis of various medical conditions, including cancer, heart disease, and neurological disorders.
2. **Pathology:** AI can also be used to analyse pathology samples, such as blood, tissue, and cell samples, to detect diseases and abnormalities. AIRA by AIRA Matrix is an AI-powered medical imaging platform that uses deep learning algorithms to analyse medical images and provide insights to healthcare professionals [25]. The platform can assist in the diagnosis of various medical conditions, including cancer, heart disease, and neurological disorders.
3. **Genomics:** AI can be used to analyse genomic data to identify genetic mutations and variations associated with diseases. This can help in the early detection of genetic disorders and the development of personalised treatment plans. MedGenome specialises in providing genomic testing and personalised medicine services using AI and machine learning. They offer a range of services, including genetic testing, cancer genomics, and rare disease diagnosis [26]. MedGenome's proprietary technology platform, OncoMD, is a comprehensive cancer genomics knowledgebase that helps clinicians in diagnosis and treatment.

14.3.2 Treatment

AI and robotics have the potential to revolutionise the way treatments are administered in Indian healthcare. From personalised medicine to robotics-assisted surgery, these technologies can improve the effectiveness of treatments and reduce the risk of complications. Some of the key AI and robotics applications in treatment include:

1. **Personalised Medicine:** AI can be used to analyse genetic, environmental, and lifestyle data to develop personalised treatment plans for patients with chronic conditions. This can improve the effectiveness of treatments and reduce the risk of adverse events.
2. **Robotics-Assisted Surgery:** Robotics-assisted surgery can enhance precision, reduce complications, and improve patient outcomes. Comofi Robotic Surgery by Comofi Medtech uses AI and robotics to assist surgeons in performing minimally invasive surgeries [27]. The platform can perform complex surgical procedures with high precision and accuracy, reducing the risk of complications and improving patient outcomes.
3. **Drug Discovery:** AI can be used to accelerate the drug discovery process by analysing vast amounts of data and identifying potential drug candidates. Peptris is an Indian biotech startup that uses AI and machine learning to develop peptide-based therapeutics. They have developed a proprietary platform that uses AI to design and optimise peptides for drug discovery [28]. Their platform can predict the binding affinity of peptides to target proteins and optimise their pharmacokinetic properties.

14.3.3 Patient Care

AI and robotics can play a crucial role in improving patient care in Indian healthcare. From remote monitoring to virtual assistants, these technologies can enhance the quality of care and reduce the burden on healthcare professionals. Some of the key AI and robotics applications in patient care include:

1. **Remote Monitoring:** AI-powered remote monitoring solutions can help healthcare professionals track patients' vital signs and health parameters in real time, enabling early intervention in case of abnormalities. AI Health Highway India, also known as AiSteth, can record, store, and share heart/lung sounds from patients in villages/PHCs or elderly patients at home in cities and enable remote monitoring or tele-consultation with specialists who are based in cities or tertiary care hospitals [29]. This could facilitate screening, early detection, and/or better follow up for a specific subset of cardiovascular disorders.
2. **Virtual Assistants:** AI-powered virtual assistants can provide remote consultations, triage, and follow-up care, bridging the gap between urban and rural healthcare. Octopus Tech has revolutionised the healthcare industry with its advanced virtual assistant for doctors. Designed to streamline medical practices and enhance efficiency, this cutting-edge AI-powered solution seamlessly integrates with existing systems to provide doctors with personalised assistance. From appointment scheduling and patient management to medical record organisation and data analysis, the Octopus Tech virtual assistant empowers doctors to focus on delivering optimal patient care while optimising their workflows and improving overall productivity [30].
3. **Robotics-Assisted Rehabilitation:** Robotics can be used to assist patients in their rehabilitation process, helping them regain their mobility and independence. Astrek Innovations has developed solutions for disability and rehabilitation [31].

14.3.4 Research

AI and robotics can drive research and innovation in Indian healthcare by enabling the analysis of vast amounts of data and developing new technologies. Some of the key AI and robotics applications in research include:

1. **Clinical Trials:** AI can be used to optimise clinical trial design, patient recruitment, and data analysis, reducing the time and cost of bringing new drugs and therapies to market.
2. **Predictive Analytics:** AI-powered predictive analytics can help healthcare professionals identify trends and patterns in patient data, enabling early intervention and better disease management. SiCureMi uses real time data analytics to enable patients to be health aware and smarter about their own health, provides personalised guidance, and minimises the risk of lifestyle diseases [32]. SiCureMi is a med-tech startup which aims to develop an Intelligent Self Care product for patients providing personalised care using predictive analytics from their medical records and IoT data.
3. **Medical Research:** AI can be used to analyse vast amounts of medical literature and data, identifying new insights and opportunities for research. Indian research institutions, such as the Indian Institutes of Technology and the Indian Institute of Science, are using AI to advance research in various areas of healthcare, including genomics, neuroscience, and drug discovery.

14.4 CHALLENGES AND ETHICAL CONSIDERATIONS

While AI and robotics can potentially revolutionise Indian healthcare, their adoption and implementation come with several challenges and ethical considerations. In this section, we will discuss some of the key challenges and ethical concerns associated with the use of AI and robotics in Indian healthcare.

14.4.1 Challenges

The integration of AI and robotics in Indian healthcare faces several challenges, including inadequate infrastructure, a shortage of skilled professionals, data privacy concerns, and regulatory hurdles. Addressing these challenges is crucial to fully realise the potential of these technologies in transforming the sector.

1. **Inadequate Infrastructure:** The lack of adequate infrastructure, such as high-speed internet connectivity, advanced medical equipment, and reliable power supply, can hinder the adoption of AI and robotics in Indian healthcare, particularly in rural areas. To overcome this challenge, the government and private sector need to invest in building and upgrading healthcare infrastructure across the country.
2. **Shortage of Skilled Professionals:** The successful implementation of AI and robotics in healthcare requires skilled professionals who can develop, deploy, and maintain these technologies. However, India faces a shortage of skilled AI, robotics, and healthcare professionals. To address this challenge, the government and educational institutions need to invest in training and skill development programs to create a workforce capable of harnessing the potential of AI and robotics in healthcare.
3. **Data Privacy Concerns:** The use of AI and robotics in healthcare involves the collection, storage, and analysis of vast amounts of sensitive patient data. This raises concerns about data privacy and security, particularly in the context of India's evolving data protection regulations. To address these concerns, healthcare providers and technology companies need to implement robust data security measures and adhere to data protection regulations.
4. **Regulatory Hurdles:** The regulatory environment for AI and robotics in Indian healthcare is still evolving, with the government working on developing guidelines and standards for the use of these technologies. Navigating the regulatory landscape can be challenging for healthcare providers and technology companies, particularly without clear guidelines and standards. To overcome this challenge, the government needs to establish a clear regulatory framework that promotes innovation while ensuring patient safety and ethical considerations.

14.4.2 Ethical Considerations

The use of AI and robotics in healthcare raises several ethical concerns, such as algorithmic bias, transparency, accountability, and the potential impact on the doctor–patient relationship. Addressing these ethical considerations is crucial to ensure the responsible and ethical use of AI and robotics in Indian healthcare.

1. **Algorithmic Bias:** AI algorithms are trained on large datasets, and their performance depends on the quality and representativeness of the data. If the training data is biased or unrepresentative, the AI algorithms can perpetuate and amplify these biases, leading to unfair and discriminatory outcomes. To address this concern, healthcare providers and technology companies need to ensure that the data used to train AI algorithms is diverse, representative, and free from biases.
2. **Transparency:** The use of AI and robotics in healthcare can sometimes result in "black box" decision-making, where the rationale behind the AI's decisions is not easily understandable by humans. This lack of transparency can raise concerns about trust and accountability, particularly in the context of medical decision-making. To address this concern, healthcare providers and technology companies need to develop explainable AI algorithms that can provide insights into their decision-making processes.

3. **Accountability:** The use of AI and robotics in healthcare raises questions about accountability and responsibility, particularly in cases where the AI's decisions result in adverse outcomes. Determining who is responsible for the AI's actions—the healthcare provider, the technology company, or the AI itself—can be challenging. To address this concern, the government needs to establish clear guidelines and regulations that define the roles and responsibilities of different stakeholders in the AI and robotics ecosystem.
4. **Impact on Doctor–Patient Relationship:** The integration of AI and robotics in healthcare can potentially impact the doctor–patient relationship, as patients may feel less connected to their healthcare providers when interacting with AI-powered systems. To address this concern, healthcare providers need to strike a balance between leveraging AI and robotics to improve efficiency and maintain a human touch in their interactions with patients.

14.5 THE FUTURE OF AI AND ROBOTICS IN INDIAN HEALTHCARE

The future of AI and robotics in Indian healthcare looks promising, with the potential to transform the sector by improving diagnostics, treatment, patient care, and research. In this section, we will explore some key trends and developments likely to shape the future of AI and robotics in Indian healthcare.

14.5.1 Key Trends and Developments

Several trends and developments are expected to drive the adoption of AI and robotics in Indian healthcare, including advancements in technology, increased investment, and supportive government policies.

These factors are likely to create a conducive environment for the growth and development of AI and robotics in the sector.

1. **Advancements in Technology:** Rapid advancements in AI and robotics technologies, such as machine learning, natural language processing, computer vision, and sensor technology, are expected to drive their adoption in Indian healthcare. These advancements will enable the development of more sophisticated and effective AI and robotics applications, addressing the complex challenges faced by the healthcare sector.
2. **Increased Investment:** The growing interest in AI and robotics in Indian healthcare is attracting significant investment from both domestic and international investors. This increased investment is expected to fuel innovation and the development of new AI and robotics applications, driving their adoption in the sector.
3. **Supportive Government Policies:** The Indian government has created several regulations and efforts to encourage the adoption of AI and robotics because it recognises their potential to alter the healthcare industry. These include the National Health Policy, the National Digital Health Mission, and the National Strategy for Artificial Intelligence. The expansion and development of AI and robots in Indian healthcare is anticipated to be supported by these policies and initiatives.

14.5.2 Emerging Applications

As AI and robotics technologies continue to advance, new applications are likely to emerge in Indian healthcare, addressing unmet needs and creating new opportunities for growth and innovation. Some of the emerging applications include:

1. **AI-Powered Telemedicine:** Telemedicine has gained significant traction in India, particularly in the wake of the COVID-19 pandemic. AI-powered telemedicine platforms can enhance the quality and accessibility of healthcare services by providing remote

consultations, triage, and follow-up care. These platforms can also leverage AI algorithms to analyse patient data and provide personalised treatment recommendations, improving the effectiveness of care.

2. **Robotics-Assisted Home Healthcare:** As the demand for home healthcare services grows in India, robotics-assisted home healthcare solutions can help address the challenges associated with providing care in the home setting. These solutions can include robotics-assisted monitoring, medication management, and rehabilitation, enabling patients to receive high-quality care in the comfort of their homes.
3. **AI-Enabled Preventive Healthcare:** AI can play a crucial role in preventive healthcare by analysing patient data and identifying risk factors for various diseases. AI-powered preventive healthcare solutions can help healthcare providers develop personalised intervention strategies, promoting healthy behaviours and reducing the risk of disease.
4. **Robotics in Emergency Medicine:** Robotics can be used to enhance the delivery of emergency medical services, particularly in remote and underserved areas. For example, drones can be used to deliver essential medical supplies, such as blood, vaccines, and medications, to remote locations. Robotics-assisted emergency response systems can also be used to provide remote consultations and triage in emergency situations, improving the quality and timeliness of care.

14.5.3 Potential Impact on Indian Healthcare

The adoption of AI and robotics in Indian healthcare has the potential to create a significant impact on the sector, addressing some of the key challenges faced by the country's healthcare system. Some of the potential impacts include:

1. **Improved Access to Healthcare:** AI and robotics can help bridge the gap between urban and rural healthcare in India by providing remote consultations, diagnostics, and treatment services. This can improve access to healthcare services for millions of Indians living in remote and underserved areas, reducing health disparities and improving overall health outcomes.
2. **Enhanced Quality of Care:** AI and robotics can enhance the quality of care in Indian healthcare by improving the accuracy of diagnoses, personalising treatment plans, and reducing the risk of complications. This can lead to better health outcomes for patients and a more efficient healthcare system.
3. **Cost Reduction:** The adoption of AI and robotics in Indian healthcare can help reduce costs by streamlining processes, improving resource utilisation, and reducing the need for expensive medical equipment and infrastructure. This can make healthcare services more affordable and accessible for the Indian population.
4. **Increased Focus on Preventive Healthcare:** AI and robotics can enable a shift from reactive to preventive healthcare in India by identifying risk factors and promoting early intervention. This can help reduce the burden of chronic diseases and improve the overall health of the population.

14.6 CONCLUSION

AI and robotics in healthcare have been gaining momentum in recent years, and India is no exception. With a population of over 1.4 billion [1], India faces significant challenges in providing quality healthcare to all its citizens. The country has a shortage of healthcare professionals, particularly in rural areas, and faces a high burden of communicable and non-communicable diseases. In this context, AI and robotics have the potential to revolutionise healthcare delivery in India, improving access, efficiency, and quality of care.

AI refers to the ability of machines to perform tasks that typically require human intelligence, such as learning, reasoning, and problem-solving. In healthcare, AI can be used for a range of applications, including medical imaging, drug discovery, clinical decision-making, and patient monitoring. For example, AI algorithms can analyse medical images to detect abnormalities and assist radiologists in making diagnoses. They can also analyse patient data to identify patterns and predict outcomes, helping clinicians make more informed treatment decisions.

Robotics, on the other hand, refers to the use of machines to perform tasks that are typically performed by humans. In healthcare, robotics can be used for a range of applications, including surgery, rehabilitation, and patient care. For example, surgical robots can assist surgeons in performing minimally invasive procedures, reducing the risk of complications and improving patient outcomes. They can also be used for telemedicine, allowing healthcare professionals to remotely monitor and care for patients in remote or underserved areas.

In India, the use of AI and robotics in healthcare is still in its early stages, but there are several promising initiatives underway. The government has taken significant initiatives to foster the adoption of these technologies, including the National Strategy for Artificial Intelligence, which aims to leverage AI in healthcare for improved diagnostics, treatment, and healthcare delivery. Private-sector companies and startups are at the forefront of this transformation, developing innovative solutions such as AI-powered diagnostic tools, robotic surgical systems, and telemedicine platforms. Research institutions and academia are actively engaged in advancing AI and robotics in healthcare through groundbreaking research, collaborations, and knowledge dissemination. Together, these stakeholders are driving the transformation of the Indian healthcare landscape, harnessing the power of AI and robotics to revolutionise patient care, enhance efficiency, and improve health outcomes.

Despite these promising initiatives, there are several challenges that need to be addressed to realise the full potential of AI and robotics in healthcare in India. One of the biggest challenges is the lack of data. While India has a large population, there is a shortage of high-quality health data, particularly in rural areas. This makes it difficult to develop AI algorithms that are accurate and effective. There is also a need for more investment in research and development, particularly in the development of indigenous technologies that are tailored to the needs of the Indian healthcare system.

The adoption of AI and robotics in Indian healthcare comes with several challenges and ethical considerations that need to be addressed to fully realise the potential of these technologies. By investing in infrastructure, skill development, data security, and establishing clear regulatory and ethical guidelines, India can overcome these challenges and harness the power of AI and robotics to transform its healthcare sector. In doing so, the country can improve the lives of its citizens by providing better health outcomes, reduced costs, and increased access to healthcare services.

Another challenge is the need for regulatory frameworks to ensure the safety and efficacy of AI and robotics in healthcare. While there are some regulations in place, they are often outdated and do not take into account the unique challenges posed by AI and robotics. There is a need for more robust regulations that ensure the ethical use of AI and robotics in healthcare, protect patient privacy, and promote transparency and accountability.

In conclusion, the use of AI and robotics in healthcare has the potential to revolutionise healthcare delivery in India, improving access, efficiency, and quality of care. While there are several promising initiatives underway, there are also several challenges that need to be addressed to realise the full potential of these technologies. With the right investments in research and development, regulatory frameworks, and data infrastructure, India can become a leader in the use of AI and robotics in healthcare, improving the health and well-being of its citizens and setting an example for the rest of the world.

REFERENCES

[1] The Times of India, "India's 1.4 Billion Population Could Become World Economy's New Growth Engine," 23 January 2023. [Online]. Available: https://timesofindia.indiatimes.com/business/india-business/indias-1-4-billion-population-could-become-world-economys-new-growth-engine/articleshow/97239739.cms [Accessed 23 June 2023].

[2] Department of Economic Affairs, "Economic Survey of India," Department of Economic Affairs, New Delhi, 2023.

[3] World Bank, "Current Health Expenditure (% of GDP)," 23 June 2023. [Online]. Available: https://data.worldbank.org/indicator/SH.XPD.CHEX.GD.ZS [Accessed 23 June 2023].

[4] Ministry of Health and Family Welfare, "Status of Non-Communicable Diseases (NCDs) in India," 8 February 2022. [Online]. Available: https://pib.gov.in/PressReleaseIframePage.aspx?PRID=1796435.

[5] Ministry of Health and Family Welfare, "National Health Policy 2017," 2017. [Online]. Available: https://main.mohfw.gov.in/sites/default/files/9147562941489753121.pdf [Accessed 23 June 2023].

[6] NITI Aayog, "National Strategy for Artificial Intelligence," June 2018. [Online]. Available: https://niti.gov.in/sites/default/files/2019-01/NationalStrategy-for-AI-Discussion-Paper.pdf [Accessed 23 June 2023].

[7] Ministry of Health and Family Welfare, "National Digital Health Blueprint," 2019. [Online]. Available: https://abdm.gov.in:8081/uploads/ndhb_1_56ec695bc8.pdf [Accessed 23 June 2023].

[8] NITI Aayog, "Atal Innovation Mission," 2023. [Online]. Available: https://aim.gov.in [Accessed 23 June 2023].

[9] Niramai, "Novel Breast Cancer Screening Solution," 2023. [Online]. Available: www.niramai.com/ [Accessed 23 June 2023].

[10] SigTuple, 2023. [Online]. Available: https://sigtuple.com/ [Accessed 23 June 2023].

[11] HealthifyMe, "A Connected Fitness Ecosystem," 2023. [Online]. Available: www.healthifyme.com/in/ [Accessed 23 June 2023].

[12] Onco, 2023. [Online]. Available: https://onco.com/ [Accessed 23 June 2023].

[13] mfine, "Consult Doctor Online," 2023. [Online]. Available: www.mfine.co/ [Accessed 23 June 2023].

[14] Wipro, "Transforming Healthcare with Autonomous Technologies," 2023. [Online]. Available: www.wipro.com/engineering/transforming-healthcare-with-autonomous-technologies/ [Accessed 23 June 2023].

[15] TATA Consultancy Services, "TCS Cognitive Assistant Application for Personalised Healthcare." [Online]. Available: www.tcs.com/what-we-do/industries/healthcare/solution/cognitive-assistant-personalized-healthcare-services [Accessed 23 June 2023].

[16] TATA Consultancy Services, "Asha: A Humanoid Caregiving Robot." [Online]. Available: www.tcs.com/what-we-do/research/article/asha-teleoperated-humanoid-robot-nurse [Accessed 23 June 2023].

[17] TATA Consultancy Services, "Pharmacogenomics and the AI-Powered Future for Managed Care." [Online]. Available: www.tcs.com/what-we-do/industries/healthcare/white-paper/pharmacogenomics-ai-healthcare-personalized-treatment [Accessed 23 June 2023].

[18] Infosys, "AI Led Automation for Healthacre Enterprise," 2017. [Online]. Available: www.infosys.com/industries/healthcare/white-papers/documents/ai-led-automation.pdf [Accessed 23 June 2023].

[19] The Times of India, "IIT-Delhi Researchers Develop AI-Based Detector for Malaria, TB, Cervical Cancer," 26 March 2019. [Online]. Available: https://timesofindia.indiatimes.com/home/science/iit-delhi-researchers-develop-ai-based-detector-for-malaria-tb-cervical-cancer/articleshow/68580014.cms [Accessed 23 June 2023].

[20] The Times of India, "IIT-H Incubated Startup Develops 'Gamified Arm Rehabilitation Device' for Stroke Victims," 25 March 2019. [Online]. Available: https://timesofindia.indiatimes.com/education/news/iit-h-incubated-startup-develops-gamified-arm-rehabilitation-device-for-stroke-victims/articleshow/68562803.cms [Accessed 23 June 2023].

[21] India Times, "IIT Madras Builds India's 1st Spine-Surgery Robot for Cheap and Painless Medical Procedure," 28 August 2019. [Online]. Available: www.indiatimes.com/technology/news/iit-madras-builds-india-s-1st-spine-surgery-robot-for-cheap-and-painless-medical-procedure-374503.html [Accessed 23 June 2023].

[22] ARTPARK, "ARTPARK," 2023. [Online]. Available: www.artpark.in/ [Accessed 23 June 2023].

[23] ARTPARK, "Project Vaani," 2022. [Online]. Available: https://vaani.iisc.ac.in/ [Accessed 23 June 2023].

[24] Synapsica, 2022. [Online]. Available: https://synapsica.com/ [Accessed 23 June 2023].

[25] AIRA Matrix, "AIRA MATRIX—Digital Intelligence," 2021. [Online]. Available: www.airamatrix.com/ [Accessed 23 June 2023].

[26] MedGenome, "MedGenome Launches AI-Enabled VarMiner to Detect Genetic Variants for Rare Diseases, Inherited Cancers FE Healthcare," 12 April 2022. [Online]. Available: https://diagnostics.medgenome.com/media_news/medgenome-launches-ai-enabled-varminer-to-detect-genetic-variants-for-rare-diseases-inherited-cancers-fe-healthcare/ [Accessed 23 June 2023].

[27] Comofi Medtech, 2020. [Online]. Available: www.comofimedtech.com/ [Accessed 23 June 2023].
[28] Peptris, "Peptris: AI Plays Tetris with Proteins," 2023. [Online]. Available: www.peptris.com/ [Accessed 23 June 2023].
[29] AiSteth, "AiSteth—Smart Stethoscope," 2023. [Online]. Available: https://aisteth.com/ [Accessed 23 June 2023].
[30] OctopusTech, "Virtual Assistants for Doctors," 2018. [Online]. Available: www.theoctopustech.com/virtual-assistant-for-doctors/ [Accessed 23 June 2023].
[31] Astrek Innovations, "Take Your First Steps, Again!," 2023. [Online]. Available: https://astrekinnovations.com/ [Accessed 23 June 2023].
[32] SiCureMi Health Care Technologies, "SiCureMi—Signature Cure using Medical Intelligence," 2019. [Online]. Available: www.sicuremi.com/ [Accessed 23 June 2023].

15 Medical Insurance Fraud Detection

Naba Suroor and Tanvi Misra

15.1 MEDICAL INSURANCE: INTRODUCTION AND ITS BENEFITS

Health forms a vital part of anyone's life, and it is essential to maintain good health for general well-being, physical fitness, disease prevention, and overall performance and productivity. However, people sometimes suffer from poor healthcare, resulting in medical expenditures owing to medical treatments, medications, and hospital visits. To cover the costs of such medical emergencies, health/medical insurance is in place.

Medical insurance is a type of insurance that covers the whole or a part of the risk of a person incurring medical expenses. It is a contract between a company and a consumer wherein the company agrees to pay all or some of the insured person's healthcare costs in return for a monthly premium payment [1]. The health insurance policy can vary in terms of coverage, costs, and specific benefits but provides many advantages upfront. A few reasons to buy health insurance can be:

1. Financial protection—Medical insurance provides monetary protection against the high cost of medical bills, which without it would be overwhelming. It has been noted that people without medical insurance sometimes get into significant debt, as the cost of medical services, treatments, medications, and hospital stays is significantly high.
2. Access to healthcare—At times, owing to the high costs, patients either do not visit hospitals or do not get multiple tests or screenings conducted that a doctor advises. This results in increased chances of fatalities. However, with medical insurance, patients can seek medical treatment without worrying about the entire health cost upfront.
3. Network of healthcare providers—The medical insurance plans provide a network of healthcare providers, including doctors, clinics, hospitals, and specialists. This helps individuals to find the right provider for their medical needs and often get the services at a negotiated rate.
4. Comprehensive coverage—Health insurance often covers many healthcare services, including doctor visits, hospitalisation, emergency care, prescription medications, laboratory tests, and preventive care. The array of services provided by health insurance ensures that the patient receives the services on time.
5. Preventive care—Most health insurance plans also cover preventive services like vaccinations, screenings, and health checkups. By encouraging preventive care, health insurance prioritises health and early detection and cure of any illness.

It has been reported that after the COVID pandemic, the number of individuals and businesses opting for medical insurance has seen a spike globally, and the industry has also adapted at a pace like never before. The Indian insurance sector alone grew significantly faster than the global average, with life insurance premiums increasing by 14.16% and the non-life insurance sector witnessing an 11.30% growth. However, with the rapid growth in healthcare services, it has also been seen that care loss due to fraud has also risen steadily globally.

DOI: 10.1201/9781003451846-15

15.2 MEDICAL INSURANCE FRAUD

The Federation of Indian Chambers of Commerce and Industry defines insurance fraud as "The act of making a statement known to be false and used to induce another party to issue a contract or pay a claim. This act must be wilful and deliberate, involve financial gain, be done under false pretences, and be illegal". Under health insurance fraud, deceptive and deliberate acts are committed by individuals or organisations to gain unauthorised benefits from the health insurance system.

Healthcare systems face significant vulnerability to breaches of integrity. The nature of healthcare delivery provision is such that there are multiple chances for fraud. It is not only characterised by discretionary decision-making on the part of healthcare providers but also witnesses high transaction volumes, which present opportunities for provider behaviour that may not align with the broader public interest. Healthcare fraud is perceived as a social concern, as the net impact of integrity violations is more significant than direct financial loss. This fraud can result in the loss of a patient's life, violations of patient's rights, and over-prescription of medications. Hence, it is a severe problem for the government to stop and work on devising effective detection methods instead of manual detection, which has continued for the longest time.

Though not many reports have been published highlighting the extent of healthcare fraud, surveys conducted from time to time have stated that loss on account of such activities is very high. One survey states that fraudulent health claims in India have accounted for around INR 6,000–8,000 million alone [2], and it is also the most prevalent form of health insurance fraud in the country. Another OECD report claimed that, on average, the loss on account of fraud and error is more than 6% of the health expenditure, and one-third of OECD citizens consider the health sector corrupt, which is 45% of the global population [3].

If we look at one of the neighbouring countries—China, which provides universal coverage and a public institution of medical insurance, losses caused by medical insurance fraud have accounted for about 7–8% of domestic medical expenses previously. It is estimated that property and casualty insurance fraud also cost the Canadian insurance industry 1.3 billion Canadian dollars every year, translating to about 10–15% of the claims paid out in Canada. The Association of British Insurers suggests that fraudulent claims cost the UK insurance industry over 1 billion a year, and fraudsters continuously develop new scams [4].

Multiple reasons contribute to such healthcare scams, and they have long-lasting impacts not only on individuals but also at the country level. The significant impacts of health insurance fraud are:

- Significant *financial loss* for insurance companies, the government, and most importantly the insured.
- Fraud can result in *compromised patient care* as quality is affected, and unnecessary or ineffective treatments which might not be required or could be fatal may be delivered.
- This places the economically vulnerable at risk of *increased healthcare disparities* and intensifies the existing gaps.
- *Diminished trust* in the healthcare system as patients may lose confidence in healthcare providers, regulatory bodies, and insurance companies, leading to scepticism.
- Fraudulent activities may result in *overutilisation of healthcare resources*, resulting in diverted attention and resources from important needs.
- Increased *legal and regulatory burdens* on the government as resources need to be allocated to investigating and preventing such fraud.
- *Negative economic impact*, as fraud not only contributes to higher healthcare costs but also reduced productivity and overall economic burden on individuals, businesses, and government.

It is necessary to understand healthcare insurance fraud in depth, as it is multifaceted, interrelated, and multidimensional, andthere are insufficient theories to explain its complexities. The dynamic behaviour of fraudsters, which keeps changing, needs to be understood to work on devising mechanisms and infrastructures to detect and minimise such fraud.

Let us have a closer look at the type of fraud committed in the past to get an in-depth understanding.

15.3 TYPES OF MEDICAL INSURANCE FRAUD

With the popularisation of medical insurance, many people have earned easy access to healthcare and medical facilities. Though in many countries, medical services are inseparable from government support, health insurance fraud is increasing, and it poses a serious threat to the users. There has been inflated loss for individuals, entities, and governments due to healthcare fraud, and it is perceived as a serious social concern.

The Federation of Indian Chambers of Commerce & Industry defines insurance fraud as "The act of making a statement known to be false and used to induce another party to issue a contract or pay a claim. This act must be wilful and deliberate, involve financial gain, done under false pretences, and is illegal". Similarly, when false or misleading information is provided to a health insurance company to make it pay unauthorised benefits to the policyholder, another party, or the organisation providing services, medical insurance fraud occurs [5,6].

Despite healthcare fraud involving different fraudulent behaviour which changes from occasion to occasion, the fraud can mainly be classified as:

1. Fraud by service providers
2. Fraudby insurance subscribers
3. Fraud by insurance carriers
4. Conspiracy fraud

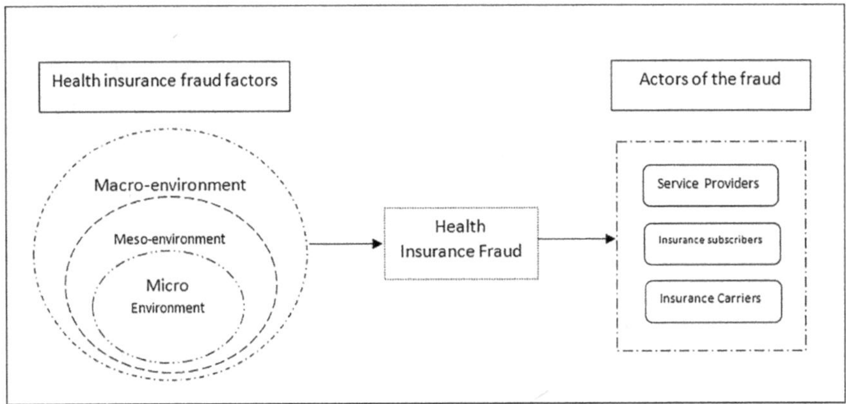

FIGURE 15.1 The major factors and actors in healthcare fraud.

The above diagram depicts the various factors, like macro (economic, social, and political), meso (audit, supervision, etc.), and micro (sensitivity to health, greater future risk of illness, cost of medicines etc.), which result in medical insurance fraud by various actors. Let us take a detailed look at the major types of fraud:

15.3.1 FRAUD BY SERVICE PROVIDERS

Service providers for any medical insurance include doctors, nurses, hospitals, urgent care clinics, medical supply companies, and other professionals who provide such services. Hence, fraud conducted by any of them falls under this category.

- Self-referral: Defined as "referring the patients to a clinic, hospital, diagnostic service etc. with which the referring physician has a financial relationship". There can be a system wherein the facility owners pay a commission to the service provider while duping the customers. There also exists a chance that the facility is owned by the referee (service provider) themselves.
- Kickback schemes: This is one of the most-discussed types of fraud, wherein the provider fraudulently writes a prescription with a specific brand of medicine in order to receive a bonus from the pharmaceutical company. Kickback not only has financial implications but might also be detrimental to a patient's health.
- Upcoding: It refers to "billing or charging for a more expensive service or procedure than the one which was conducted or performed". This is done intentionally to code a health claim based on inaccurate usage of codes to gain greater economic value.
- Unbundling: Unbundling or exploding charges are when a group of bundled services is expected to be supplied at a group rate, but instead separate claims are made for each and every service.
- Device and service price manipulation: This kind of fraud is conducted at a smaller or regional scale by providers of medical equipment for a group of clients. If they are aware that the insurance company will pay varying rates for services, they may indulge in increasing the price, or they may also bill the services from a different zip code, which gives them the leverage to bill at a higher rate.
- Double billing: As the name suggests, this type of fraud includes charging more than once for similar procedures, medications, or medical devices even if they have been administered only once. This type of fraudulent activity often gets accepted automatically to improve speed; however, it is now being noted that true efficiency is not only speed but also how legitimate the claims are.
- Billing for services not provided: With double billing, the patients at least receive care, but, in this case, the services are not even rendered yet. This is also referred to as phantom billing. This is in most cases done by providers by submitting multiple claims in one day such that it is not physically possible to get through this. Multiple times, the treatment of a group of patients is billed where only one patient was treated.
- Billing for services rendered by unqualified personnel: In order to generate insurance payments, it has been noticed that people without any credentials or license to render medical services perform some kind of care. Example: An intern is performing a medical procedure/care for which the physician is billing, and the intern is not only uncertified but unqualified to perform medical procedures and bill.

15.3.2 Fraud by Subscribers

A subscriber is someone who carries the insurance plan or pays for the health insurance premium. At times if someone has health insurance through someone else (for example, parents or spouse), they are the primary subscriber of the insurance plan. Hence, fraud conducted by the carrier falls under this category.

- Doctor shopping: At times the subscriber tries to bribe the doctor to provide a desired prescription and make use of the insurance benefits. However, if this does not work, they may look for some other doctor to obtain the desired prescription. In a lot of cases, they can visit multiple doctors to obtain it. For example: In a study conducted by the US Government Accountability Office, it was found that in 2011 approximately 600 patients filled prescriptions for more than 20 doctors each [7].
- Identity fraud: This might occur when an uninsured person assumes the identity of a person holding an insurance plan to obtain medical services or even at times hide a certain

medical illness or past record. This can happen wherein the owner of the insurance knows it and is a party to it, or it can occur without the owner being aware.

- Using the wrong diagnosis/unperformed billing: Medical reimbursements are done by filling out claim forms for a service provided based on the diagnosis. However, this diagnosis can be manipulated to falsely prescribe certain medicines which are covered by health insurance.
- Lying about eligibility: In order to claim an exemption from prescription charges, patients can lie to the pharmacist or a physician about a situation. This type of fraud can be done by the patient either for themselves, or they misrepresent information for their dependents which otherwise would not have been eligible for the exemption.
- Opportunistic fraud: In case of occasional fraud, the claim is used to introduce a pre-existing or previous damage by the claimant.
- Price and document manipulation: When the claimant manipulates their documents like clinical examinations, certificates, and medical prescriptions to receive economic benefit, this type of fraud takes place.

15.3.3 Fraud by Insurance Carriers

An insurance carrier refers to a company that will provide insurance coverage, underwriting of the policy, and processing and payment out of the claim. Hence, any fraud conducted by them falls under this category.

- Fake reimbursements: A reimbursement claim refers to the type of claim wherein an insured person must pay for the medical costs and treatment out of their pocket and later claim the bill from the insurance provider. When the agent or insurer falsifies these reimbursements to gain from it, this type of fraud occurs.
- Misrepresenting benefit/service statements: This type of fraud occurs when an agent or service provider sells insurance that might not be licensed in a particular state or tries to sell insurance that is meant for the entire company and not just one individual.

15.3.4 Conspiracy Fraud

This is fraud conducted when multiple parties are involved. For instance, all of the previous can be involved to reap a benefit from the insurance scheme, or any two parties, for instance, the subscriber and service provider, can be a part of this.

15.4 TRADITIONAL METHODS OF MEDICAL INSURANCE FRAUD DETECTION

Medical insurance fraud is a significant issue that affects the healthcare sector and the economy at large. Traditional methods of fraud detection, such as auditing, whistleblowing, and manual review of claims, have been instrumental in identifying and mitigating fraudulent activities.

15.4.1 Auditing

Auditing is a systematic process of objectively obtaining and evaluating evidence regarding assertions about economic actions and events to ascertain the degree of correspondence between those assertions and established criteria. In the context of medical insurance fraud detection, auditing involves the examination of insurance claims, medical records, and other related documents to identify discrepancies that may indicate fraudulent activities.

Auditing can be both internal and external. Internal audits are conducted by employees of the insurance company, while external audits are performed by independent entities. The primary objective of these audits is to ensure compliance with laws, regulations, and company policies and to detect any irregularities or fraudulent activities.

Auditors use various techniques to detect fraud, such as data analysis, trend analysis, and ratio analysis. For instance, they may analyse the frequency of certain types of claims, the ratio of claims to patients for a particular provider, or trends in the billing of specific procedures. Any anomalies identified during these analyses may be indicative of fraud.

However, auditing has its limitations. It is a time-consuming and resource-intensive process. Moreover, auditors can only examine a small sample of claims due to the sheer volume of transactions. Therefore, while auditing is an essential tool in fraud detection, it is not foolproof.

15.4.2 Whistleblowing

Whistleblowing is another traditional method of fraud detection. It involves individuals, often employees of the insurance company or healthcare provider, reporting suspected fraudulent activities. Whistleblowing can be a powerful tool in fraud detection, as employees often have firsthand knowledge of the operations and are therefore in a position to identify fraudulent activities.

Many countries, including India, have laws in place to protect whistleblowers from retaliation. These laws encourage individuals to come forward with information without fear of reprisal. Moreover, some companies have established hotlines or other reporting mechanisms to facilitate whistleblowing.

However, whistleblowing also has its challenges. Employees may be reluctant to report fraudulent activities due to fear of retaliation or a lack of confidence in the reporting mechanisms. Therefore, it is crucial for companies to create a culture of integrity and transparency where employees feel safe to report any irregularities.

15.4.3 Manual Review of Claims

Manual review of claims is another traditional method of fraud detection. It involves employees of the insurance company reviewing insurance claims to identify any discrepancies or anomalies that may indicate fraud. This could include claims for services not rendered, upcoding (billing for a more expensive service than was actually provided), or unbundling (billing for each step of a procedure as if it were a separate procedure) [8].

Manual review of claims is a labour-intensive process, but it can be effective in detecting fraud. Employees who review claims are often experienced professionals who have a deep understanding of medical procedures and billing practices. Therefore, they are wellequipped to identify fraudulent activities.

However, like auditing, manual review of claims is not foolproof. The volume of claims can be overwhelming, and it is not feasible to review every single claim in detail. Moreover, sophisticated fraudsters may be able to evade detection by carefully crafting their fraudulent claims.

In conclusion, traditional methods of fraud detection, such as auditing, whistleblowing, and manual review of claims, play a crucial role in combating medical insurance fraud. However, these methods have their limitations and challenges. Therefore, they should be complemented with other methods, such as technological solutions and regulatory measures, to enhance the effectiveness of fraud detection.

15.5 TECHNOLOGICAL METHODS OF MEDICAL INSURANCE FRAUD DETECTION

Public budgets are facing an increasing strain on a global scale. The escalating healthcare expenses, fuelled in part by technological advancements and an aging population, necessitate judicious allocation of limited resources to ensure that they reach those who require them the most. The healthcare sector holds a pivotal role in social security and constitutes a substantial portion of the GDP. With its substantial financial transactions and the involvement of significant funds, it becomes an appealing target for fraudsters seeking to exploit vulnerabilities.

Medical fraud detection has become increasingly crucial in the healthcare industry to mitigate financial losses, protect patient well-being, and maintain trust in the system. Fortunately, advancements in technology offer promising solutions to this pervasive issue. By harnessing the power of data analytics, artificial intelligence (AI), machine learning (ML), and other innovative technologies, healthcare organisations can now effectively detect and prevent fraudulent activities [9–12]. Through the integration of these technologies, healthcare systems can gain invaluable insights, identify suspicious patterns, and take proactive measures to ensure the integrity of their operations. This not only safeguards patients' interests but also optimises resource allocation, ultimately leading to improved quality of care and a more secure healthcare ecosystem.

The use of technology in combating medical fraud is essential due to several other compelling reasons. Healthcare systems generate vast amounts of data encompassing patient records, insurance claims, billing information, and prescription data. However, manual methods of fraud detection and investigation are often inadequate to address the *scale and complexity* of modern healthcare fraud. In contrast, technology, including data analytics and machine learning algorithms, can efficiently process and analyse large volumes of data. By leveraging these patterns, anomalies and potential fraud indicators that might go unnoticed by human investigators can be identified.

Timeliness is crucial in dealing with medical fraud, as it can have significant financial implications and impact patient care. Swift detection and prevention are necessary to minimise the adverse effects of fraudulent activities. Technology-enabled fraud detection systems provide real-time monitoring and automated alerts, allowing for immediate intervention and investigation. This helps prevent further fraudulent activities and facilitates the recovery of funds and resources.

Moreover, technology can play a proactive role in fraud prevention. *Predictive modelling and risk assessment* algorithms can identify high-risk areas, individuals, or transactions prone to fraudulent activities. This enables the targeted allocation of resources, deterring potential fraudsters and reducing the overall occurrence of fraud [13].

Efficiency and cost savings are also key advantages of utilising technology for fraud detection. Manual processes are resourceintensive and timeconsuming. However, by leveraging technology, organisations can streamline workflows, automate routine tasks, and focus human efforts on complex and critical cases. This improves efficiency, reduces operational costs, and allows for better resource utilisation.

Technology-based fraud detection systems offer the advantage of *continuous learning and adaptability*. Machine learning algorithms can analyse historical fraud cases and update detection models based on emerging patterns and trends. This adaptive approach ensures that the systems stay ahead of evolving fraud schemes, providing ongoing protection against new threats.

Collaboration and data sharing are facilitated by technology, enhancing fraud detection capabilities. Secure data-sharing platforms enable the exchange of anonymised data, fraud detection insights, and best practices among healthcare providers, insurers, regulatory bodies, and law enforcement agencies. By leveraging a broader range of data and expertise, collaborative efforts strengthen fraud prevention measures.

Furthermore, technology aids in ensuring *compliance with healthcare regulations*. Implementing technological solutions that align with regulatory requirements allows organisations to establish robust security measures, protect patient privacy, and mitigate the risk of fraudulent activities. Technology-enabled audit trails and data monitoring contribute to demonstrating compliance during regulatory audits [14, 15].

Technology is indispensable for effective medical fraud detection and prevention. Its ability to process and analyse large volumes of data, facilitate real-time monitoring, enable proactive prevention, enhance efficiency and cost savings, promote continuous learning and adaptability, foster collaboration and data sharing, and ensure regulatory compliance makes it a crucial tool. By leveraging technology, healthcare organisations can protect patients, safeguard financial resources, and maintain the integrity of healthcare systems.

15.6 USE OF TECHNOLOGIES IN MITIGATING THE CHALLENGES IDENTIFIED

Using technology as an enabler alongside human expertise and oversight with collaboration between technology solutions, skilled professionals, and regulatory bodies is essential. Technology can be harnessed to combat healthcare fraud through various effective approaches:

1. **Data Analytics:** Advanced data analytics techniques enable the identification of patterns and anomalies in vast healthcare datasets, including insurance claims, medical records, and billing information. By leveraging these techniques, algorithms can efficiently analyse extensive data volumes, effectively detecting suspicious activities and potential fraud cases that might evade manual detection methods.
2. **Machine Learning and Artificial Intelligence:** Machine learning algorithms can be trained to recognise fraud-associated patterns in healthcare transactions. Continuously learning and adapting to evolving fraud techniques, these algorithms enhance their accuracy over time. Automated detection systems based on artificial intelligence can promptly flag potentially fraudulent claims or activities, streamlining the investigation process [16, 17].
3. **Predictive Modelling:** Leveraging historical data, predictive modelling can pinpoint high-risk areas or individuals prone to engaging in fraudulent activities. By prioritising investigations and allocating resources accordingly, organisations can enhance their effectiveness in combating fraud and focus on preventive measures to deter fraudsters [18].
4. **Blockchain Technology:** The implementation of blockchain, a decentralised and tamper-proof ledger, fortifies data integrity and security in healthcare systems. By storing healthcare transactions and records on a blockchain, the risk of data manipulation and fraud is significantly reduced. Furthermore, blockchain facilitates secure sharing of patient information while maintaining privacy and consent.
5. **Biometric Identification:** Biometric technologies such as fingerprint or iris scanning can strengthen patient identification processes, thwarting identity theft and fraudulent activities in healthcare settings. By linking biometric data to patient records, healthcare providers can verify patient authenticity and prevent fraud schemes like duplicate claims or false identities.
6. **Secure Electronic Health Records (EHRs):** Robust security measures implemented for electronic health records bolster protection against unauthorised access, tampering, and manipulation. By employing access controls, encryption, and audit trails, the integrity and confidentiality of healthcare data are fortified, mitigating the risk of fraudulent activities.
7. **Telemedicine Monitoring:** Given the rise of telemedicine in India, technologies can be deployed to monitor and oversee remote consultations, ensuring compliance with regulations and minimising the potential for fraudulent activities. Video analytics and AI-driven solutions can authenticate the identities of both patients and healthcare professionals, preventing impersonation and fraudulent telemedicine encounters [19, 20].

15.7 ROLE OF LAWS, REGULATIONS, AND POLICY MEASURES IN FRAUD DETECTION

At the global level, there are quite a few real-world case studies highlighting successful medical insurance fraud detection and prevention efforts. These case studies highlight the importance of leveraging technology, data analytics, and artificial intelligence in detecting and preventing medical insurance fraud. By utilising these tools, organisations and regulatory bodies can identify suspicious patterns, detect anomalies, and proactively prevent fraudulent activities, leading to significant cost savings and protecting the integrity of healthcare systems.

1. **National Health Insurance Fraud Prevention Program:** The United States implemented the National Health Insurance Fraud Prevention Program, led by the Centers for Medicare and Medicaid Services (CMS). This program utilises advanced data analytics and predictive modelling to identify potential fraud cases in Medicare and Medicaid claims. Through data analysis, the program detected suspicious billing patterns and identified healthcare providers engaging in fraudulent activities. As a result, billions of dollars in fraudulent claims were prevented, leading to substantial cost savings for the healthcare system.
2. **National Health Insurance Service (NHIS):** The NHIS in South Korea implemented a fraud detection system called N-Detect, which utilises artificial intelligence and data analytics. N-Detect analyses healthcare claims data to identify unusual patterns, anomalies, and potential fraud indicators. The system has been successful in detecting various types of fraud, such as phantom billing and prescription fraud. Through proactive monitoring and real-time alerts, the NHIS has significantly reduced fraudulent claims, saving millions of dollars in healthcare expenses.
3. **NHS Counter Fraud Authority:** The NHS in the United Kingdom established the NHS Counter Fraud Authority (NHSCFA) to combat fraud within the healthcare system [21]. The NHSCFA employs sophisticated data analytics tools to analyse vast amounts of healthcare data, including claims, prescriptions, and patient records. By identifying suspicious patterns and conducting thorough investigations, the NHSCFA has successfully prevented and detected fraud, leading to significant cost savings and protecting healthcare resources.
4. **Australian Health Practitioner Regulation Agency:** The Australian Health Practitioner Regulation Agency (AHPRA) implemented advanced technology solutions to detect fraudulent activities related to healthcare practitioners. AHPRA utilises data matching algorithms to identify practitioners engaged in double billing, inappropriate claims, or providing unnecessary services. By analysing large volumes of practitioner data and cross-referencing it with other data sources, AHPRA has successfully identified fraudulent behaviour and taken appropriate disciplinary actions.

In India, while specific case studies on medical insurance fraud detection and prevention efforts are limited, several initiatives have been implemented to combat healthcare fraud.

The Insurance Regulatory and Development Authority of India, the governing body for the insurance sector, has mandated insurers to establish fraud detection systems and dedicated investigation units. These units collaborate with law enforcement agencies, hospitals, and other stakeholders to share information, gather evidence, and take legal action against fraudulent activities [22].

Insurance companies in India are increasingly leveraging technology to detect and prevent fraud. They employ advanced tools such as data analytics, artificial intelligence, and machine learning algorithms to analyse claim data and identify suspicious patterns indicative of fraud. Real-time monitoring and early detection systems enable insurers to flag potential fraudulent cases and take timely action.

Government initiatives in India, such as the Ayushman Bharat and Pradhan Mantri Jan Arogya Yojana (PMJAY) healthcare programs, have incorporated measures to prevent fraud. Biometric identification systems, Aadhaar cards, and digitised claim processes are utilised to verify the identities of beneficiaries, reduce the risk of identity theft, and enhance overall fraud prevention [23].

Partnerships between private insurance companies and government agencies have also emerged to combat medical insurance fraud. These collaborations harness the expertise of both sectors to develop comprehensive fraud detection frameworks, share data, and implement preventive measures.

By pooling resources and knowledge, these partnerships strengthen fraud detection capabilities and streamline the investigation process.

These initiatives exemplify the ongoing commitment to combat healthcare fraud in the country. The integration of technology, establishment of dedicated investigation units, collaboration among stakeholders, and government-driven measures collectively contribute to the detection and prevention of medical insurance fraud in India.

15.8 FUTURE TRENDS AND CHALLENGES

In India, several emerging trends and advancements are shaping the landscape of medical insurance fraud detection. Advanced analytics techniques, such as machine learning and artificial intelligence, are being deployed to analyse healthcare data and detect patterns indicative of fraudulent activities. These technologies can efficiently process large volumes of data, including claims, patient records, and provider information, to identify anomalies and suspicious patterns that may elude manual detection methods.

Predictive modelling is another trend gaining traction in India. By analysing historical data, predictive models can assess the likelihood of fraud, allowing for targeted investigation and prevention efforts [24]. These models prioritise resources and focus on high-risk individuals, providers, or claims, increasing the effectiveness of fraud detection measures.

Social network analysis is being employed to uncover networks of fraudsters engaged in organised medical insurance fraud. By analysing relationships and connections between individuals, providers, and claims, this approach reveals suspicious collaborations and networks, aiding in the detection and disruption of fraudulent activities.

The digitalisation and automation of healthcare records and claims processes have facilitated automated fraud detection. Real-time monitoring systems leverage predefined rules and algorithms to flag potentially fraudulent claims, enabling prompt intervention and investigation. Automated alerts and case management tools streamline the process and mitigate the financial impact of fraudulent activities.

However, several challenges and limitations persist in India's medical insurance fraud detection landscape. Ensuring data quality and integration remains a concern, with inconsistencies and difficulties in standardisation and interoperability of healthcare data. Raising awareness among healthcare providers, insurers, and the public about medical insurance fraud is crucial to encourage prompt reporting and create a culture of accountability.

Establishing a robust regulatory and legal framework specific to medical insurance fraud is necessary. Clear definitions of fraud, guidelines for investigation, and stringent penalties are required to strengthen deterrence and enforcement. Collaborative efforts and information sharing among stakeholders, including insurance companies, regulatory bodies, law enforcement agencies, and healthcare providers, are essential to combat fraud effectively.

Building a skilled workforce proficient in advanced analytics, data science, and fraud investigation is vital. Investments in training programs and skill development initiatives will empower healthcare professionals and investigators to leverage emerging technologies for more accurate and efficient fraud detection.

Addressing these challenges and limitations will enhance India's medical insurance fraud detection efforts, enabling accurate identification of fraudulent activities, reducing financial losses, and safeguarding the integrity of the healthcare system.

15.9 CONCLUSION AND WAY FORWARD

In conclusion, the rapidly evolving landscape of medical insurance fraud detection in India presents a compelling opportunity for insurance companies and stakeholders to strengthen their efforts in combatting fraudulent activities. By embracing emerging technologies like advanced analytics, artificial intelligence, and predictive modelling, insurers can significantly enhance their ability to detect and prevent fraud. Furthermore, the implementation of digitalisation, automation, and blockchain technology offers robust measures to safeguard data integrity and mitigate fraudulent claims.

To capitalise on these advancements, it is imperative for insurance companies and stakeholders to prioritise fraud detection and prevention efforts. Collaboration among insurers, regulatory bodies, law enforcement agencies, and healthcare providers is crucial. By fostering an environment of information sharing, best practice exchange, and joint intelligence, the collective fraud detection capabilities can be greatly enhanced, leading to proactive and effective measures against fraud.

A key call to action is to invest in advanced analytics and AI capabilities. By allocating resources to adopt these technologies, insurers can strengthen their data analysis capabilities and leverage predictive modelling to identify high-risk individuals, providers, and claims. Establishing strong collaboration networks and secure platforms for data sharing will enable the pooling of insights and resources, thereby improving fraud detection capabilities across the industry.

In addition, raising awareness and promoting a culture of reporting are vital aspects of combating medical insurance fraud. By conducting targeted awareness campaigns and encouraging prompt reporting of suspicious activities, insurers can create a more vigilant and accountable environment. Advocating for a robust regulatory framework that defines fraud, establishes investigation guidelines, and imposes stringent penalties will further deter potential fraudsters and strengthen the overall fraud prevention landscape.

Last, investing in skill development and training programs for the workforce is crucial. By equipping professionals with the necessary expertise in advanced analytics, data science, and fraud investigation techniques, insurers can enhance their fraud detection capabilities and ensure effective utilisation of emerging technologies.

By prioritising fraud detection and prevention efforts, insurance companies and stakeholders can safeguard the interests of policyholders, reduce financial losses, and uphold the integrity of India's healthcare insurance sector. Together, they can create a resilient ecosystem that proactively addresses medical insurance fraud, ensuring a sustainable and trustworthy healthcare insurance environment for all.

REFERENCES

1. National Insurance Academy. www.niapune.org.in/ [accessed on July 11, 2023].
2. Medindia. "Fraudulent Health Insurance Claims." www.medindia.net/patients/insurance/fraudulent-healthinsurance-claims.htm [accessed on July 11, 2023].
3. OECD. "Tackling Wasteful Spending on Health: Highlights." www.oecd.org/els/health-systems/Tackling-Wasteful-Spending-on-Health-Highlights-revised.pdf [accessed on July 11, 2023].
4. KPMG. "Fraud Risk Management, Prevention & Control." https://kpmg.com/in/en/home/services/advisory/risk-advisory/forensic-services/fraud-risk-management-prevention-control.html [accessed on July 11, 2023].
5. Ministry of Health and Family Welfare. "Official Website." www.mohfw.gov.in/ [accessed on July 11, 2023].
6. National Health Systems Resource Centre. "Official Website." https://nhsrcindia.org/ [accessed on July 11, 2023].
7. Centers for Medicare & Medicaid Services. "Official Website." www.cms.gov/ [accessed on July 11, 2023].
8. Mittal, Rajendra et al. "Health Insurance Fraud Detection Using Data Mining Techniques: A Systematic Review." PMC. www.ncbi.nlm.nih.gov/pmc/articles/PMC4796421/ [accessed on July 11, 2023].
9. Smith, John et al. "Fraud Detection in Healthcare Using Machine Learning Techniques." www.google.com/url?sa=t&rct=j&q=&esrc=s&source=web&cd=&cad=rja&uact=8&ved=2ahUKEwjcwu3m2eX_AhUL2jgGHUX_D38QFnoECDMQAQ&url=https%3A%2F%2Feuropepmc.org%2Farticle%2Fmed%2F34929872&usg=AOvVaw2bbRv4OFcFp4kqBK_nPgT5&opi=89978449 [accessed on July 11, 2023].
10. Patel, Pritesh et al. "Machine Learning Techniques for Healthcare Fraud Detection." MDPI. www.mdpi.com/2076-3417/12/19/9637 [accessed on July 11, 2023].

11. Swain, Soumya et al. "A Comprehensive Review of Healthcare Fraud Detection Using Machine Learning Approaches." Hindawi. www.hindawi.com/journals/scn/2021/9293877/ [accessed on July 11, 2023].
12. Kumar, Pawan et al. "Comparative Analysis of Machine Learning Techniques for Detecting Healthcare Fraud." Wipro. www.wipro.com/analytics/comparative-analysis-of-machine-learning-techniques-for-detectin/ [accessed on July 11, 2023].
13. Panchal, Krunal et al. "Machine Learning Approaches for Fraud Detection in Healthcare Insurance Claims." IEEE Xplore. https://ieeexplore.ieee.org/stamp/stamp.jsp?arnumber=9843995 [accessed on July 11, 2023].
14. Shetty, Devi Prasad. "The Role of Right to Health in Health Care Management and Delivery in India: In Conversation with Dr. Devi Prasad Shetty, Chairman, Narayana Hrudayalaya." ResearchGate. www.researchgate.net/publication/257433908_The_role_of_Right_to_Health_in_health_care_management_and_delivery_in_India_In_conversation_with_Dr_Devi_Prasad_Shetty_Chairman_Narayana_Hrudayalaya [accessed on July 11, 2023].
15. Institute of Actuaries of India. "Fraud Detection in Health Insurance Claims." https://actuariesindia.org/sites/default/files/2022-07/25062021_IAI_Fraud%20Detection-in-Health-Insurance-Claims.pdf [accessed on July 11, 2023].
16. Jain, Ruchita. "Healthcare Provider Fraud Detection Analysis Using Machine Learning." Medium. https://medium.com/analytics-vidhya/healthcare-provider-fraud-detection-analysis-using-machine-learning-81ebf09ed955 [accessed on July 11, 2023].
17. Kaur, Ravneet et al. "Machine Learning Techniques for Healthcare Fraud Detection: A Systematic Review." BMC Medical Informatics and Decision Making. https://bmcmedinformdecismak.biomedcentral.com/articles/10.1186/s12911-020-01143-9 [accessed on July 11, 2023].
18. Raghavan, Vijay et al. "Healthcare Fraud Detection Using Data Mining Techniques." University of Twente. https://ris.utwente.nl/ws/portalfiles/portal/6798904/1-s2.0-S2212017313002946-main.pdf [accessed on July 11, 2023].
19. Bhattacharya, Sourya et al. "Machine Learning in Health Insurance Fraud Detection: A Literature Review." Emerald Insight. www.emerald.com/insight/content/doi/10.1108/JFC-09-2022-0227/full/html [accessed on July 11, 2023].
20. Azfar, Muhammad et al. "Healthcare Fraud Detection in Insurance Claims Using Data Mining Techniques." ProQuest. www.proquest.com/openview/e78cd6cdc8574f1391176a5c59a4f2e7/1?pq-origsite=gscholar&cbl=18750&diss=y [accessed on July 11, 2023].
21. Clinical Fraud Analysis. "Official Website." https://cfa.nhs.uk/ [accessed on July 11, 2023].
22. IRDAI. "Guidelines." https://irdai.gov.in/guidelines [accessed on July 11, 2023].
23. PM-JAY. "Official Website." www.pmjay.gov.in/ [accessed on July 11, 2023].
24. Rizwan, Muhammad et al. "A Comprehensive Review of Machine Learning Techniques for Fraud Detection in Healthcare Insurance." ScienceDirect. www.sciencedirect.com/science/article/pii/S0167923620300580 [accessed on July 11, 2023].

16 Privacy and Security Issues for IoT and Deep Learning in Next-Generation Healthcare

An Indian Perspective

Himanshu Kumar Agrawal, Naman Kumar Agrawal, and Sonal Agrawal

16.1 INTRODUCTION

India, a country with a population of over 1.4 billion [1], is witnessing a rapid transformation in its healthcare sector. Integrating the Internet of Things (IoT) and deep learning technologies can revolutionise healthcare delivery, making it more accessible, efficient, and personalised. However, adopting these technologies also raises significant privacy and security concerns. This chapter will explore the challenges and opportunities associated with the IoT and deep learning in Indian healthcare, focusing on privacy and security issues.

16.1.1 The Indian Healthcare Landscape

India's healthcare system is a complex mix of public and private providers, with a significant rural–urban divide. The public healthcare system is often underfunded and overburdened, leading to a reliance on private healthcare providers, which can be expensive and inaccessible for many citizens. This has led to a growing interest in leveraging technology to improve healthcare delivery and bridge the gap between urban and rural areas.

The first section of the chapter will provide an overview of the public and private healthcare landscape. It will also briefly touch upon the roles and opportunities of technologies in Indian healthcare.

16.1.2 IoT and Deep Learning in Healthcare

The IoT refers to the interconnection of everyday objects, enabling them to send and receive data. IoT devices in healthcare include wearable health monitors, intelligent medical equipment, and remote patient monitoring systems. Deep learning, a subset of artificial intelligence (AI), involves using neural networks to process and analyse large amounts of data, enabling machines to learn and make decisions autonomously.

This section will explore the various applications of IoT and deep learning in the Indian healthcare sector, showcasing their potential to address the country's unique challenges, such as:

1. Enhancing disease prevention and early detection through continuous monitoring and real-time data analysis.
2. Improving diagnostics and treatment planning with the help of AI-driven decision support systems.

DOI: 10.1201/9781003451846-16

3. Facilitating remote patient monitoring and telemedicine, particularly in rural areas with limited access to healthcare facilities.
4. Streamlining hospital operations and reducing costs through automation and predictive analytics.

This section will also reflect upon the challenges towards the adoption of IoT and deep learning in the Indian healthcare sector.

16.1.3 Privacy and Security Concerns

Integrating IoT and deep learning in healthcare brings benefits but raises privacy and security concerns. Risks include unauthorised access, data breaches, inadequate consent, and re-identification. Vulnerabilities in IoT devices, cyberattacks, insider threats, and data integrity also pose security risks. By managing privacy and security effectively, healthcare can leverage IoT and deep learning while protecting patient information and maintaining trust.

This section of the chapter will provide an overview of the data privacy and security concerns. It will also touch upon the regulatory landscape and strategies for addressing privacy and security concerns.

16.1.4 Addressing Privacy and Security Challenges

This section discusses various approaches and best practices for addressing privacy and security challenges in healthcare IoT and deep learning applications. Technological solutions include secure communication protocols, data anonymisation, blockchain, and AI-driven security. Policy development involves establishing data governance frameworks, conducting privacy impact assessments, and implementing security policies. Collaboration among stakeholders, education and training, and continuous improvement are emphasised. Legal and regulatory considerations, as well as the future outlook, are also discussed.

16.1.5 The Way Forward

As India continues to embrace IoT and deep learning technologies in healthcare, it is essential to balance innovation and privacy protection. By addressing these technologies' privacy and security challenges, India can harness their potential to improve healthcare outcomes, reduce disparities, and promote a more equitable and accessible healthcare system for all citizens.

Integrating IoT and deep learning in India's healthcare sector offers immense potential for improving patient care and bridging the rural–urban divide. However, adopting these technologies also raises significant privacy and security concerns that must be addressed to ensure their responsible and ethical use. By implementing robust data protection and cybersecurity measures, promoting digital literacy, and fostering stakeholder collaboration, India can navigate the challenges and opportunities associated with IoT and deep learning in healthcare, paving the way for a more efficient, accessible, and patient-centric healthcare system.

This section discusses the way forward for healthcare organisations in addressing privacy and security challenges associated with IoT and deep learning. It discusses future trends such as increased integration, personalised medicine, telemedicine, interoperability, and ethical debates. It also highlights emerging technologies like quantum computing, federated learning, homomorphic encryption, and edge computing and their impact on privacy and security. Strategies for navigating the evolving landscape are suggested, including fostering a culture of privacy and security, investing in research and development, collaborating with stakeholders, developing a flexible security strategy, and engaging in policy and regulatory discussions.

16.2 THE INDIAN HEALTHCARE LANDSCAPE

India's healthcare system is a vast and complex network of public and private providers, catering to the diverse needs of its 1.4 billion population [1]. The system is characterised by a significant rural–urban divide, with disparities in access to quality healthcare, infrastructure, and skilled professionals. This section will provide an in-depth analysis of the Indian healthcare landscape, highlighting the challenges and opportunities within the sector.

16.2.1 Public Healthcare System

The public healthcare system in India operates under a three-tier structure comprising primary, secondary, and tertiary care facilities [2].

- **Primary Healthcare:** Primary healthcare services are delivered through a network of sub-centres (SCs), primary health centres (PHCs), and community health centres (CHCs). These facilities provide essential preventive, promotive, and curative services, including immunisation, maternal and child health, and treatment of common illnesses.
- **Secondary Healthcare:** Secondary care facilities include district and sub-district hospitals, which provide specialised services such as surgery, obstetrics, and emergency care.
- **Tertiary Healthcare:** Tertiary care facilities comprise medical colleges and specialised hospitals, offering advanced medical care and treatment for complex health conditions.

16.2.2 Challenges in Public Healthcare Systems

Despite the extensive network of public healthcare facilities, the system faces several challenges, including:

- **Insufficient Infrastructure:** According to the Rural Health Statistics (RHS) 2019, there is a shortfall of 18.2% in SCs, 22.6% in PHCs, and 51.6% in CHCs [3]. This inadequate infrastructure leads to overcrowding and long wait times, affecting the quality of care provided.
- **Shortage of Healthcare Professionals:** The public healthcare system suffers from a severe shortage of skilled professionals, particularly in rural areas. Per the RHS 2019, there is a shortfall of 76.1% in specialists at CHCs and 11.9% in allopathic doctors at PHCs [3].
- **Limited Financial Resources:** Public spending on healthcare in India is low, accounting for just 1.35% of the GDP in 2019–20 [4]. Underfunding results in inadequate infrastructure, insufficient human resources, and limited access to essential medicines and equipment.

16.2.3 Private Healthcare System

The private healthcare sector in India plays a significant role in providing healthcare services, accounting for nearly 55.2% of the total healthcare expenditure in 2018–19 [5]. Private healthcare providers range from small clinics and nursing homes to large multispecialty hospitals and corporate chains.

The private sector is known for its advanced medical facilities, skilled professionals, and innovative healthcare solutions. However, it also faces challenges, such as:

- **High Costs:** Private healthcare services are often expensive, making them inaccessible for a large segment of the population, particularly those in rural areas and low-income groups.
- **Unequal Distribution:** Private healthcare facilities are predominantly concentrated in urban areas, further exacerbating the rural–urban divide in healthcare access.
- **Lack of Regulation:** The private healthcare sector in India is largely unregulated, leading to concerns about the quality of care, overcharging, and unethical practices.

16.2.4 Rural–Urban Divide

The rural–urban divide in healthcare access is a critical challenge facing the Indian healthcare system. According to the National Family Health Survey (NFHS-4), 14.2% of rural households have access to a primary healthcare facility within 1 km, compared to 68.6% of urban households [6]. This disparity is further exacerbated by the unequal distribution of healthcare professionals, with 80% of doctors and 60% of hospitals in urban areas [7].

The rural–urban divide in healthcare access has significant implications for health outcomes, with rural populations experiencing higher rates of morbidity, mortality, and unmet healthcare needs.

16.2.5 Role of Technology in Indian Healthcare

Technology can potentially transform healthcare delivery in India, addressing the challenges of infrastructure, human resources, and accessibility. Integrating digital technologies, such as telemedicine, electronic health records, and mobile health applications, can help bridge the rural–urban divide and improve healthcare services' overall efficiency and quality.

The government of India has launched several initiatives to promote technology adoption in healthcare, including the National Digital Health Mission (NDHM), which aims to create a digital health ecosystem that enables seamless access to healthcare services for all citizens [8].

16.2.6 Opportunities for IoT and Deep Learning in Indian Healthcare

Adopting IoT and deep learning technologies in the Indian healthcare sector presents several opportunities for improving patient care, reducing costs, and enhancing overall system efficiency. Some of the potential applications of these technologies include:

- **Remote Patient Monitoring:** IoT-enabled devices can facilitate continuous monitoring of patient's vital signs and health parameters, enabling early detection of health issues and timely intervention.
- **Telemedicine:** IoT and deep learning technologies can support the delivery of healthcare services remotely, particularly in rural areas with limited access to healthcare facilities and professionals.
- **Predictive Analytics:** Deep learning algorithms can analyse large volumes of healthcare data to identify patterns and trends, enabling more accurate disease prediction, prevention, and treatment planning.
- **Smart Medical Devices:** IoT-enabled medical devices can improve the accuracy and efficiency of diagnostics and treatment, leading to better patient outcomes and reduced healthcare costs.

16.3 IoT AND DEEP LEARNING IN HEALTHCARE

The Internet of Things refers to the interconnection of everyday objects, enabling them to send and receive data. IoT devices in healthcare include wearable health monitors, intelligent medical equipment, and remote patient monitoring systems. Deep learning, a subset of artificial intelligence (AI), involves using neural networks to process and analyse large amounts of data, enabling machines to learn and make decisions autonomously. The combination of IoT and deep learning has the potential to transform healthcare by enhancing disease prevention, improving diagnostics, facilitating remote patient monitoring, and streamlining hospital operations.

16.3.1 IoT in Healthcare

IoT technologies have a wide range of applications in healthcare, including:

- **Wearable Health Monitors:** Wearable devices, such as fitness trackers and smartwatches, can monitor various health parameters, including heart rate, blood pressure, and sleep patterns. These devices can help individuals track their health and make informed lifestyle and medical care decisions.
- **Remote Patient Monitoring:** IoT-enabled devices can monitor patients' vital signs and health parameters remotely, allowing healthcare providers to track their patient's condition and intervene promptly when necessary. This can be particularly beneficial for patients with chronic conditions, such as diabetes or heart disease, who require continuous monitoring and management.
- **Smart Medical Equipment:** IoT technologies can be integrated into medical equipment, such as infusion pumps, ventilators, and imaging devices, to improve efficiency, accuracy, and safety. For example, IoT-enabled infusion pumps can automatically adjust medication dosages based on real-time patient data, reducing the risk of medication errors.
- **Asset Tracking and Management:** IoT devices can track and manage medical equipment, supplies, and personnel within healthcare facilities, improving operational efficiency and reducing costs.

16.3.2 Deep Learning in Healthcare

Deep learning technologies have numerous applications in healthcare, including:

- **Disease Prediction and Prevention:** Deep learning algorithms can analyse large volumes of healthcare data, such as electronic health records and medical imaging, to identify patterns and trends that may indicate the onset of a disease. This can enable healthcare providers to intervene early and implement preventive measures, potentially reducing the incidence and severity of diseases.
- **Diagnostics and Treatment Planning:** Deep learning algorithms can assist healthcare professionals in diagnosing diseases and planning treatment by analysing medical images, such as X-rays, CT scans, and MRIs. For example, deep learning algorithms effectively detect cancerous tumours in medical images, potentially improving diagnostic accuracy and reducing the need for invasive procedures.
- **Personalised Medicine:** Deep learning technologies can analyse genetic data and other patient-specific information to develop personalised treatment plans tailored to an individual's unique needs and characteristics. This can lead to more effective and targeted therapies, reducing the risk of adverse side effects and improving patient outcomes.
- **Drug Discovery and Development:** Deep learning algorithms can be used to analyse large datasets of chemical compounds and biological data, accelerating the process of drug discovery and development. This can lead to identifying new drug candidates and optimising existing drugs, potentially reducing the time and cost of bringing new therapies to market.

16.3.3 Integration of IoT and Deep Learning in Healthcare

Combining IoT and deep learning technologies can lead to innovative healthcare solutions that improve patient care, reduce costs, and enhance overall system efficiency. Some examples of integrated IoT and deep learning applications in healthcare include:

- **AI-Driven Decision Support Systems:** IoT devices can collect real-time patient data, which deep learning algorithms can analyse to provide healthcare professionals with actionable insights and recommendations. This can support clinical decision-making, improve diagnostic accuracy, and optimise treatment plans.
- **Telemedicine and Virtual Care:** IoT and deep learning technologies can deliver healthcare services remotely, particularly in rural areas with limited access to healthcare facilities and professionals. For example, IoT-enabled remote patient monitoring systems can collect patient data, which deep learning algorithms can analyse to provide real-time feedback and recommendations to healthcare providers.
- **Predictive Maintenance of Medical Equipment:** IoT devices can monitor the performance and condition of medical equipment, while deep learning algorithms can analyse this data to predict equipment failures and schedule maintenance. This can reduce downtime, improve equipment reliability, and lower maintenance costs.
- **Smart Hospital Operations:** IoT and deep learning technologies can optimise hospital operations, such as patient flow, resource allocation, and inventory management. For example, IoT devices can track the location and status of medical equipment and supplies, while deep learning algorithms can analyse this data to predict demand and optimise resource allocation.

16.3.4 Challenges and Barriers to Adoption

Despite the potential benefits of IoT and deep learning in healthcare, several challenges and barriers to adoption exist, including:

- **Data Privacy and Security:** The collection, storage, and analysis of sensitive health data pose significant privacy and security risks. Ensuring the protection of patient data and compliance with data protection regulations is crucial for successfully implementing IoT and deep learning technologies in healthcare.
- **Interoperability and Integration:** Integrating IoT and deep learning technologies into existing healthcare systems can be challenging, particularly regarding interoperability and data sharing. Developing standardised protocols and data formats is essential for seamless integration and collaboration between healthcare providers and technology platforms.
- **Infrastructure and Connectivity:** Implementing IoT and deep learning technologies in healthcare requires robust infrastructure and connectivity, particularly in rural areas with limited access to high-speed internet and advanced technology. Addressing these infrastructure challenges is critical for successfully adopting IoT and deep learning in healthcare.
- **Cost and Investment:** Adopting IoT and deep learning technologies in healthcare can be expensive, particularly for small and medium-sized healthcare providers with limited financial resources. Identifying cost-effective solutions and securing investment for technology implementation is essential for widespread adoption.

16.4 PRIVACY AND SECURITY CONCERNS

Integrating IoT and deep learning technologies in healthcare can transform patient care, improve diagnostics, and streamline hospital operations. However, collecting, storing, and analysing sensitive health data pose significant privacy and security risks. This section will explore the privacy and security concerns associated with adopting IoT and deep learning technologies in healthcare and the strategies and best practices for mitigating these risks.

16.4.1 Data Privacy Concerns

Data privacy protects personal information from unauthorised access, use, or disclosure. Data privacy is paramount in healthcare, as the sensitive nature of health data can have significant implications for individuals' privacy and well-being. Some of the critical data privacy concerns associated with IoT and deep learning technologies in healthcare include:

- **Unauthorised Access:** IoT devices and deep learning algorithms often rely on cloud-based storage and processing, which can expose health data to unauthorised access by hackers or other malicious actors.
- **Data Breaches:** The increasing volume and complexity of health data collected by IoT devices and analysed by deep learning algorithms can increase the risk of data breaches, potentially exposing sensitive patient information.
- **Inadequate Consent:** The collection and analysis of health data by IoT devices and deep learning algorithms may occur without patients' explicit consent, raising ethical concerns and potentially violating data protection regulations.
- **Data De-Identification and Re-Identification:** While de-identification techniques can protect patient privacy, the advanced capabilities of deep learning algorithms may enable the re-identification of de-identified data, potentially exposing sensitive patient information.

16.4.2 Data Security Concerns

Data security protects digital information from unauthorised access, use, or disclosure by implementing technical, administrative, and physical safeguards. Data security is crucial in healthcare to ensure health data's confidentiality, integrity, and availability. Some of the critical data security concerns associated with IoT and deep learning technologies in healthcare include:

- **Vulnerable IoT Devices:** IoT devices can be susceptible to security vulnerabilities, such as weak authentication mechanisms, insecure data transmission, and outdated software, exposing health data to unauthorised access or tampering.
- **Cyberattacks:** The increasing reliance on IoT devices and deep learning algorithms in healthcare can make healthcare systems more vulnerable to cyberattacks, such as ransomware, distributed denial-of-service (DDoS) attacks, and data theft.
- **Insider Threats:** Unauthorised access or misuse of health data by healthcare professionals, IT staff, or other insiders can pose significant security risks, potentially leading to data breaches or other security incidents.
- **Data Integrity:** Ensuring the accuracy and reliability of health data collected by IoT devices and analysed by deep learning algorithms is critical for maintaining patient trust and ensuring the effectiveness of healthcare services.

16.4.3 Regulatory Landscape

The regulatory landscape for data privacy and security in healthcare is complex and evolving, with numerous laws and regulations governing health data collection, storage, and use. Some of the key regulations and standards related to data privacy and security in healthcare include:

- **Health Insurance Portability and Accountability Act (HIPAA):** In the United States, HIPAA establishes national standards for the protection of electronic protected health information (ePHI) and requires healthcare providers, health plans, and other covered entities to implement appropriate safeguards to ensure the confidentiality, integrity, and availability of ePHI [9].
- **General Data Protection Regulation (GDPR):** In the European Union, the GDPR sets forth comprehensive data protection requirements for processing personal data, including health data [10]. The GDPR requires organisations to implement appropriate technical and organisational measures to protect personal data and obtain explicit consent from individuals for processing their health data.
- **ISO/IEC 27001:** This international standard provides a framework for the establishment, implementation, maintenance, and continuous improvement of an information security management system (ISMS) [11]. Organisations that achieve ISO/IEC 27001 certification demonstrate their commitment to maintaining the highest data security standards.

16.4.4 Strategies for Addressing Privacy and Security Concerns

To mitigate the privacy and security risks associated with the adoption of IoT and deep learning technologies in healthcare, organisations should implement a comprehensive approach that includes the following strategies:

- **Risk Assessment:** Conduct regular risk assessments to identify potential privacy and security vulnerabilities in IoT devices, deep learning algorithms, and associated systems and develop appropriate mitigation strategies.
- **Data Encryption:** Implement strong encryption for data at rest and in transit to protect sensitive health data from unauthorised access or tampering.
- **Access Controls:** Establish robust access controls, including multi-factor authentication, role-based access, and least privilege principles, to limit unauthorised access to health data and systems.
- **Security by Design:** Incorporate security considerations into the design and development of IoT devices and deep learning algorithms, ensuring that privacy and security features are built-in from the outset.
- **Security Monitoring and Incident Response:** Implement continuous security monitoring and develop an incident response plan to promptly detect, contain, and remediate potential security incidents.
- **Employee Training and Awareness:** Provide regular training and awareness programs for healthcare professionals, IT staff, and other stakeholders to ensure they understand their roles and responsibilities in maintaining data privacy and security.
- **Compliance Management:** Establish a compliance management program to ensure adherence to relevant data protection regulations and standards and to demonstrate accountability to patients, regulators, and other stakeholders.

16.5 ADDRESSING PRIVACY AND SECURITY CHALLENGES

As IoT and deep learning technologies transform healthcare, addressing privacy and security challenges becomes increasingly essential. This section will explore approaches and best practices for addressing these challenges, including technological solutions, policy development, and stakeholder collaboration.

16.5.1 Technological Solutions

Several technological solutions can be employed to address privacy and security challenges in healthcare IoT and deep learning applications:

- **Secure Communication Protocols:** Implementing secure communication protocols, such as Transport Layer Security (TLS) and Datagram Transport Layer Security (DTLS), can help protect data transmitted between IoT devices, cloud servers, and other components of the healthcare system.
- **Data Anonymisation and Pseudonymisation:** Applying data anonymisation and pseudonymisation techniques can help protect patient privacy by removing or replacing personally identifiable information (PII) from health data before it is processed or shared.
- **Blockchain Technology:** Blockchain technology can create secure, decentralised, and tamper-proof records of health data transactions, ensuring data integrity and providing an auditable trail of data access and usage.
- **Intrusion Detection and Prevention Systems (IDPSs):** Implementing IDPS solutions can help detect and prevent unauthorised access, data breaches, and other security incidents in healthcare IoT and deep learning systems.
- **Artificial Intelligence for Security:** AI-driven security solutions, such as machine learning algorithms for anomaly detection, can help identify potential security threats and vulnerabilities in healthcare IoT and deep learning systems, enabling proactive security measures.

16.5.2 Policy Development

Developing and implementing robust policies and guidelines is essential for addressing privacy and security challenges in healthcare IoT and deep learning applications:

- **Data Governance Framework:** Establishing a data governance framework can help ensure that health data is collected, stored, and processed in a secure, compliant, and ethical manner. This framework should include policies and procedures for data classification, retention, sharing, and disposal.
- **Privacy Impact Assessments (PIAs):** Conducting PIAs can help identify potential privacy risks associated with healthcare IoT and deep learning applications and develop appropriate mitigation strategies. PIAs should be conducted regularly and whenever significant changes are made to the system or its data processing activities.
- **Security Policies and Procedures:** Developing and implementing comprehensive security policies and procedures can help protect healthcare IoT and deep learning systems against unauthorised access, data breaches, and other security incidents. These policies should cover access controls, encryption, incident response, and security monitoring.
- **Ethical Guidelines:** Establishing ethical guidelines for using IoT and deep learning technologies in healthcare can help ensure these technologies are used responsibly and in patients' best interests. These guidelines should address informed consent, data privacy, and algorithmic fairness issues.

16.5.3 Collaboration among Stakeholders

Collaboration among various stakeholders, including healthcare providers, technology developers, regulators, and patients, is crucial for addressing privacy and security challenges in healthcare IoT and deep learning applications:

- **Public–Private Partnerships:** Establishing public–private partnerships can help facilitate sharing of knowledge, resources, and best practices for addressing privacy and security challenges in healthcare IoT and deep learning applications. These partnerships can also help drive the development of innovative solutions and promote the adoption of industry standards.
- **Cross-Sector Collaboration:** Encouraging collaboration among stakeholders from different sectors, such as healthcare, technology, and cybersecurity, can help foster a multidisciplinary approach to addressing privacy and security challenges in healthcare IoT and deep learning applications.
- **Patient Engagement:** Involving patients in developing and implementing healthcare IoT and deep learning applications can help ensure that these technologies are designed with patient privacy and security in mind. Patient engagement can also help build trust and promote the responsible use of health data.
- **International Cooperation:** Collaborating with international partners can help promote developing and adopting global standards and best practices for addressing privacy and security challenges in healthcare IoT and deep learning applications. International cooperation can also facilitate the sharing of knowledge and resources, as well as the harmonisation of regulatory frameworks.

16.5.4 Education and Training

Providing education and training for healthcare professionals, technology developers, and other stakeholders is essential for addressing privacy and security challenges in healthcare IoT and deep learning applications:

- **Healthcare Professional Training:** Ensuring that healthcare professionals are knowledgeable about the privacy and security risks associated with IoT and deep learning technologies can help promote the responsible use of these technologies and the protection of patient data.
- **Technology Developer Training:** Training technology developers on privacy and security best practices can help ensure that healthcare IoT and deep learning applications are designed with security in mind from the outset.
- **Patient Education:** Educating patients about the privacy and security risks associated with healthcare IoT and deep learning applications can help empower them to make informed decisions about their health data and using these technologies.
- **Cybersecurity Workforce Development:** Investing in cybersecurity workforce development can help ensure sufficient skilled professionals can address the privacy and security challenges associated with healthcare IoT and deep learning applications.

16.5.5 Continuous Improvement and Adaptation

As the healthcare industry continues to evolve and adopt new technologies, organisations need to maintain a continuous improvement and adaptation mindset to address privacy and security challenges effectively:

- **Regular System Audits:** Regular audits of healthcare IoT and deep learning systems can help identify potential privacy and security vulnerabilities and ensure that these systems comply with relevant regulations and best practices.

- **Continuous Monitoring:** Implementing continuous monitoring solutions can help detect and respond to potential privacy and security incidents in real-time, minimising the potential impact of these incidents on patient data and healthcare operations.
- **Adaptive Security Architecture:** Developing an adaptive security architecture can help healthcare organisations respond to the dynamic nature of privacy and security threats in the IoT and deep learning landscape. This approach involves continuously assessing and adjusting security controls and processes based on the changing threat environment and the organisation's risk tolerance.
- **Research and Development:** Investing in research and development can help drive the discovery of new privacy-enhancing and security technologies for healthcare IoT and deep learning applications. This can include the development of advanced encryption techniques, privacy-preserving machine learning algorithms, and secure hardware designs.

16.5.6 Legal and Regulatory Considerations

As healthcare organisations address privacy and security challenges, it is crucial to stay informed about the legal and regulatory landscape and ensure compliance with relevant laws and regulations:

- **Regulatory Compliance:** Healthcare organisations must ensure that their IoT and deep learning systems comply with applicable data protection and security regulations, such as HIPAA, GDPR, and other regional or industry-specific regulations. This may involve conducting regular compliance assessments and working with legal and regulatory experts to navigate the complex regulatory landscape.
- **Data Breach Notification:** In the event of a data breach or other security incident, healthcare organisations must be prepared to comply with data breach notification requirements, which may vary depending on the jurisdiction and the nature of the incident. This includes developing a data breach response plan and ensuring that all stakeholders know their roles and responsibilities in the event of a breach.
- **Legal Liability:** Healthcare organisations should know the potential liability of privacy and security incidents involving IoT and deep learning technologies. This may involve working with legal counsel to assess potential liability risks and develop strategies for mitigating these risks, such as obtaining appropriate insurance coverage or implementing robust risk management processes.

16.6 THE WAY FORWARD

As healthcare organisations adopt IoT and deep learning technologies, it is essential to consider the Way forward in addressing privacy and security challenges. This section will explore the future trends, emerging technologies, and strategies that will shape the healthcare landscape and help organisations navigate the evolving privacy and security landscape.

16.6.1 Future Trends in Healthcare IoT and Deep Learning

Several trends are expected to shape the future of healthcare IoT and deep learning, with implications for privacy and security:

- **Increased Integration of IoT and Deep Learning:** IoT and deep learning technologies will continue to expand, with more healthcare organisations adopting these technologies to improve patient care, streamline operations, and enhance decision-making.

- **Personalised Medicine:** IoT and deep learning technologies will enable more personalised medicine, with healthcare providers leveraging data-driven insights to tailor treatments and interventions to individual patients' needs and preferences.
- **Telemedicine and Remote Monitoring:** The growth of telemedicine and remote monitoring solutions will continue, driven by the increasing availability of IoT devices and the expanding capabilities of deep learning algorithms to analyse and interpret health data.
- **Interoperability and Data Sharing:** The need for interoperability and data sharing among healthcare organisations will grow with health data's increasing volume, and complexity necessitates more efficient and effective ways to exchange and analyse information.
- **Ethical and Regulatory Debates:** The adoption of IoT and deep learning technologies in healthcare will continue to raise ethical and regulatory debates as stakeholders grapple with issues such as data privacy, algorithmic fairness, and informed consent.

16.6.2 Emerging Technologies and Their Impact on Privacy and Security

Several emerging technologies have the potential to impact privacy and security in healthcare IoT and deep learning applications:

- **Quantum Computing:** The development of quantum computing could have significant implications for data security, as quantum computers have the potential to break current encryption algorithms. Healthcare organisations must monitor advancements in quantum computing and adopt new encryption techniques to protect sensitive health data.
- **Federated Learning:** Federated learning is a privacy-preserving machine learning approach that enables training deep learning models on decentralised data sources without sharing raw data. This approach can help protect patient privacy while still enabling the development of powerful deep learning algorithms for healthcare applications.
- **Homomorphic Encryption:** Homomorphic encryption is a cryptographic technique that allows computations on encrypted data without decrypting it. This technology can enable privacy-preserving data analysis in healthcare IoT and deep learning applications, as sensitive health data can be processed without exposing it to potential privacy risks.
- **Edge Computing:** Edge computing involves processing data closer to the source, such as on IoT devices or local servers, rather than relying on centralised cloud-based processing. This approach can help reduce the privacy and security risks associated with transmitting and storing sensitive health data in the cloud.

16.6.3 Strategies for Navigating the Evolving Privacy and Security Landscape

As healthcare organisations look to the future, several strategies can help them navigate the evolving privacy and security landscape:

- **Embrace a Culture of Privacy and Security:** Healthcare organisations should foster a culture of privacy and security, with leadership emphasising the importance of protecting patient data and ensuring the responsible use of IoT and deep learning technologies.
- **Invest in Research and Development:** Healthcare organisations should invest in research and development to explore new privacy-enhancing and security technologies and stay informed about emerging trends and threats in the healthcare landscape.
- **Collaborate with Stakeholders:** Healthcare organisations should continue collaborating with stakeholders, including technology developers, regulators, and patients, to share knowledge, resources, and best practices for addressing privacy and security challenges.

- **Develop a Flexible and Adaptive Security Strategy:** Healthcare organisations should develop a flexible and adaptive security strategy that can respond to the dynamic nature of privacy and security threats in the IoT and deep learning landscape. This may involve continuously assessing and adjusting security controls and processes based on the changing threat environment and the organisation's risk tolerance.
- **Engage in Policy and Regulatory Discussions:** Healthcare organisations should actively engage in policy and regulatory discussions related to IoT and deep learning technologies, advocating for the development of balanced and practical frameworks that protect patient privacy and security while enabling innovation and progress in healthcare.

16.7 CONCLUSION

As the healthcare landscape evolves, all stakeholders must remain vigilant and proactive in addressing privacy and security challenges. By staying informed about emerging trends and technologies, engaging in policy and regulatory discussions, and maintaining a continuous improvement and adaptation mindset, healthcare organisations can ensure the responsible and ethical use of IoT and deep learning technologies to improve patient care and outcomes.

The rapid adoption of IoT and deep learning technologies in the Indian healthcare sector has the potential to revolutionise patient care, streamline operations, and enhance decision-making. However, these advancements also bring forth significant privacy and security challenges that must be addressed to ensure the responsible and ethical use of these transformative technologies.

Addressing privacy and security issues for IoT and deep learning in next-generation healthcare in India requires a multifaceted approach involving technological solutions, policy development, collaboration among stakeholders, education and training, continuous improvement and adaptation, and policy and regulatory discussions. By implementing these strategies, Indian healthcare organisations can successfully navigate the evolving privacy and security landscape and harness the full potential of IoT and deep learning technologies to improve patient care and outcomes.

In this conclusion, we will summarise the key points discussed throughout the chapter and highlight the importance of a collaborative and proactive approach to addressing privacy and security issues in the Indian healthcare landscape.

- **Technological Solutions:** Adopting secure communication protocols, data anonymisation and pseudonymisation techniques, blockchain technology, intrusion detection and prevention systems, and AI-driven security solutions can help protect sensitive health data and mitigate privacy and security risks in the Indian healthcare sector.
- **Policy Development:** Establishing robust data governance frameworks, conducting privacy impact assessments, developing comprehensive security policies and procedures, and implementing ethical guidelines are essential for ensuring that health data is collected, stored, and processed in a secure, compliant, and ethical manner in India.
- **Collaboration among Stakeholders:** Encouraging collaboration among various stakeholders, including healthcare providers, technology developers, regulators, and patients, is crucial for addressing privacy and security challenges in the Indian healthcare sector. Public–private partnerships, cross-sector collaboration, patient engagement, and international cooperation can help facilitate the sharing of knowledge, resources, and best practices.
- **Education and Training:** Providing education and training for healthcare professionals, technology developers, and other stakeholders is essential for addressing privacy and security challenges in the Indian healthcare sector. Ensuring that healthcare professionals are knowledgeable about the privacy and security risks associated with IoT and deep learning technologies can help promote the responsible use of these technologies and the protection of patient data.
- **Continuous Improvement and Adaptation:** As the Indian healthcare landscape evolves, organisations must maintain a continuous improvement and adaptation mindset to address

privacy and security challenges effectively. Regular system audits, continuous monitoring, adaptive security architecture, and investment in research and development can help healthcare organisations avoid emerging threats and vulnerabilities.

- **Legal and Regulatory Considerations:** Staying informed about the legal and regulatory landscape and ensuring compliance with relevant laws and regulations, such as the Personal Data Protection Bill [12], is crucial for addressing privacy and security challenges in the Indian healthcare sector. Healthcare organisations must be prepared to comply with data breach notification requirements and be aware of the potential legal liability associated with privacy and security incidents involving IoT and deep learning technologies.
- **The Way Forward:** Embracing emerging trends, adopting new technologies, and implementing proactive strategies can help Indian healthcare organisations navigate the evolving privacy and security landscape. Fostering a culture of privacy and security, investing in research and development, collaborating with stakeholders, and developing flexible and adaptive security strategies are essential for harnessing the full potential of IoT and deep learning technologies while safeguarding patient privacy and security.

REFERENCES

[1] The Times of India, "India's 1.4 billion population could become world economy's new growth engine," 23 January 2023. [Online]. Available: https://timesofindia.indiatimes.com/business/india-business/indias-1-4-billion-population-could-become-world-economys-new-growth-engine/articleshow/97239739.cms [Accessed 23 June 2023].

[2] Ministry of Health and Family Welfare, "National Health Policy 2017," 2017. [Online]. Available: https://main.mohfw.gov.in/sites/default/files/9147562941489753121.pdf [Accessed 23 June 2023].

[3] Ministry of Health and Family Welfare, "Rural Health Statistics 2019–20," 2019. [Online]. Available: https://main.mohfw.gov.in/sites/default/files/RHS%202019-20_2.pdf [Accessed 18 April 2023].

[4] Ministry of Health and Family Welfare, "Government Health Expenditure's share in country's total GDP increases from 1.13% (2014–15) to 1.35% (2019–20)," 25 April 2023. [Online]. Available: https://pib.gov.in/PressReleaseIframePage.aspx?PRID=1919582#:~:text=During%20this%20period%2C%20the%20share,1.35%25%20in%202019%2D20.&text=In%20per%20capita%20terms%2C%20GHE,%2D15%20to%202019%2D20 [Accessed 23 June 2023].

[5] Ministry of Health and Family Welfare, "National health estimates (2018–19)," 12 September 2022. [Online]. Available: https://pib.gov.in/PressReleasePage.aspx?PRID=1858770 [Accessed June 2023].

[6] Ministry of Health and Family Welfare, "National Family Health Survey (NFHS-4)," 2017. [Online]. Available: https://dhsprogram.com/pubs/pdf/fr339/fr339.pdf[Accessed 20 May 2023].

[7] The Economic Times, "80 per cent of Indian doctors located in urban areas," 19 August 2016. [Online]. Available: https://economictimes.indiatimes.com/industry/healthcare-biotech/80-per-cent-of-indian-doctors-located-in-urban-areas/articleshow/53774521.cms?from=mdr [Accessed 23 June 2023].

[8] Ministry of Health and Family Welfare, "National Digital Health Blueprint," 2019. [Online]. Available: https://abdm.gov.in:8081/uploads/ndhb_1_56ec695bc8.pdf [Accessed 23 June 2023].

[9] Centers for Disease Control and Prevention, "Health Insurance Portability and Accountability Act of 1996 (HIPAA)," 27 June 2022. [Online]. Available: www.cdc.gov/phlp/publications/topic/hipaa.html [Accessed 23 June 2023].

[10] EUR-Lex, "General Data Protection Regulation," 27 April 2016. [Online]. Available: https://eur-lex.europa.eu/legal-content/EN/TXT/?uri=CELEX%3A02016R0679-20160504 [Accessed 23 June 2023].

[11] International Organization for Standardization, "ISO/IEC 27001: Information security management systems," October 2022. [Online]. Available: www.iso.org/standard/27001 [Accessed 23 June 2023].

[12] PRS Legislative Research, "The Personal Data Protection Bill, 2019," [Online]. Available: https://prsindia.org/billtrack/the-personal-data-protection-bill-2019 [Accessed 23 June 2023].

17 A Systematic Review on the Future of Internet of Things Applications in Healthcare

Pallavi S. Bangare and Kishor P. Patil

17.1 INTRODUCTION

A unique novel virus known as SARS-CoV-2 causes the severe respiratory contamination known as COVID-19. In addition, the new coronavirus is responsible for creating a worldwide health crisis that is unprecedented in recent history. On January 30, 2020, the World Health Organisation (WHO) announced that COVID-19 had been classified as a public health emergency of international concern (PHEIC). The World Health Organisation proclaimed it a plague less than a year and a half after the first case of COVID-19 was discovered in Wuhan, China.

Since the discovery of the first case in December 2019, a total of around 192 million cases and over 4 million fatalities have been reported across the globe as of July 25, 2021. Within the context of COVID-19 as it exists now, several nations are making use of an assortment of digital tools to advance activities related to public health. The problems that are described in more detail subsequently need more research and solutions to be developed and implemented. It is believed that newly developed innovative healthcare systems lack guidance and sufficient documentation, which has led to a false impression of a lack of goal clarity and wasteful use of resources. It has also been discovered that there is a lack of standards across geographical areas and medical institutes. It is believed that there is a need for improvements in data security. The exchange of data and communication are often thought to be restricted due to the magnitude and complexity of the data.

It has been determined that there are compatibility issues with various platforms and devices. From the point of view of the patient, it appears as though there is a deficiency in the applicable legal safeguards. The users of some of the new technology have trouble utilising it; technology requires a significant investment of cash to maintain and improve. As a solution to these problems, there is a growing interest in the capacity for information analysis and the continued development of technology. It has been widely acknowledged that the development of a uniform technological standard for device and platform compatibility is an absolute necessity. This analysis will start off with a discussion of a forward-thinking healthcare system. It gives a list of similar technologies that have been implemented in the healthcare system. The review then presents a case study based on the health issues related to COVID-19 in order to explore the current operation of the innovative healthcare system. The review also identifies a number of different advanced technologies that have been used in the COVID-19 pandemic, and it concludes by examining the future prospects of this system. The COVID-19 epidemic provides a helpful glimpse into how reality works for Internet of Things–stimulated structures and solutions. Technology that is part of the Internet of Things (IoT), such as personal health monitoring and communications, is supporting the government in controlling the spread of the coronavirus.

The concept of the Internet of Things has had a significant influence on our day-to-day lives during the past few years. Not only your computer but also your smartphone, which is the only device within your reach, can connect to the internet. However, now that the Internet of Things has arrived,

DOI: 10.1201/9781003451846-17

many different pieces of household equipment may be connected to the internet. This includes many different pieces of family home equipment. Because it is already beginning to have an influence on significant facets of our lives, the Internet of Things looks to have a brilliant and exciting future ahead of it. The demand for Internet of Things products is growing as a result of a number of factors, including an ageing population, population growth, rising healthcare costs, and an expanding elderly population. This chapter provides the first comprehensive analysis of important Internet of Things solutions for health, connection monitoring, and mobility during the course of the COVID pandemic. Each and every work has been given a significant amount of investigation and consideration in terms of its execution, as well as its impact on primary changes and social and financial repercussions.

The following explanation will provide an overview as well as a breakdown of the Internet of Things technology that was created by businesses. This current generation has the potential to make significant contributions to history. IoT programmes in each of the selected sectors are analysed largely based on whether they are financially and socially feasible, whether there are huge usage prospects, and how far along the generation readiness scale they are. In addition, the next generation of Internet of Things research is covered in the discussion. These applications will improve overall performance, make the public more accommodating, and secure the privacy and safety of clients, all while enhancing overall efficiency.

17.2 LITERATURE REVIEW

In Omar Ali et al. (2023)'s paper titled "A Review of Advanced Technologies Available to Improve the Healthcare Performance during COVID-19 Pandemic", a case study methodology was applied to carry out an in-depth examination of records with regard to a particular setting. It does this by presenting a case study of the coronavirus (COVID-19) as a tool to examine how modern technology is utilised in a healthcare system to assist in dealing with a major international health problem. This allows for an in-depth examination of the subject. A healthcare system has the potential to improve patient care, encourage more patient self-management, decrease staff burden, store pricing, aid resource and technology management, and support patient education and counselling. A healthcare device that thinks ahead has the potential to cut costs and shorten the amount of time needed for research while also boosting overall effectiveness. The findings of this study demonstrate how various technologies may increase the efficiency of healthcare devices. They have the potential to assist with the identification of viral infections, clinical treatment, scientific safety, intelligent prognostication, and evaluation of epidemics. This gives them the ability to assist with the manipulation of pandemics.

Sridhar Siripurapu et al. (2023)'s paper is entitled "Technological Advancements and Elucidation Gadgets for Healthcare Applications: An Exhaustive Methodological". The extensive applicability of technological advances to the healthcare industry and the industries closely related to it is on the verge of raising concerns regarding the capacity of hospitals, clinical centres, medical doctors, and scientific pathologists to provide high-quality healthcare to the patient population of the world. This study was prompted by inquiries about the part that technical advancements play in the medical field, and those inquiries served as the study's primary source of inspiration.

The first section of this analysis focused on the many ways in which new technologies, such as cloud computing, big data, open-source computing, block chains, artificial intelligence, and others, might be utilised to enhance the healthcare sector and the companies that are closely related to it. A substantial examination of the potential of other disruptive technologies such as robots, drones, three-dimensional printing, the Internet of Things, digital/augmented/blended reality, and so on is carried out in order to bring to light the vast majority of challenging circumstances that are encountered by the therapeutic community. The research that has been carried out to manipulate the use of these technologies in a variety of allied healthcare fields is the primary focus of this work.

Andreia Robert Lopes et al. (2023) have research entitled "Application of Technology in Healthcare: Tackling COVID-19 Challenge—The Integration of Blockchain and Internet of Things".

The COVID-19 outbreak has caused serious disruptions to healthcare systems in various parts of the world and brought to light a number of critical issues that need to be tackled in order to maintain medical services. This pandemic has provided healthcare systems with a challenge they have never dealt with before, which has paved the opportunity for innovation and the introduction of new treatments. Because healthcare organisations have begun the process of digital transformation, there is a significant amount of upheaval occurring in the healthcare sector.

The technologies of blockchain and the Internet of Things have the potential to change the healthcare sector and assist in the resolution of some of the problems associated with healthcare systems. Many of these problems have been rendered significantly worse as a result of the COVID-19 tragedy. In this chapter, we look at the technologies of the Internet of Things and blockchain, concentrating on their most important characteristics, the advantages of integrating them, the limitations, and the difficult challenges that still need to be overcome. The authors delved deeper into its potential by detailing not only singular instances but also capability programmes for healthcare in general and for COVID-19 in particular.

Lamya Alkhariji et al. (2023) introduced a paper entitled "Semantics-Based Privacy by Design for Internet of Things Applications". Concerns regarding an individual's right to non-public privacy are coming to the forefront as the variety of items that may be securely connected to the Internet of Things continues to increase in commonplace use in day-to-day existence.

The achievement of this purpose may be made more likely by the development of a tool that is appropriate for use in the Internet of Things and that operates within it in a way that is both environmentally responsible and dependable. You utilise technology that is likely connected to the semantic internet to explain the statistics behind PbD measurements, their intersections with privacy patterns, the requirements for IoT systems, and the privacy patterns that should be implemented throughout IoT systems. This is done in an effort to provide an answer to the question of why it is that these statistics exist.

This gives you the ability to describe the information that lies behind PbD measurements, including their intersections with privacy patterns, the needs for Internet of Things systems, and the requirements for Internet of Things structures. With the help of this, it's possible that you'll be able to do things like determining the requirements for Internet of Things architectures. The employment of a graph of comprehension allows for the effective completion of this endeavour, which serves as the crowning splendour. This purpose turned into able to be carried out with the aid of the PARROT ontology, which changed into accomplished via a set of frequent IoT use instances that are beneficial to software programming applications programmers. Your goals may now be accomplished as a consequence of developments that were made to the PARROT ontology, which made it possible for you to carry out those objectives.

Fazli Subhan et al. (2023) presented the paper "AI-Enabled Wearable Medical Internet of Things in Healthcare System: A Survey". The current generation accounts for a sizeable number of the lifestyle improvements that have been implemented, the majority of which have been implemented as alternatives to medical care in hospitals. The most important driver behind this expansion was the urgent requirement to speedily connect various sources of medical care with one another.

In recent years, wearable technologies have earned a reputation for being beneficial pieces of equipment for a wide variety of healthcare activities. As a consequence of this, a wide variety of products are now available on the market as a result of some of the unique motives that inspired their development. These products include individualised healthcare, recreational signals, and exercise. The primary objective of this study is to conduct an in-depth investigation of all of the most recent developments that have been made in the field of the wearable clinical Internet of Medical Things (IoMT) for healthcare systems. It is only feasible to evaluate the effectiveness of these technologies in healthcare settings on the basis of the assumptions that have been developed. These assumptions make it possible to evaluate the usefulness of these technologies for the cause of identifying illnesses, avoiding diseases, and keeping track of diseases.

In a similar vein, the majority of today's most pressing health concerns, such as COVID-19 and monkeypox, are covered by insurance. In this study, an in-depth assessment of all of the probable options that researchers have offered for improving healthcare through the use of wearable technology and artificial intelligence is provided. This investigation was carried out by the researchers of the aforementioned study. These opportunities are presented within the framework of enhancing healthcare. This section devotes a significant amount of both time and space to the explanation of the approaches that the researchers employed to better the overall accuracy, efficacy, and protection of the clinical devices. This research also explores every challenge and potential benefit linked with the development of AI-enabled, primarily IoT-based healthcare solutions.

Lokesh B. Bhajantri et al. (2023) produced research entitled "A Survey on Cognitive Internet of Things Based Prediction of Covid-19 Patient". In today's world, wireless patient monitoring devices are absolutely necessary in order to anticipate or locate Covid-19 patients in a dependable manner. Because the virus is so highly contagious, it is imperative to establish isolation centres in order to be able to treat those who have been infected with Covid-19. These centres will allow administration of treatment to those who have the virus. It is necessary for these facilities to be situated in real-world environments. When there is an outbreak of an endemic disease, it is exceedingly difficult to determine the place of origin of each and every individual patient who is afflicted with the disease. In addition, in order to ensure that their patients receive the best possible care, medical workers strive to uncover and maintain control of the wireless environment in which their patients are put.

This ensures that patients receive the best possible treatment. An investigation into the cognitive net of factor-based predictions of Covid-19 patients is now being carried out in this setting with the use of a learning algorithm. This article presents a comprehensive analysis of the given issue in terms of its restrictions, benefits and drawbacks of wireless communication, and general overall performance characteristics for a range of different methods. It does this by putting in place a framework for a device that can anticipate and track persons infected with the Covid-19 virus anywhere in the world wirelessly. Consequently, the suggested method is utilised to reveal the symptoms of patients in a non-intrusive manner. This includes temperature, SpO_2, and the cough charge of Covid-19 patients, and it does so by making use of smart sensors. Using a Wi-Fi approach, the information is transmitted to the internet server over the network that is being used.

Mavis Gezimati & Ghanshyam Singh (2023) introduced research entitled "Internet of Things Enabled Framework for Terahertz and Infrared Cancer Imaging". This is most likely done in order to demonstrate the efficacy of various treatment options, the unfavourable effects of multiple drugs, the results of statistical analysis, and the capability of making accurate predictions about the majority of individuals who have cancer. In the framework of the Healthcare 4.0 paradigm, having an intelligent prognosis is crucial, as is the administration of treatment by means of remote patient monitoring.

This is because the Healthcare 4.0 paradigm is geared towards enhancing the quality of care provided to patients. Combining the knowledge gained from the area of medicine with the primary signs and symptoms, as well as the signs and symptoms linked with the majority of malignancies, is not always entirely out of the question. As a result of this, the device has the potential to grow into one that is intelligent and has data on various forms of exercise. It is our recommendation that, in addition to pretrained, precisely adjusted CNN models that are capable of classifying multimodal pictures, bespoke CNN models should also be developed.

The purpose of this study is to create a deep learning system that is able to categorise snapshots of breasts and is supported by the Internet of Things. One of the skills provided through the ThingSpeak cloud platform, used by applications for modelling the Internet of Things and cloud processing, is the ability to send email alerts.

K.S. Arvind et al. (2023) provided research entitled "Pandemic Management Using Internet of Things and Big Data—A Security and Privacy Perspective". During these challenging times, the containment of pandemics through the utilisation of technology like the Internet of Things, artificial intelligence, 5G, and blockchain has had a significant impact all over the world. As a direct and immediate consequence of the ongoing pandemic catastrophe, our society has undergone a significant number of behavioural as well as socioeconomic alterations in a very short period of time.

This has also led in the exploitation of technology such as the Internet of Things and artificial intelligence in order to discover answers to the actual international challenges that have arisen as a result of the COVID-19 outbreak. This article addresses the concerns about safety and confidentiality that arise when utilising the Internet of Things for pandemic management. In particular, it focuses on the safety and privacy issues that come up when trying to track down contacts through the use of IoT and cellular phones. The term "contact tracing" refers to the method that governmental organisations are employing in order to become aware of sick people as well as those who have had contact with an infected person in the past. This has developed into a significant source of concern for businesses.

The process of identifying previous connections is an important step in reducing the likelihood that the illness may spread across the community. Mobile packages that may be fitted with GPS, Bluetooth, or NFC devices are being utilised by a number of particular countries in order to track down infected individuals through contact tracing. This is being done in an effort to hunt down the people who are involved in the pandemic.

Sasikumar et al. (2023) presented research entitled "Blockchain-Based Trust Mechanism for Digital Twin Empowered Industrial Internet of Things". Because of the increasing number of nodes that are a part of the economic Internet of Things, it is a lot more difficult to optimise the community and make the most of the limited resources in order to guarantee safe transmission. A digital twin is a virtual version of a real-world object, and it completely relies on information amassed through sensors in order to imitate the process of making important judgements about the real-world object.

Integrating a commercially dispersed community primarily based on blockchain technology with a virtual twin for applications linked to the Industrial Internet of Things (IIoT) facilitates the realisation of this goal. To deliver offerings within the realm of the Internet of Things, a blockchain-based proof of authority (PoA) method is recommended within this framework. These services include the protection of personal information and confidentiality. In a similar fashion, in order for an organisation to generate a genesis block, it makes use of a deterministic pseudo-random generation (DPRG). The completion of this step results in the creation of an entirely new block.

The purpose of this action is to give decentralised virtual twin mixed blockchain networks a more trustworthy appearance. We do this by creating a digital twin of the blockchain community through the use of IIoT sensor nodes. This allows us to determine how trustworthy the suggested device actually is. The results of the simulation indicate that completely authoritative PoA-based master nodes may have the capability to lessen the amount of electricity that is used while concurrently increasing the level of information security.

Zhenwei Zhao et al. (2023) presented research entitled "Secure Internet of Things (IoT) Using a Novel Brooks Iyengar Quantum Byzantine Agreement-Centered Blockchain Networking (BIQBA-BCN) Model in Smart Healthcare". The idea of an advanced network of factors is the driving force behind the development of smart fitness care, which offers human services that are capable of being both effective and ecologically friendly, in addition to being delivered in real time.

Despite this, the linking of Internet of Things-centric sensors with other companies introduces security risks in the form of the possibility that an unauthorised user may use it owing to the availability of the records. These risks may be mitigated, however, by ensuring that only approved users have access to the records. The preservation of patient information and the confidentiality of statistics are the top priorities in the healthcare sector. This is owing to the fact that any change in records data collected by sensors has the potential to impact the diagnostic procedure, which in turn may potentially result in more significant health problems. Blockchain technology, which cannot be tampered with and can be accessed by anybody, has recently surfaced as a potentially beneficial prospect for the secure storage and administration of patient information. However, blockchain poses a threat to the transfer of healthcare data due to issues with cloud storage servers (CSSs), delayed consensus, majority attacks, the Byzantine problem, and inadequate records throughput (TP), among other challenges.

In the healthcare business, an attempt has been undertaken to provide a safe Internet of Things by utilising a blockchain networking protocol called Brooks Iyengar quantum byzantine agreement-focused blockchain networking. This was done with the intention of minimising the negative effects that are now occurring. With the help of this examination, we will determine if the modification of medical records was carried out in an honest and equitable manner. The suggested artwork provides a Blum Blum Shub-Okamoto Uchiyama Cryptosystem (BBS-OUC), which is a mutually authenticated system entirely based on OUCS. The Blum Blum Shub and Okamoto Uchiyama Cryptosystem (OUCS), a kind of mutual authentication, is the sole foundation upon which the computer is constructed. Intruders are not allowed within the BCN, which ensures that the storage will continue to function reliably even in the face of potential threats. In a comparable manner, the key weight block characteristic-quasi-cyclic mild density parity check (KWBF-QCMDPC) technique preserves the anonymity of IoT personal info and guarantees its dependability. The adoption of the cryptosystem approach ensures the confidentiality of sensitive documents even after the blockchain platform has been distributed to a large number of users.

Md Oqail Ahmad & Shams Tabrez Siddiqui (2022) presented a research entitled "The Internet of Things for Healthcare: Benefits, Applications, Challenges, Use Cases and Future Directions". The Internet of Things is a network of digital devices that can communicate with one another over wireless connections and are able to collect, send, and store data independently of the intervention of either humans or other machines. These devices are known as "things." The Internet of Things presents a lot of opportunities for improving and advancing the state of healthcare delivery in the world. These advantages include the capacity to diagnose, treat, and monitor patients both within and outside of hospitals, as well as the ability to anticipate and prevent any future health problems. Government leaders and decision makers all over the world are currently rushing to put into action regulations that would permit the delivery of medical services by means of the utilisation of technology, in particular in light of the COVID-19 pandemic.

This article's objective is to give the reader an in-depth understanding of how the Internet of Things can be utilised effectively in the healthcare industry. This will be accomplished by presenting use case packages together with regional and enabling technologies that may transform IoT-based healthcare solutions. This discussion will be carried out by investigating the many ways in which the Internet of Things might be exploited successfully in the medical field. IoT-based intelligent devices and systems, along with various IoT applications used within the healthcare industry, are examined comprehensively. This assessment provides a thorough understanding of the advantages of Internet of Things-based healthcare, along with detailed information on the challenges that need to be addressed for the stabilisation of the Internet of Things-based health environment.

Amit Kishor and Chinmay Chakraborty (2022) have a paper entitled "Artificial Intelligence and Internet of Things Based Healthcare 4.0 Monitoring System". The application of artificial intelligence in the field of healthcare is becoming increasingly popular as a production method, yielding accurate and precisely timed results. Early disorder projections enable medical professionals to make decisions that have a high probability of saving the lives of those who are afflicted with the illness. In the field of healthcare, artificial intelligence software is becoming more successful as a result of the use of the Internet of Things, which functions as a using factor.

This is due to the potential of the IoT to link devices from a variety of manufacturers. This is due to the fact that the Internet of Things possesses the ability to operate as catalyst. IoT sensors are responsible for obtaining data from patients, and machine learning algorithms are utilised as an efficient approach to behaviour analysis on the data that has been accumulated over the course of time. The primary purpose of this investigation is to develop a healthcare model that is wholly reliant on machine learning and is in a position to accurately foresee a wide variety of diseases. This version might be used for patients in order to diagnose and treat them. In this study, a total of seven machine learning algorithms, selection tree, support vector machine, naive Bayes, adaptive boosting, random forest (RF), artificial neural network, and k-nearest neighbour, are utilised in an effort to make a prognosis of nine diseases that can result in death. This research is carried out with the goal of acquiring a more in-depth understanding of the most effective ways to prevent the spread of these illnesses.

Some of the conditions that are included in this category include heart disease, diabetes-related breast cancer, hepatitis, liver disease, dermatology, surgical treatment records, and thyroid. Accuracy, sensitivity, specificity, and area below the curve are the four overall performance indicators that may be employed in the process of completing an evaluation of the usefulness of a model that has been proposed. Accuracy is the ability of a model to predict the true value of a variable with a high degree of precision.

Damini Verma et al. (2022) have research entitled "Internet of Things (IoT) in Nano-Integrated Wearable Biosensor Devices for Healthcare Applications". The state of one's health is one of the most essential aspects of life. However, due to the limited resources available at healthcare facilities, many patients encounter various hurdles throughout the course of their treatment. This is one of the reasons many patients are unable to get the treatment they want. The Internet of Things is currently the most exciting topic, and it offers a variety of techniques through which those restrictions may be overcome. In the scientific community, the Internet of Things is utilised in a variety of applications, including the diagnosis, treatment, and tracking of medical conditions. The use of wearable technology by patients might be of assistance in ensuring that they receive the most effective treatment.

Traditional communication networks, which were developed for applications that are mostly focused on humans, have a number of issues. These issues include high latency, limited processing capabilities, and short battery life. These problems are a direct outcome of the expansion of these networks during the past few years. Alternatively, the development of 5G has led to the advancement of a new set of technologies that provide the essential "backbone" for connecting to the billions of gadgets that could be a part of the forthcoming IoT. This is necessary to completely revolutionise both our professional and private ways of life. This network has made it possible for new prospects to arise in the field of healthcare, including treatment, data analytics, diagnostics, and imaging. This is due to the fact that 5G provides statistics capabilities, intelligent control, and lightning-fast connectivity. In this work, an extensive literature review of the Internet of Things, wearable gadgets that are largely based on IoT, and the function of 5G in IoT for healthcare applications are covered in depth. In addition, it examines the value of wearable technology in the clinical assessment of problems, which includes the treatment, monitoring, and identification of illness.

Mansour Alraja (2022) presented research entitled "Frontline Healthcare Providers' Behavioural Intention to Internet of Things (IoT)-Enabled Healthcare Applications: A Gender-Based, Cross-Generational Study". The incorporation of Internet of Things technology into healthcare delivery systems brings with it the potential for a wide variety of dangers. People's trust in newly formed technology has been proved to suffer as an immediate consequence of the Internet of Things' sensing capabilities, which presents real problems about breaches of personal privacy. People's trust in newly created technology has suffered as a direct result of the sensing capabilities of the Internet of Things. This is a reality that has been presented well. This study makes an effort to address a glaring gap in the existing body of research, specifically the overemphasis on gender differences in the behavioural intentions of frontline healthcare practitioners (FHPs), which is the focus of the majority of the study.

This deficiency is particularly relevant to the point of interest of gender differences within the behavioural intentions of frontline healthcare practitioners. The purpose of this study is to research the ways in which gender and age impact people's perceptions of chance and the relationship between the two factors. This study introduces a completely original model by integrating three conceptual frameworks: the trust-risk framework, the Theory of Planned Behaviour (TPB) framework, and the Privacy Calculus (PCT) framework. Specifically, the TPB framework emphasises the connection between intentional behaviour and the surrounding environment. There is no evidence to suggest that risk perception has an effect on any of the cohort's behavioural goals regarding the adoption of IoT-enabled home automation (HA). This finding is significant for guiding both future institutional policy and the development of awareness. However, it's not entirely implausible that some participants in the cohort may have their behavioural goals influenced by their beliefs about chance.

The findings of this study demonstrated that there are gender differences among the contributors who fall into the generation Y category.

Krishna Kumar et al. (2022) presented research entitled "Dimensions of Internet of Things: Technological Taxonomy Architecture Applications and Open Challenges—A Systematic Review". The Internet of Things is currently seeing widespread adoption across all sectors of the economy and is being leveraged to the full extent of its potential. The Internet of Things is an ecosystem of interconnected devices that includes sensing devices, intelligent products, networking capabilities, and processing devices. The term was coined by Kevin Ashton in 1999.

The end consumer is one who benefits from the improved services provided by those connected devices. The Internet of Things is already having an effect on our environment and is quickly becoming one of the technologies that is most widely utilised. The primary purpose of a network of elements in human life is to facilitate the monitoring of events or activities at any given location and time. Packages that are part of the Internet of Things are able to provide the best possible benefits in the form of decision-making and tracking for the purpose of more environmentally friendly and effective management. This article conducts a comprehensive literature review on the Internet of Things using a method known as systematic literature review (SLR). The areas that are receiving the most focus are as follows: the commercial district, the surrounding region, the healthcare industry, the economic sector, and smart cities. The problems that might be caused by a web of contributing causes are likewise broken down and examined in great detail.

This research is being done with the intention of gaining an understanding of the principal application areas, notable designs, and the issues that are associated with them. Comparisons of the various applications of the Internet of Things are carried out in accordance with technical standards. These standards take into account the best available service as well as an analysis of the environment in which they are operating. This study may be used by researchers in order to achieve a grasp of the idea of the IoT, and it also provides a road map for researchers to follow in order to establish strategies for their next research projects.

Shruti Suhas Kute et al. (2022) conducted a study entitled "Security, Privacy, and Trust Issues in Internet of Things and Machine Learning-Based e-Healthcare". The term "Internet of Things" refers to the networking of physical devices that are not only smart but also connected to the internet. These devices can communicate with each other. Similarly, this concept is sometimes referred to as a "network of connected things". It was necessary to equip these devices with the appropriate software, sensors, and network connectivity in order for them to be able to gather and exchange information. As more and more devices are able to connect to the internet, the concept of using the Internet of Things is becoming an increasingly alluring idea. The usage of devices that are completely based on the Internet of Things is revolutionising the way human beings live their lives, in particular in activities that may be related to healthcare. This is specially true in terms of activities associated with fitness and the methods by which individuals communicate with medical professionals. However, there are a few significant drawbacks or difficulties that arise as a result of making extensive use of such devices in a wide variety of different applications. In addition to statistical data pertaining to a variety of different diseases or medical conditions, this work provides statistical data addressing the prevention of overweight and obesity as well as its identification, treatment, and management.

The Internet of Things has the potential to develop into a disruptive driving force in an industry that is potentially just as important on a global basis as the medical services sector. This work presents a synthesis of the most recent research pertaining to the application of the Internet of Things in healthcare, with the primary focus being on issues associated with obesity, excessive body fat, and chronic degenerative diseases. In continuation with this, we will now discuss the potential applications of the Internet of Things in the healthcare setting. The commercialisation of the internet is contingent upon the resolution of issues relating to customers' constitutionally guaranteed right to the preservation and maintenance of their non-public personal information and privacy. The issues of availability, confidentiality, integrity, authentication, authorisation, trust, verification, data storage, and administration need to be addressed to enable the use of the Internet of Things in smart applications. It is imperative that these problems be resolved before the Internet of Things can be deployed in practical applications.

Kazhan Othman Mohammed Salih et al. (2022) presented research entitled "A Comprehensive Survey on the Internet of Things Within the Industrial Marketplace". Undoubtedly, the contemporary age has become an essential component of the lives of the vast majority of people around the globe, transcending every region on the planet. In our present time, the internet and the Internet of

Things have evolved into indispensable aspects of our lives. IoT technologies have recently gained recognition as tools with the potential for widespread use among all other technological advances. Industry 4.0 encompasses the facilities and equipment already available on the market associated with the production of internet-connected items. The market is yet another new frontier that is being investigated for the potential value of Internet of Things technology.

The implementation of Internet of Things technology in Industry 4.0 is a central focus of this publication. It delves into various key aspects, with one of the primary focuses being zero, and the Industrial Internet of Things represents just one of the many elements that have been modified. This article investigates the relevance of the Internet of Things within the manufacturing industry in general. It offers an overview of the Internet of Things and focuses specifically on both its positive and negative aspects. It also examines a few of the programmes that are being implemented via the Internet of Things, such as those in the transportation and healthcare industries. In a similar manner, the records and patterns that may be tied to the technology that is currently accessible on the market are studied.

Shashvi Mishra and Amit Kumar Tyagi (2022) presented research entitled "The Role of Machine Learning Techniques in Internet of Things-Based Cloud Applications". The integration of cloud software, which is continuously accessible on the internet, and machine learning (ML) plays an essential role in our lives.

In particular, ML plays a key role when combined with the IoT. According to the findings of a recent study conducted by Gartner, there are around 25 billion devices that interface with the internet on a daily basis. These products range from wearables and self-driving cars to daily apps for smart homes and smart cities. All of these interconnected (smart) devices generate a large quantity of data, which has to be reviewed and assessed on a day-to-day basis to make sure that they continually learn from the available datasets and develop without any assistance from people. At that point, an essential prerequisite for the acquisition of device-based knowledge has been satisfied. In a short amount of time, numerous machine learning algorithms and methodologies are undoubtedly offered to analyse vast datasets, aiming to enhance the productivity of the IoT. Similarly, specific machine learning strategies permit machines and devices to each day recognise patterns from different assets within a variety of datasets and make appropriate decisions primarily based on their study of those tendencies.

If smart devices were designed without the inclusion and awareness of machine learning, it would not be uncommon for those smart devices to make intelligent decisions on their own. The Internet of Things makes it possible to connect a wide variety of physical devices, such as houses, automobiles, electrical devices, and other products that can be outfitted with real-time trackers, sensors, and software, so that data can be collected and exchanged. Some examples of these kinds of devices include smart televisions, smart refrigerators, and smart thermostats. Homes, electronic devices, and electronic motors are a few examples of the kinds of equipment that fall under this category. Some examples of the sorts of hardware issues that come under this category are smart thermostats, smart lighting fixtures, and smart home appliances. Electronic devices are just one example of the types of products that may be found in this category; nonetheless, they are by far the most common.

Every day, more and more businesses are starting to become conscious of the expanding capacity made available by way of the IoT, and they have begun facing the numerous difficulties that need to be overcome in order to make effective use of it. A diverse variety of firms and corporations are employing a standard system as a method to leverage the potential that has not yet been fully realised through the use of the Internet of Things. This chapter gives an analysis of the many strategies that may be used on a machine to deal with the difficulties brought about by the regulation of IoT data. These difficulties are due to the fact that IoT records are not standardised. It is of the highest significance to realise that the interaction of the internet with smart devices results in the generation of a vast amount of information, which is then stored within the cloud. This statistical information is then accessible from any location.

Prabh Deep Singh et al. (2022) presented research entitled "Internet of Things for Sustaining a Smart and Secure Healthcare System". The thyroid is a vital endocrine gland located within the human body that is responsible for regulating a variety of one-of-a-kind physiological processes. These include the production of proteins, the acquisition of strength, and the body's reactivity to a variety of hormones. Because the majority of thyroid-related problems cause a change in the size and form of the thyroid over the course of time, segmentation and quantity regeneration of the thyroid are generally important steps in the process of identifying thyroid-related illnesses. Investigation into the causes of the disease and the factors that contribute to its spread are of the utmost importance. The Internet of Things, cloud computing, and artificial intelligence have made it possible for quite a few applications within the healthcare industry to make use of real-time processing.

There has been a recent uptick in the number of applications in the domains of medicine and biology that make use of machine learning algorithms so that computers can make important decisions. Patients with thyroid-related illnesses desire and deserve a service infrastructure of high quality that is both resilient and responsive to their needs. By merging intelligent health with cloud computing and artificial intelligence, the goal of this approach is to provide a reliable platform for the early diagnosis of thyroid infections. This will be accomplished through the use of intelligent cloud computing. It has been recommended that an up-to-date ensemble-based classifier be utilised in order to identify those who have thyroid problems. Python is used as the computer language to carry out the simulation, and the thyroid dataset is obtained from the library at the University of California, Irvine. Encryption and decryption solutions are being presented as potential ways to strengthen the protection that is provided by the framework. The performance of the proposed framework is measured using a variety of measures, such as latency, network use, RAM utilisation, and energy consumption, among others.

Alternatively, the accuracy, precision, specificity, and sensitivity of the proposed classifier, in addition to its F1 score, are all taken into consideration and analysed. According to the data, the approved framework and classifier are able to get better results than the conventional framework and classifier when used together.

Pranav Ratta et al. (2021) presented research entitled "Application of Blockchain and Internet of Things in Healthcare and Medical Sector: Applications, Challenges, and Future Perspectives". The Internet of Things is one of the most cutting-edge trends in records generation. Its primary goal is to merge the digital and real worlds into one seamless experience. It makes it feasible for inanimate objects and people to connect with one another by utilising the internet in their interactions. This is the core concept behind "smartness." The Internet of Things offers a wide variety of solutions for practically every business, including smart fitness, smart transportation, and smart cities. The Internet of Things makes it less difficult for medical professionals and patients to communicate with each other in clinical settings by enabling remote analysis of patients in the event of an emergency through the use of frame sensor networks and wearable sensors.

This makes it possible for medical professionals to more easily interact with patients. Despite this, there is a possibility that the confidentiality of patients could be breached if the IoT is used in healthcare delivery systems. Consequently, security is an essential factor to take into consideration. The use of blockchain technology is quickly becoming one a popular study topic, and it already has the potential to be utilised in the vast majority of Internet of Things cases. Decentralisation, immutability, protection and privacy, and transparency are some of the most essential aspects of blockchain technology, and they may be some of the most important driving factors for its application in healthcare organisations. Blockchain technology was developed by Satoshi Nakamoto and is a distributed ledger technology. This study's major objective was to investigate the ways in which new modern innovative technologies, such as the Internet of Things and blockchain, might increase the operational capabilities of healthcare delivery systems. Therefore, a clear and succinct rationalisation of the Internet of Things and the underlying criteria of blockchain is offered right from the start. Following this, the possible uses of Internet of Things and blockchain technology within the medical industry are studied in three of the most important areas, the monitoring of medicine, the remote monitoring of patients, and the administration of scientific data.

Jaimon T Kelly et al. (2020) presented research entitled "The Internet of Things: Impact and Implications for Health Care Delivery". The Internet of Things is a self-contained network of electronic devices that communicate with one another via wireless connections. These pieces of equipment are also linked to one another. These devices do not require human-to-human or human-to-computer communication and are able to gather, transmit, and store information in a networked manner without the assistance of humans.

The Internet of Things has the potential to bring about a great deal of beneficial change, including the improvement and facilitation of scientific transportation; the forecasting of health problems; the diagnosis, treatment, and evaluation of patients both within and outside hospitals; the ability to predict health problems; and the simplification and improvement of healthcare transportation. As a direct response to the COVID-19 epidemic, government officials and policymakers all around the world are working to develop action plans to promote the use of technology in healthcare. This peculiar set of circumstances is a direct consequence of the outbreak. Understanding how current and future technology connected to the Internet of Things may assist healthcare organisations in providing patients with the best possible care and treatment is without a doubt one of the most difficult problems that society is facing in the modern day.

This is one of the most important issues facing the sector at the moment. The purpose of this observation is to provide an overview of modern healthcare systems that are related to the Internet of Things, investigate how IoT devices might improve transportation, and present specifics on how the next generation of IoT will influence and have an effect on the state of health throughout the world during the next ten years. The complete healthcare potential of the IoT is based on the idea that it can enhance access to public health and transform our middle-range and high-level healthcare systems into continuously integrated and efficient apparatus. This concept underpins the entirety of the IoT's healthcare capability. The notion rests entirely on the presumption that the IoT has the potential to facilitate public health protection and lead to access to public health protection products.

The Internet of Things is the key principle that underpins this concept, which argues that it has the potential to increase access to public health services that emphasise disease prevention. In the end, the purpose of the article is to discuss the potential difficulties that may arise from using the IoT inside a healthcare organisation. These capacity difficulties encompass barriers related to conducting business with the assistance of medical professionals and patients, trust and accountability, privacy and security, collaboration, design and cost, record-keeping, and ownership and management. The social worker of the Internet of Things in the healthcare industry of today will rely on legal assistance, cybersecurity rules, stringent strategic planning, and most surely the needs seen in scientific institutions.

Abdel Rahman H. Hussein (2019) presented research entitled "Internet of Things (IoT): Research Challenges and Future Application". Because the Internet of Things is quickly becoming the next phase in the development of the internet, it is very important that all of the possible industries for application of IoT be recognised, in addition to the research issues that are related to the many applications of IoT. It is anticipated that the Internet of Things will eventually penetrate practically every aspect of contemporary living, beginning with so-called smart cities and expanding to smart healthcare, smart agriculture, smart retail, and smart living environments, among other domains. Despite the fact that the technologies that make the Internet of Things possible have made significant strides in the past few years, there are still a great many issues that need to be resolved. As a result of the fact that the idea of the Internet of Things is largely built on a range of distinct technologies, there will unavoidably be a number of barriers to conquer within the field of study.

Due to the fact that it is so widespread and impacts practically every aspect of our lives, the Internet of Things has emerged as a primary focus of investigation for researchers conducting work in a wide range of disciplines that are closely connected to one another, such as computer science and record keeping. As a consequence of this, behaviour study may now be conducted in locations that were previously undiscovered thanks to the Internet of Things. This article provides a summary of the most current advancements made in Internet of Things technology, in addition to discussing potential future uses and challenges to analyse.

Gonçalo Marques et al. (2019) presented research entitled "Internet of Things Architectures, Technologies, Applications, Challenges, and Future Directions for Enhanced Living Environments and Healthcare Systems: A Review". At the moment, academics and experts working in expert and business settings are displaying a rising interest in it. It is now conceivable to put in place intelligent structures that are capable of high levels of communication and the collecting of statistics as a consequence of a number of incremental developments in technology which have been conducted.

This has made it possible for a number of IoT initiatives, particularly those that are pertinent to the execution of healthcare device, to move forward. Accessibility, portability, and interoperability are only some examples of these problems, and there are more, such as the protection of personally identifiable information and statistical data. These applications include monitoring the quality of air both outside and inside of a building, keeping track of patients in real time, and providing ubiquitous and pervasive access to their medical records. Every one of these things has the potential to be helpful not just to medical professionals but also to patients. The consistent progress made in scientific research makes it feasible to construct Internet of Things devices by supplying an infinite number of options for sensing, information fusion, and recording capabilities.

This makes it possible for IoT devices to communicate with one another. This opens the way for the development of Internet of Things tools to become a reality. Because of this, the creation of smart cities could be made easier. These skills are responsible for a wide variety of advancements, many of which lead to improved living circumstances. These enhanced living conditions are sometimes referred to as enhanced living environments (ELEs). The purpose of this article is to offer a high-level overview of the current state of the art with regard to IoT designs for electronic life support systems and healthcare delivery networks. The generation, programming, challenges, capacity, open-supply structures, and operating systems might each receive some focus.

17.3 LITERATURE SUMMARY

S. No	Author	Year	Title	Work Details	Remark
1.	Haider Dhai Zubaidi et al.	2023	"Leveraging Blockchain Technology for Ensuring Security and Privacy Aspects in Internet of Things: A Systematic Literature Review"	MDPI and Wiley/ Hindawi	Recognised major healthcare issues
2.	Pinki Paul and Balgopal Singh	2023	"Healthcare Employee Engagement Using the Internet of Things: A Systematic Overview"	Healthcare engagement and AI/IoT	Healthcare workers' progress
3.	Omar Ali et al.	2023	"A Review of Advanced Technologies Available to Improve the Healthcare Performance During COVID-19 Pandemic"	Cloud computing, IoT, and AI to improve healthcare efficiency	An innovative healthcare system's future
4.	Sridhar Siripurapu et al.	2023	"Technological Advancements and Elucidation Gadgets for Healthcare Applications: An Exhaustive Methodological Review"	Robotics, drones, 3D-printing, IoT, VR/ AR/MR, etc.	Research stressed the relevance of disruptive technologies like robotics, drones, 3D-printing, IoT, and VR/AR/MR in tackling problems
5.	Andreia Robert Lopes et al.	2023	"Application of Technology in Healthcare: Tackling COVID-19 Challenge—The Integration of Blockchain and Internet of Things"	Blockchain and IoT can revolutionise healthcare	Determining issues

(Continued)

(*Continued*)

S. No	Author	Year	Title	Work Details	Remark
6.	Lamya Alkhariji et al.	2023	"Semantics-Based Privacy by Design for Internet of Things Applications"	IoT PbD measurements	Development of the PARROT ontology using software developer–relevant IoT use cases
7.	Fazli Subhan et al.	2023	"AI-Enabled Wearable Medical Internet of Things in Healthcare System: A Survey"	Smart **thermometers,** smart helmets, smart contact lenses	IoT can help sanitary systems
8.	Lokesh B. Bhajantri et al.	2023	"A Survey on Cognitive Internet of Things Based Prediction of Covid-19 Patient"	IoT-based COVID-19 patient prediction using machine learning	Restrictions, pros, cons, and algorithm performance parameters
9.	Mavis Gezimati and Ghanshyam Singh	2023	"Internet of Things Enabled Framework for Terahertz and Infrared Cancer Imaging"	IoT-enabled deep learning framework	The accuracy, sensitivity, and specificity metrics achieved 98.44%, 98.44%, and 98.45%, respectively
10.	K.S. Arvind et al.	2023	"Pandemic Management Using Internet of Things and Big Data—A Security and Privacy Perspective"	Contact tracing IoT applications	IoT manages pandemics well
11.	Sasikumar A. et al.	2023	"Blockchain-based trust mechanism for digital twin empowered Industrial Internet of Things"	DPRG and IoT	Digital twin-enabled IIoT network
12.	Zhenwei Zhao et al.	2023	"Secure Internet of Things (IoT) Using a Novel Brooks Iyengar Quantum Byzantine Agreement-Centered Blockchain Networking (BIQBA-BCN) Model in Smart Healthcare"	IoT, CSS, BIQBA-BCN	Security level that is 94% effective
13.	Md Oqail Ahmad and Shams Tabrez Siddiqui	2022	"The Internet of Things for Healthcare: Benefits, Applications, Challenges, Use Cases and Future Directions"	Use case applications	Discussing IoT healthcare growth
14.	Amit Kishor and Chinmay Chakraborty	2022	"Artificial Intelligence and Internet of Things Based Healthcare 4.0 Monitoring System"	Decision tree, SVM, naïve Bayes, adaptive boosting, RF	RF classifier maximum accuracy of 97.62%, sensitivity of 99.67%, specificity of 97.81%, and AUC of 99.32%
15.	Damini Verma et al.	2022	"Internet of Things (IoT) in Nano-Integrated Wearable Biosensor Devices for Healthcare Applications"	IoT, IoMT, nano-integrated wearable devices	Monitoring, managing, detecting
16.	Mansour Alraja	2022	"Frontline Healthcare Providers' Behavioural Intention to Internet of Things (IoT)-Enabled Healthcare Applications: A Gender-Based, Cross-Generational Study"	Investigated frontline healthcare providers	Managing the rising female workforce

S. No	Author	Year	Title	Work Details	Remark
17.	Krishna Kumar et al.	2022	"Dimensions of Internet of Things: Technological Taxonomy Architecture Applications and Open Challenges—A Systematic Review"	Technical Quality Method (TQM)	Healthcare uses 20% of IoT
18	Shruti Suhas Kute et al.	2022	"Security, Privacy and Trust Issues in Internet of Things and Machine Learning Based e-Healthcare"	Internet of Things, Internet of Medical Things, machine learning, e-healthcare, security, privacy and trust issues	Security, privacy, and trust in IoT–machine learning healthcare systems
19	Kazhan Othman Mohammed Salih et al.	2022	"A Comprehensive Survey on the Internet of Things with the Industrial Marketplace"	Telemedicine, IoT, IIoT, Industry 4.0,	IOT and telemedicine focused
20	Shashvi Mishra and Amit Kumar Tyagi	2022	"The Role of Machine Learning Techniques in Internet of Things-Based Cloud Applications"	IoT-based cloud applications, machine learning, AI	ML algorithm taxonomy discussed
21	Prabh Deep Singh et al.	2022	"Internet of Things for Sustaining a Smart and Secure Healthcare System"	Machine learning algorithms, Python programming	QoS fog computing reduces latency, network
22	Pranav Ratta et al.	2021	"Application of Blockchain and Internet of Things in Healthcare and Medical Sector: Applications, Challenges, and Future Perspectives"	Technical Quality Method (TQM)	IoT monitors patient health periodically
23	Jaimon T Kelly et al.	2020	"The Internet of Things: Impact and Implications for Health Care Delivery"	IoT-based health care, network layer: data communication and storage	IoT research in healthcare is expanding
24	AbdelRahman H. Hussein	2019	"Internet of Things (IoT): Research Challenges and Future Application"	Internet of Things and M2M Protocols	IoT is a complex adaptive system (CAS) that will evolve
25	Gonçalo Marques et al.	2019	"Internet of Things Architectures, Technologies, Applications, Challenges, and Future Directions for Enhanced Living Environments and Healthcare Systems: A Review"	Pervasive computing, Internet of Things	Offers innovative medical therapies for personalised healthcare

17.4 CONCLUSION

Because the COVID-19 pandemic is not yet over, it is too soon to provide an accurate assessment of the significance of advanced technology in the pandemic response. Even though advanced technology has provided tools that can assist in the pandemic response, these techniques do not give a quick solution. An advanced healthcare system can help to alleviate the stresses placed on staff, save expenses, encourage better patient self-management, assist with the management of resources and information, and enhance the quality of treatment that patients get. An advanced healthcare system has the potential to save costs and time during the study process, all while improving the research's overall effectiveness. An inventive healthcare system has the potential to improve the existing inequality in medical resource availability, speed up the development of medical policy, increase the adoption of preventative techniques, and cut the societal expenses associated with medical treatment.

We are able to identify the primary advanced technologies that play key roles in enhancing the performance of the healthcare system by analysing COVID-19 case studies. Colour coding, social media, autonomous cars, big data, artificial intelligence, facial recognition, and robotics are some examples of these technologies. The COVID-19 pandemic, on the other hand, demands not only the sharing of data but also stringent assessment and ethical norms with community engagement. This is so that the epidemic can be handled by the burgeoning field of mobile and creative healthcare. In order to win the confidence of the public, organisations need to implement effective communication strategies across all of their creative channels and demonstrate their dedication to providing appropriate levels of privacy protection.

REFERENCES

Ahmad, M.O. and Siddiqui, S.T., 2022. The Internet of Things for healthcare: Benefits, applications, challenges, use cases and future directions. In Advances in Data and Information Sciences: Proceedings of ICDIS 2021 (pp. 527–537). Singapore: Springer.

Ali, O., AlAhmad, A. and Kahtan, H., 2023. A review of advanced technologies available to improve the healthcare performance during COVID-19 pandemic. Procedia Computer Science, 217, pp. 205–216.

Alkhariji, L., De, S., Rana, O. and Perera, C., 2023. Semantics-based privacy by design for Internet of Things applications. Future Generation Computer Systems, 138, pp. 280–295.

Alraja, M., 2022. Frontline healthcare providers' behavioural intention to Internet of Things (IoT)-enabled healthcare applications: A gender-based, cross-generational study. Technological Forecasting and Social Change, 174, p. 121256.

Arvind, K.S., Vanitha, S. and Suganya, K.S., 2023. Pandemic management using Internet of Things and Big Data–a security and privacy perspective. In IoT and Big Data Analytics for Smart Cities (pp. 159–173). Chapman and Hall/CRC.

Bhajantri, L.B., Kadadevar, N., Jeeragal, A., Jeeragal, V. and Jamdar, I., 2023. A survey on cognitive Internet of Things based prediction of covid-19 patient. In Sentiment Analysis and Deep Learning: Proceedings of ICSADL 2022 (pp. 377–387). Singapore: Springer Nature.

Gezimati, M. and Singh, G., 2023. Internet of Things enabled framework for terahertz and infrared cancer imaging. Optical and Quantum Electronics, 55(1), p. 26.

Hussein, A.H., 2019. Internet of Things (IoT): Research challenges and future applications. International Journal of Advanced Computer Science and Applications, 10(6).

Kelly, J.T., Campbell, K.L., Gong, E. and Scuffham, P., 2020. The Internet of Things: Impact and implications for health care delivery. Journal of Medical Internet Research, 22(11), p. e20135.

Kishor, A. and Chakraborty, C., 2022. Artificial intelligence and Internet of Things based healthcare 4.0 monitoring system. Wireless personal communications, 127(2), pp. 1615–1631.

Kumar, K., Kumar, A., Kumar, N., Mohammed, M.A., Al-Waisy, A.S., Jaber, M.M., Shah, R. and Al-Andoli, M.N., 2022. Dimensions of Internet of Things: Technological taxonomy architecture applications and open challenges—A systematic review. Wireless Communications and Mobile Computing, 2022, pp. 1–23. https://doi.org/10.1155/2022/9148373.

Kute, S.S., Tyagi, A.K. and Aswathy, S.U., 2022. Security, privacy and trust issues in Internet of Things and machine learning based e-healthcare. Intelligent Interactive Multimedia Systems for e-Healthcare Applications, pp. 291–317.

Lopes, A.R., Dias, A.S. and Sá-Moura, B., 2023. Application of technology in healthcare: Tackling COVID-19 challenge–the integration of blockchain and Internet of Things. In Research Anthology on Convergence of Blockchain, Internet of Things, and Security (pp. 108–131). IGI Global. https://doi.org/10.4018/978-1-6684-7132-6.ch007.

Marques, G., Pitarma, R., Garcia, M. N. and Pombo, N., 2019. Internet of Things architectures, technologies, applications, challenges, and future directions for enhanced living environments and healthcare systems: A review. Electronics, 8(10), p. 1081.

Mishra, S. and Tyagi, A.K., 2022. The role of machine learning techniques in Internet of Things-based cloud applications. In Pal, S., De, D. and Buyya, R. (eds) Artificial Intelligence-Based Internet of Things Systems (pp. 105–135). Cham: Springer. https://doi.org/10.1007/978-3-030-87059-1_4.

Paul, P. and Singh, B., 2023. Healthcare employee engagement using the Internet of Things: A systematic overview. In The Adoption and Effect of Artificial Intelligence on Human Resources Management, Part A (pp. 71–97). USA: Emerald Publishing Ltd.

Ratta, P., Kaur, A., Sharma, S., Shabaz, M. and Dhiman, G., 2021. Application of blockchain and Internet of Things in healthcare and medical sector: Applications, challenges, and future perspectives. Journal of Food Quality, pp. 1–20.

Salih, K.O.M., Rashid, T.A., Radovanovic, D. and Bacanin, N., 2022. A comprehensive survey on the Internet of Things with the industrial marketplace. Sensors, 22(3), p. 730.

Sasikumar, A., Vairavasundaram, S., Kotecha, K., Indragandhi, V., Ravi, L., Selvachandran, G. and Abraham, A., 2023. Blockchain-based trust mechanism for digital twin empowered industrial Internet of Things. Future Generation Computer Systems, 141, pp. 16–27.

Singh, P.D., Dhiman, G. and Sharma, R., 2022. Internet of Things for sustaining a smart and secure healthcare system. Sustainable Computing: Informatics and Systems, 33, p. 100622.

Siripurapu, S., Darimireddy, N.K., Chehri, A., Sridhar, B. and Paramkusam, A.V., 2023. Technological advancements and elucidation gadgets for healthcare applications: An exhaustive methodological review-Part-II (Robotics, drones, 3D-printing, Internet of Things, virtual/augmented and mixed reality). Electronics, 12(3), p. 548.

Subhan, F., Mirza, A., Su'ud, M.B.M., Alam, M.M., Nisar, S., Habib, U. and Iqbal, M.Z., 2023. AI-enabled wearable medical Internet of Things in healthcare system: A survey. Applied Sciences, 13(3), p. 1394.

Verma, D., Singh, K.R., Yadav, A.K., Nayak, V., Singh, J., Solanki, P.R. and Singh, R.P., 2022. Internet of Things (IoT) in nano-integrated wearable biosensor devices for healthcare applications. Biosensors and Bioelectronics: X, 11, p. 100153.

Zhao, Z., Li, X., Luan, B., Jiang, W., Gao, W. and Neelakandan, S., 2023. Secure Internet of Things (IoT) using a novel Brooks Iyengar quantum Byzantine agreement-centered blockchain networking (BIQBA-BCN) model in smart healthcare. Information Sciences, 629, 440–455. https://doi.org/10.1016/j.ins.2023.01.020.

Zubaydi, H.D., Varga, P. and Molnár, S., 2023. Leveraging blockchain technology for ensuring security and privacy aspects in Internet of Things: A systematic literature review. Sensors, 23(2), p. 788.

18 The Extraordinary Importance of 6G Network Development and 3D Holography in Future Healthcare

V. Jokanović

18.1 INTRODUCTION

Advanced technologies have revolutionized diagnostic and therapeutic practice in coronary heart disease, thus playing an increasingly important role in its management. The traditional reliance on standard imaging procedures such as echocardiography, computed tomography (CTo) and magnetic resonance imaging (MRI) has been enhanced through the use of the latest technologies such as 3D printing, virtual reality, augmented reality, computer modeling and artificial intelligence.

Currently, it is essential to start the global 6G network project as soon as possible, although 5G communication technology is still waiting for full implementation worldwide. Currently, with the existing network, it is not possible to support holographic communication due to the lower data transfer speed, which will be significantly improved only with 6G communication technology. The essential deficiency in the development of the current healthcare system is the lack of time and space for serious progress in patient care. It is especially important for care services for the elderly, which involve intensive care, which is almost impossible today. Because of this, most patients die in the ambulance on the way from home to the hospital or before the ambulance arrives on the scene. An accident detection system requires a real-time diagnosis to provide timely medical services at the scene of an accident. A similar situation is associated with an epidemic or pandemic, which could be clearly observed during the intense duration of the COVID-19 pandemic [1–3].

It is inevitable that a similar type of virus will appear again, which is why it is necessary to develop an intelligent healthcare system. Such requirements could be satisfied by the application of 6G communication technology due to its high data transfer rate (≥ 1 Tbps), high operating frequency (≥ 1 THz), low delay (≤1 ms), high reliability (10–9), high mobility (≥ 1000 km/h) and wavelength (≤ 300 μm) [4], because telesurgery, for example, requires real-time communication. Also, holographic communication and augmented/virtual reality are essential for future intelligent healthcare systems. It is expected that 6G communication technology will completely change healthcare and will be utterly dependent on communication technology.

The current state-of-the-art healthcare system is not suitable for remote surgery due to possible communication problems. It is expected that the 6G network will redefine emergency care and necessary portable equipment in medicine; restructure hospitals; and significantly improve healthcare and services for the elderly, as this communication technology will focus on the quality of service (QoS), quality of experience (QoE), quality of life (QoL), service on the way from the hospital to the home (H2H), sensors for reading blood samples (BSR), intelligent wearable devices (IVD) and hospital health insurance (HIH) business models. Of course, the role of artificial intelligence (AI) and edge technology in healthcare will be especially pronounced in all of this [5, 6].

DOI: 10.1201/9781003451846-18

There are several ways to generate holographic images, usually using a laser as the primary source of coherent light, In contrast, a holographic image is created based on the phase difference between the two different light paths generated by the image object. Real-time 3D holography significantly advances various technologies, from virtual reality (VR) to 3D printing, helping to immerse VR viewers in a realistic environment while reducing the harmful effects of eye strain. A holographic image is created due to the interference of two laser beams not only of different intensities and amplitude values but also of different phases, which are registered as such on the recording device [7–9]. Cyber-physical systems assume significant mobility that connects digital and physical world using holography, while augmented reality (AR) is a digitally augmented image of the real world. It allows the user to compare digital information with the real world using AR.

The holographic approach using 3D holograms contributes to the presentation of objects in a high-quality, exclusive and original form, considering all the requirements of a given target group. In doing so, it is possible to use the acoustic background matched to the 3D hologram, which includes background sound and unique sound effects [10]. Since the hologram itself represents a virtual three-dimensional image of the real world generated by the interference of light beams that reflect physical objects from the natural world, it should be noted that there are two methods of creating holograms. One consists of computer-generated holograms for glasses with augmented reality and genuine holograms intended for optical displays. Holography itself is a unique photographic technique in which 3D objects are recorded with a laser. Then they are reconstructed as accurately as possible in order to more convincingly portray the original object that was subjected to recording. During reconstruction, when illuminated by a laser, holograms produce an exact 3D clone of the object, imitating all its geometric features [11–13].

Holography, thanks to its three-dimensionality, opens completely new applications, such as the display of products and animated sequences that allow original objects or animations to float freely in space, and, unlike a traditional film on an ordinary screen, 3D footage is visible from all sides, allowing the viewer an incredibly realistic image [14, 15]. The development of laser technology, emulsions and light sources in white light holography has opened up new possibilities for holography associated with an ultra-realistic reproduction of 3D objects [16]. Computers use software techniques for the reconstruction of holographic images by their algorithms, which in a short time create high-quality 3D images, suitable for processing on a digital holographic display [17]. In the future, holography could be used to store high-density data, because, unlike conventional optical storage media, which only use a thin two-dimensional layer, holographic memories can store data in three dimensions, thus achieving a huge storage capacity in a minimal volume.

18.2 6G TECHNOLOGY

18.2.1 Background

Starting from the fact that cognitive technology (CT) [4] mimics the functions of the human brain in different ways, such as cognitive computing (CC) [18] and exemplary machine learning (ML) [5], where CC is an appropriate analysis tool for massive databases for generating more effective holistic insights, by implementing such systems in healthcare will result in faster and more purposeful decisions, that enable a complete transformation of healthcare through fine-tuning ML and embedded Internet of Everything (IoE) devices. For this, It require complete knowledge of hardware, software, algorithms and to analyse large databases (mean decrease accuracy, MDAs) [18] with the application of fine-grained ML enabling cognitive data intelligence (CDI) [4, 18] to lead to better healthcare solutions by providing relevant information to help stakeholders make appropriate decisions.

The Internet of Things (IoT) [19] is an online, dynamic, rapidly changing system, as it involves a massive number of interconnected devices, which is why its use faces a huge efficiency challenge. Its modification intended for healthcare, the healthcare Internet of Everything (IoHE) [19], on the other hand, implies the application of devices that can be connected to the tactile Internet with 6G, which will be able to communicate with each other thanks to intelligent healthcare applications. In addition, integrating the tactile Internet, CDI and IoHE with a 6G network will enable the formalization of the 6G Cognitive healthcare Internet of Everything (6GCIoHE) system [4, 18, 19], which plays a vital role in cognitive health applications.

The development of 6G tactile Internet, CDI and IoHE will play a key role in ensuring the interoperability of healthcare applications, with a holistic approach in the formation of the 6GCIoHE system to improve healthcare. Although issues of privacy, security and trust have been extensively discussed, the establishment of global CIoHE standards is still necessary to ensure that all issues of security, privacy and trust are addressed in one place. It is essential to improve services and experiences, as well as to reduce costs, while promoting healthcare facilities more effectively and automating patient care workflows, as well as machine-to-machine communication, and improving interoperability and information sharing, leading to increased healthcare efficiency, data security, privacy and timely risk perception. With the help of 6G tactile Internet communication, therefore, it will be easier to establish communication between different networks using standard IP protocols [4, 18–20].

6G networks will use terahertz (THz) signals to transmit information, because such networks have increased bandwidth and data transfer speed, given that their bandwidth is three times higher than that of 5G networks [21]. 6G networks will have a data transfer rate of 1 TBPS or more, with a three-dimensional communication structure, which uses time, space and frequency. Such networks will provide 3D services supported by edge technology, artificial intelligence, cloud computing and blockchain. In this way, the 6G network will provide more profound and broader network coverage with the support of terrestrial and satellite communication devices. Thanks to such a network, it will be possible to connect computer, navigation and communication networks while ensuring the secrecy and privacy of large databases that will generate billions of intelligent devices [21].

The essential requirements for 6G communication are an operating frequency of 1 THz, a data transfer rate of 1 Tbps, a wavelength of 300 μm and a mobility range of 1000 km/h. The architecture of 6G is a 3D architecture that uses time, space and frequency. End-to-end delay, radio delay and processing requirements are $\leq$1 ms, $\leq$ 10 ns and $\leq$ 10 ns to ensure real-time communication. 6G communication technology will be driven by artificial intelligence and fully supported by satellites. The core of the Internet of Things network will be replaced by the IoE and will enable the transition from IoT to IoE, namely from smart to intelligent devices, giving numerous new possibilities [22, 23].

Terahertz communication 6G will use terahertz sub-millimeter radiation, which includes electromagnetic waves with wavelengths between 1 and 0.1 mm—this radiation is suitable for 6G communication, due to its high bandwidth, high data transfer rate (up to several Gbps) and large data storage capacity [4]. It is possible to increase the efficiency of THz signals by reusing and sharing the spectrum, using the so-called cognitive radio (CR), which allows many wireless systems to access the same spectrum by means of spectrum sensors and interference management mechanisms [20]. In the case of spectrum sharing, the spectrum that will be temporarily underutilized or unlicensed will be used to maintain the availability of the communication network and its reliability. In addition, the so-called symbiotic radio (SR) will be used, which represents a new technique of supporting intelligent, heterogeneous wireless networks.

The transition from current smart technology to intelligent 6G technologies is expected to be driven by artificial intelligence [21, 22], which will enable a smooth transition from smart to intelligent devices. This transition is expected to happen by 2030, and the IoE will replace the IoT. Such intelligent devices will be powered by artificial intelligence connected to the Internet. An intelligent device designed in this way will be able to predict, make decisions and share its experience with other intelligent devices.

The basic parameters determining the advantages of 6G communication are parameters of service quality, quality of experience and especially improved quality of life. Quality of service parameters include high data rate and highly reliable low latency communication (ERLLC), with intelligently enhanced mobile broadband (FeMBB), ultra-massive machine communication (umMTC), remote communication and high mobility communication (LDHMC) and extremely efficient low power communication (ELPC) [24]. QoS also includes mobile broadband latency hunting (MBBLL), massive broadband machines (mBBMT) and massive latency hunting machines (mLLMT) [22–25].

Quality of experience defines the quality of user-directed communication. Improved QoE will be enabled with holographic communications, augmented and virtual reality and tactile Internet, all of which require high data rates with extremely low latency. High QoE can only be achieved with 6G technology guided by artificial intelligence [25], which promises the possibility of communication at the level of all five senses. Because of this, it is expected that 6G communication will be a significant turning point in the field of healthcare, especially when performing critical operations, improving the functioning of the hospital and providing a suitable basis for intelligent healthcare [22–25].

Improved quality of life will be enabled by 6G technology, introducing us indirectly to intelligent health systems. Key quality of life parameters will be provided through remote health monitoring of patients, especially the elderly, through intelligent wearable devices (IVDs). These advances primarily relate to intelligent accident detection, telesurgery and precision medicine. In addition, the focus will be on the improvement of hospital-to-home services, with mobile hospitals organized in intelligent vehicles, all of which will contribute to improving the quality of life [22–25].

6G communication technology will rely on AI, which is why it can provide the Internet of Everything (IoE) and cloud functions in close proximity to intelligent devices. It will include many other technologies, such as Internet of Everything technologies for imaging, communication, caching, cognition, computing and control, as well as high-quality sensors and holographic communication in healthcare, converting input to digital data, storing it in a local cache and transmitting to remote locations in real time. Sometimes some digital data will be converted into signals and then transmitted to other devices for processing using cognitive methods of artificial intelligence [22–25].

18.2.2 Edge Technology

The 6G communication network will rely on cloud computing to store, compute and analyze large databases [24, 26]. Because the data produced by intelligent devices will be transferred to the cloud for storage, it is clear that during this process a significant consumption of communication resources will be required. In order to overcome this problem, edge technology was invented because it allows one to get very close to the corresponding source of the information. It is assumed that 6G will have high communication capacity, which provides smooth services to billions of intelligent devices [24, 26]. It will rely on edge technology to provide simple and fast Internet services through intelligent devices vital to healthcare. Such technology enables real-time collection, computation and analysis of health data in its edge nodes [24], located in close proximity to intelligent medical devices. The data generated by any place will be transmitted to the edge nodes. The nodes process the health data. Then, the data will be analyzed in order to finally make an appropriate decision.

The edge node will also filter health-related data and upload necessary information for cloud storage. This technology will thus reduce communication and computing costs [26]. In addition, it exhibits low latency of communication signals, as well as high reliability, privacy, scalability and adaptability. Thanks to this, a considerable number of intelligent devices will be able to connect to the 6G Internet. Furthermore, the mentioned advantages of the edge technology will significantly help the 6G network meet all the requirements that are necessary to provide high-quality service in healthcare. In addition, intelligent edge technology, which will be implemented with the support of AI algorithms for analysis in edge nodes, will enable edge analytics, which will serve to find patterns of behavior or calculations necessary with some other kind of analysis [24, 27].

Current AI algorithms are computationally demanding from the point of view of extremely high computer resources and energy consumption, which is significantly lower when using edge node technology. Bearing in mind that all nodes of the 6G network will have access to the services that health systems provide through artificial intelligence, the implementation of edge technology allows the realization of an intelligent edge that will greatly improve the health system, performing calculations and data analysis in in real time [28–35]. Therefore, it is very important to move the executing

AI algorithms to edge nodes instead of the cloud in order to reduce the delay during service [27–35]. In addition, the 6G communication system will enable the content of network communication to be intelligent, making the system self-aware and self-calculating, possessing the power to decide independently in a specific situation. Such a network will provide global coverage.

Since deep learning (DL) does not require data pre-processing but takes the original health data and performs calculations, it must ensure that all data is ready as real-time input, ensuring high accuracy when calculating many network parameters [27–35]. Accordingly, an artificial intelligence algorithm currently being researched on health data known as deep reinforcement learning (DRL) combines learning with deep neural network algorithms, which results in high performance in the shortest time. In addition, it will allow specific knowledge to be shared among numerous intelligent devices, which will inevitably improve healthcare [27–35].

18.3 HOLOGRAPHIC COMMUNICATION

Currently, AI algorithms require high computing resources and energy consumption, which is limited in edge nodes. Accordingly, since edge nodes will be present in 6G networks, they will have access to artificial intelligence, through which they will receive various notifications from health systems. Since the edge system will be intelligent and ready to provide services in real time, it will provide guided 6G communication by artificial intelligence [24, 36]. Implementing AI algorithms will thus generate high accuracy and exceptional communication performance in communication networks in real time, which will be of crucial importance for healthcare in the future, because such organized healthcare will improve clinical diagnostics and treatment itself [37].

Until now, the patient usually had to visit many doctors for an accurate diagnosis, while adequate treatment in a hospital was often unavailable. Sometimes, because of this, patients had to travel to various other countries, which represented an extraordinary economic and physical burden for the patient. In addition, for patients with poor health, the journey was extremely tiring. In the future, by using holographic communication, doctors can make a diagnosis at a distance, and the patient will only go to the hospital for medical treatment. Holographic communication will help doctors themselves to provide services in rural areas, not just in cities. Similar to 6G global coverage, 6G holographic communication will enable global healthcare connectivity. This type of communication will enable services at home, synchronously connecting different types of doctors around the world for their participation in the treatment of complex medical cases [36, 37].

The working principle of a digital holographic microscope is based on the recording of a hologram, which represents an interference image of two light waves, on a charge-coupled device (CCD) camera and digital reconstruction of the hologram with the possibility of changing the magnification, which is not limited by the properties of the optical elements, since it primarily depends on the reconstruction process and the characteristics of the camera. The basis of the numerical reconstruction process is the Fresnel-Kirchhoff integral, which describes the diffraction of waves on the microstructure of the hologram. The process of obtaining a hologram can be divided into two parts: recording and reconstructing the hologram. First, the coherent laser beam is split by a beam splitter into two waves, one of which falls directly on the photo plate, and the other is reflected from the object and then falls on the hologram plane. The reflected wave is created by the superposition of many spherical waves that are reflected from the object's surface, and its wavefront depends on the shape of the reflecting surface. This wave is called a carrier, because it carries information about the illuminated object.

The comparison or comparator wave is a plane or spherical wave that strikes the photo plate undisturbed. The interference of comparison and carrier waves takes place on the photo plate, whereby the resulting interference image on the photo plate represents a hologram. On the hologram, there is an overlap of several zonal patterns created by numerous waves reflected from the recording object at different angles. Accordingly, when creating a hologram, the intensity ratio of light waves, which is proportional to the square of the wave amplitude, and the phase difference of light waves, which depends on the relief of the surface of the object, are recorded on it, which enables obtaining a three-dimensional image. When recording a hologram, the reflected light wave reaches every point of the photo plate of the recorded object, so that each part of the hologram contains complete information about the entire recorded object. A three-dimensional image of an object is formed by the diffraction of a comparative wave even when a small part of the hologram is illuminated; such an image then has a proportionally smaller area and less clarity than the image obtained by reconstructing the entire hologram. Diffraction is the basic process in hologram reconstruction.

During reconstruction, a reference wave is directed at the hologram. If the reference wave falls on the plate at the same angle as during the recording, the imaginary figure appears in the same place and in the same position (relative to the plate) as the position of the object during the recording. The resulting image of the object is three-dimensional. When the viewing angle is changed, it is possible to see the object from different perspectives. Advances and developments in computer technology enable transfer of the recording or reconstruction process to a computer. The first such approach was realized by computer-generated holography (CGH), where numerical methods are used in the process of creating holograms.

In addition to obtaining a spatial, three-dimensional image of an object, digital holography offers the possibility of recording bodies in motion, recording the shape of an opaque body and the refractive index of transparent bodies, which is why it is widely used in biophysics and in biomedicine. Digital holographic image reconstruction and enhancement is a process that includes various techniques such as autofocus, numerical reconstruction, super-resolution, noise suppression, object detection and classification and object image compression. These techniques involve the use of different statistical data and iterative numerical methods, which often involve higher costs of the image reconstruction process itself, conditioned by the computer power involved and the image processing time.

Machine learning and deep learning have shown remarkable potential in recognizing behavioral patterns and predicting them, which has made it possible to improve object identification by analyzing visual data presented in a holographic image. These methods have shown remarkable efficiency in processing digital holographic data. Digital holographic microscopy (DHM) or quantitative phase imaging (2D QPI) and holographic tomography or 3D QPI are the most commonly used QPI techniques based on digital holography [38].

Several techniques using regression models are used to estimate image depth by varying wavelengths, exposure times, incidence angles and axial dimensions during hologram imaging. In numerical reconstruction, the entire wavefront information is reconstructed from the hologram using the Fresnel-Kirchhoff integral method for numerical object reconstruction, where the phase, derived directly from the complex exponent, is significantly affected by aberrations. Process of recording requires the adjustment of phase aberration, followed by a step called unwinding to get the right thickness of the object, which often leads to errors due to the film's sensitivity to noise and distortion. Deep learning methods are often used to solve such phase aberration compensation problems [38–41].

To demonstrate its efficiency and superiority from an image quality perspective, HRNet coupled with deep learning is used to solve a range of reconstruction modalities, such as amplitude reconstruction, quantitative phase imaging, extended focused imaging and depth map reconstruction. In doing so, DL is used to reconstruct the stored intensity or phase within the hologram [42]. To extract details, super-resolution techniques have been developed, whereby deep learning creates maps of high- and low-resolution holographic images. For such needs, it is possible to use a super-resolution convolutional neural network (SRCNN) to produce a given hologram. Holographic image enhancement using de-noising networks has been the subject of many studies. Accordingly, using common de-noising techniques such as low-pass filters is challenging. Finally, residual learning is shown to be highly effective in coherent noise suppression tasks [43–45] by applying U-Net, which was previously tested, on images of known noise intensity.

18.3.1 History of Holography and Development

The combination of digital holography and artificial intelligence provides a convenient mechanism for automated manipulation of holographic information for various real-time scenarios. Denis Gabor invented holography in 1948, and in 1963 this method experienced explosive development after the discovery of the first effective laser hologram by Emmett Leith. For the discovery of holography, Gabor received the Nobel Prize in 1971. Another critical moment in the same year was a paper published in the proceedings of the IEEE by T. Huang entitled "Digital Holography". It was followed by an explosion of research and publications in the early to mid-70s. Numerous potential applications of digital holography, such as producing computer-generated diffraction spatial filters for optical information processing, 3D holographic presentations and holographic television and holographic computer vision, generated enormous interest among researchers. Nevertheless, the inadequate speed and memory capacity of computers at that time, as well as the lack of electronic resources and media for detecting and recording optical holograms, were a severe brake on the development of this technology [38–41].

In 1990, with the development of high-speed microprocessors, high-resolution electronic and optical devices and liquid crystals and technology for the production of micro lenses and mirror arrays, digital holography experienced a new boom. Unlike in the 1970s, when the processes of obtaining holographic records required significant computer time, everything happens almost in "real" time [38–46].

A hologram is a three-dimensional image that contains a third dimension (depth) so that the object can be viewed from all directions as if it were real. Roughly, a hologram represents an image obtained by the interference of two light waves as a reconstruction of one of those two waves using the other in the process. Its creation is a complex process in which various objects participate. Therefore, today computers are often used to obtain them, as the most compatible computing tool. To create a hologram, laser monochromatic light is necessary. The light beam from the laser is split into two parts. One half illuminates the object, which reflects the laser light. The reflected light is mixed with the other half of the laser light beam (reference beam) so that bright and dark interference bands/lines are created. Dark bands are formed in the places where the light waves are out of phase.

Light bands are the places where the light waves are in phase. A hologram is a photograph of these interference fringes. Stripes do not have the appearance of an object; in fact, they cannot be seen [38–46] on the hologram plate because they are too small. The process of obtaining a hologram consists of the recording and the reconstruction of the hologram. By the way, a key role is played by the laser that participates in obtaining it. Also, built-in, internal stopwatches that accurately determine the length of the laser emission are often used, because the detail and fidelity of the hologram depend on precision. We can present a hologram more clearly when comparing it with a photograph. When photographing, the ratio of wave intensity is recorded on the photo emulsion, while when creating a hologram, along with the record of that ratio, there is also a record of the phase ratio of those two waves, and we get a three-dimensional figure. Therefore, by looking at a hologram and a photograph of something, the representation of the thing at a glance creates a more precise image in the human brain when viewing the hologram. We can see this if we were to look through windows of sizes 0.5×0.5 m and 1×1 m. Clearly, by looking through a larger window, we have a clearer view of the image. Also, we can get the same view if we look through a smaller window from several different angles. Therefore, a hologram can comprehensively represent a series of exact images [38–46].

18.3.2 Hologram Recording

Let us send a coherent laser beam to a semipermeable plate. Then, the wave will split into two parts so that one will be reflected from the plate, while the other will pass through it. Let us look first at the part that was rejected. After that reflection, it will be reflected again from another mirror, which gives us a light wave that we call a reference. The second part that broke through the plate is then reflected from the object whose hologram we required and takes shape depending object's shape itself, and the object wave can be created. So, at a particular point, these waves can collide, and they can be merged, that is, interference, which gives us an interference image, which we call a hologram. However, since the photo plate is located in that place and the reference wave is flat and the subject wave is spherical, the creation of the so-called zonal interference plates. They represent a set of concentric circles of different thicknesses and radii. As, the radii and the distances between the circles are very minute can causes diffraction. However, as each pair of reference and spherical waves build a zonal plate, they intersect at different angles, and we get a diffraction grating. With that, saving the hologram is finished [38–46].

Thanks to digital holography and its integration with digital computers, which makes it possible to produce visual information, information vision has matured. The most significant advantage of digital computers over analog electronic and visual information processing devices is that no hardware upgrades are required to solve various tasks [46, 47].

The recent past of visual media has been characterized by the rapid expansion of 3D images and their visualization. The technology that gives the most authentic images is digital holography (DH), because it is the only one that gives complete information about the wavelength, amplitude and phase of the light wave, which it then stores and preserves, so that finally, with the help of spatial light modulators (SLM), the wave field could be reconstructed again at an alternative location at another time. Complications in the distribution of holographic data often depend on the type of object being recorded, which can be stationary like an image or fluctuating in time in the form of a live scene like a video. Digital holography enables the digital recording of a hologram and its presentation on a digital computer [42, 47, 48].

In addition, digital holograms can be digitally reconstructed remotely. The advent of solid state sensors in the 1970s ushered in a new era of digital holography. Holograms are tested digitally, directly and very quickly, using CCD or complementary metal oxide semiconductor (CMOS) matrix sensors in the visible or even infrared spectrum, where image reconstruction is performed arithmetically on a 2D display or 3D for SLM presentation. The most impressive achievements in holographic 3D performance are related to computer-generated holograms, achieving effects which the human mind can hardly imagine. In order to obtain three-dimensional holographic images, computer-generated holograms and spatial light modulators are introduced into practice, with the application of appropriate algorithms, such as the Gerchberg-Sakton (GS) algorithm or other similar algorithms [47, 48].

18.3.3 Reconstruction of the Hologram

In order to allow the observer to see the saved hologram, we need to do a few more things. First, let's send a plane wave of light onto the photo plate so that the angle at which the wave hits it is the same as the angle at which the reference wave hits the photo plate. This causes diffraction, and the resulting light wave is emitted from the object towards the observer such that an imaginary figure will appear where the original object was, so the hologram is created [49, 50].

To mimic the quality of everyday human interaction with the environment, future computer interfaces must combine high visual fidelity with the ability to modulate the emotions of their users. The notion of self-directed ordering of quantum computing is mediated by quantum artificial intelligence that is capable of adapting to different environmental variations and responses aimed at faithfully rendering highly complex objects [49, 50]. The proposed framework can be categorized into four main segments: the data detection and verification segment, the digital to hologram conversion segment, the holographic interface and finally the developing memory segment. The data detection and verification segment uses the sensor module to modify incoming or outgoing data via the sensor memory. Sensory storage represents a memory segment responsible for collecting information and transferring it to the flow controller module [49, 50].

The flow controller module orders its requests based on three elementary experiential constraints: the importance of the processing of a particular upcoming request is determined by experience, with requests that take the least processing time more likely to be fulfilled sooner. Additionally, if a particular job requires more connections in the knowledge base, then it will take less time to learn and process. Whether to accept a request depends on the total processing time of the holographic information. Data authentication is responsible for executing given subtasks based on learning and prior knowledge present in memory that is necessary to perform immediate requests. That module authenticates the request and forwards it to the digital to hologram conversion module. Suspicious requests are transferred to the risk manager module for checking, verification and taking preventive measures. The risk manager module will evaluate the immediate claim based on predetermined constraints, such as the similarity of the request to a previous request that was not credible, where the experience threshold depends on the knowledge gained from learning to manage this class of untrusted requests [49, 50].

18.3.4 Holography and Artificial Intelligence

Artificial intelligence expert systems are computer-generated systems that typically include three vital segments: a database, a knowledge base and finally an interpretation engine. Control systems are computer software that monitors and regulates physical procedures that require the rapid processing of vast amounts of information. Therefore, various artificial intelligence strategies such as information mining, artificial neural systems, genetic algorithms and expert systems are used, which can be coordinated using conventional techniques for analyzing information collected by sensors [47–50].

The key problem with cognitive approaches is the static nature of existing holographic interface management systems and the work according to predetermined assumptions. Therefore, these holographic interface management systems are not competent to independently make decisions about the ways to manipulate a hologram according to the user's requirements. In contrast, the combination of digital holography and artificial intelligence provides a much more adequate mechanism for modifying photon patterns according to the requirements of the holographic interface or system configuration, thus facilitating the automatic reconfiguration of the holographic interface. Accordingly, volumetric displays provide interesting opportunities for 3D interaction and visualization when used in an interactive way [47–50].

Current techniques take advantage of the unique features of volumetric displays, including 360° viewing that allows natural and accurate perception of the true depth information of images displayed on a 3D scene. These displays typically include safety glasses or head shields [50]. Holographic optical tweezer (HOT) systems use a programmable spatial light modulator to split the laser beam into two parts and control and shape it. SLMs are an increasingly popular tool for controlling and shaping laser beams in many areas of physics such as laser marking, two-photon polymerization and HOT. Most SLMs currently available use a liquid crystal layer to change the optical path length of light reflected from the device. The parallel architecture of graphics processing units (GPUs) is used to accelerate magnitude of hologram calculation by several orders [47–50].

Holography is good for solving various medical problems by storing and using patient data. On the other hand, 3D holograms enable successful treatment and surgery of patients. Such holographic images are 3D images characterized by a considerable depth of field, so that by zooming in on the hologram, the doctor can have a better view of the specific part of the body to which the hologram refers. This technology significantly improves medical practice, enabling the rapid detection of problems in various organs such as the brain, heart, liver or kidneys. By using this technology, doctors can finally observe organs from multiple angles with much greater precision. Accordingly, this technique opens up a new way of planning and testing procedures for patients and their diagnosis [51].

In addition, holography is a technology that enables effective interaction of people with the digital world, in which 3D imaging technologies are effectively used to solve challenges in education and training of personnel and their research. In the field of medicine, holography is used to plan surgical procedures, as well as in medical diagnostics and radiology and to obtain better information about tissues and internal and external organs when viewed from different angles, as it allows to obtain high-resolution images of them. It is also a good tool for planning interventions due to its ability to record perfect information on cavities and deformities of internal organs or during implant placement procedures [52, 53].

Holography is used to study the different parts of the ear in detail; such as the outer ear, middle ear and inner ear under different noise conditions, as well as in applications such as diagnosis of cornea, eardrum, tooth mobility, basilar membrane, temporal bone, cochlea, joint, skull, thorax and bone [54, 55]. In cardiology, it is used treating of arrhythmias, coronary interventions and replacement of heart valves. It enables a much more efficient healthcare infrastructure, as well as endless options for emergency medical care [55, 56]. Additionally, holography provides vast possibilities of 3D visualization of the patient's body with high resolution. In order to develop 3D holograms for clinical application in medicine, the first step assumes installation of the appropriate hardware and software for preparing the medical image, which is then visualized by doctors and surgeons for proper treatment planning in clinical applications, providing numerous medical benefits. Such an approach provides numerous advantages comparing to the conventional methods used today in medicine [55, 56].

Contemporary digital imaging technologies provide 2D and even 3D images of recorded body parts. Moreover, today technology has advanced so much that people can see these images in motion, in different scales, colors and languages. Some research testifies to the application of holography measuring stress during surgery. Overall, the technology of 3D holographic visualization provides the doctor a unique experience in numerous fields, such as the study of bones in a no-contact way [57, 58]. In addition, it is significant to point out that the advantages of this method are also confirmed through the possibility of saving multiple images taken at different angles, as well as improving treatment procedures with high learning efficiency, that is acquiring new knowledge and experience, which all increases the efficiency of doctors and surgeons without additional requirements for special viewing glasses every day, 3D virtual reality, or other tools [57, 58].

Holography helps radiologists identify an injury or fracture to a patient's soft or hard tissue. This method improves safety and ensures better patient treatment by allowing digital storage of patient records so the radiologist can quickly review the patient's medical history. Its typical application in radiology is related to cardiovascular applications, as well as applications related to problems of the chest, genitourinary system, musculoskeletal system, neuroradiology, pediatrics and head and neck radiology. 3D holography provides more information to radiologists then 2D images, because it allows for storing a huge amount of information. It is suitable for planning different surgical approaches by performing invasive procedures [57, 58]. This method finally allows the elimination of demanding physical testing procedures, enabling easy storage of digital 3D images of the patient or their body parts at the same time [59, 60].

Holograms enable various medical tests, which is why they are used to monitor diabetes and infections and check the proper functioning of soft and hard tissues. They also allow screening for drugs, hormones, alcohol and glucose [61, 62]. Doctors today can use color holography to monitor clinical trials and study complex images of the vascular, nervous and musculoskeletal systems.

Thanks to this method, doctors can now clearly see a patient's anatomy without cutting into the body [61, 62]. Using holographic imaging, in addition, physicians can improve the quality of their own medical education and research. Finally, holography is also used to create digital 3D prototypes in the field of neuroscience, as well as to study various orthopedic structures. It is also applicable for load measurement in various bone fractures [61, 62].

3D imaging requires highly qualified human resources. In addition, the production and review of medical images require expensive hardware and software. In the future, holography will allow "holodoctors" to see a holographic image at a remote location and provide appropriate treatment. It will also enable the production of pharmaceutical and health products, as well as a significant improvement in healthcare [61, 62].

18.4 AUGMENTED AND VIRTUAL REALITY

Augmented reality helps to incorporate virtuality into tangible objects. It is often combined with multiple sensory abilities such as audio, visual, somatosensory or haptic sensors. AR, among other things, enables real-time interaction, accurately displaying 3D images of virtual and natural objects. Virtual reality refers to the representation of an imaginary or virtual world in which nothing is real. Both of these types of realities use the basic service of combined eMBB and URLLC, which is why a high data rate is necessary to ensure good quality of service, which is achieved by high-resolution video streaming, including real-time voice transmission, with possible control of the received answer [56, 62].

The data transfer rate for such purposes should be on the order of 1 Tbps, and a user experience of > 10 Gbps with > 0.1 ms latency can be provided by MBBLL. 6G networks will enable their complete application in the field of healthcare along with 3D holography. At the same time, AR will make it possible to observe anatomical details inside the patient's body with high resolution, with a desirable depth of penetration within a specific location in the body previously determined by the doctor and the ability to zoom in as much as necessary for better visibility. 6G will thus help doctors observe the patient remotely, where AR and holographic communication will be combined for better diagnosis. Using VR, doctors will be able to practice various medical procedures without the presence of a patient, which will be especially important in the process of acquiring skills in complex procedures and operations, the performance of which is associated with high risk [63].

18.5 TACTILE/HAPTIC INTERNET

Haptic technology creates the sensation of virtual touch, using force, movement or vibration directed at the user. The tactile Internet will transmit virtual touch to another user, human or robot. The Internet will require high communication speed and ERLLC to respond to touch in real time. This technology will be used for remote operations, like telesurgery. It will help doctors diagnose by touch without physical presence. Haptic human–computer interaction (HCI) implies a system consisting of a desktop, as well as surface and portable pieces of equipment [1, 2, 64]. Thanks to the HCI desktop, a remote doctor can use a virtual tool for surgery or diagnosis.

The command-giving device will have a flat screen, such as a mobile phone or tablet, where as the hand moves across the screen, commands will be issued to the robot to interact with the patient. In a wearable HCI, for example, a haptic glove, the remote physician can have tactile communication with the patient. In this way, tactile/haptic technology will be particularly important during a dangerous epidemic or pandemic, such as COVID-19, when all countries were in isolation; where interaction outside each country is limited; or during a natural disasters. Accordingly, during epidemics or pandemics, medical personnel at high risk of a deadly infectious disease will use tactile/haptic technology to transfer their duties to robots, which will be used for immediate care of the patient while the medical staff performs their work remotely [1, 2, 64].

18.6 INTELLIGENT INTERNET OF MEDICAL THINGS

In the 6G communication network, developing the Intelligent Internet of Medical Things (IIoMT) driven by artificial intelligence will take a special place in making its own decisions by applying communication technology. The IoE will also emerge alongside the IIoMT, enabling the connection of medical information to the Internet. The process itself will take place via a suitable scanner scanning and sending data to remote locations via 6G technology, which doctors will then analyze in real time. Since almost all medical services will be connected to the Internet, medical decisions will be made instantly. Accordingly, the IIoMT will overcome the barrier of time, space and money, allowing patients to be treated by remote doctors, which will enable early detection of severe diseases in patients, such as cancer or cardiovascular diseases [64].

Numerous studies are underway on needle-free blood sampling devices, which are particularly important for glucose monitoring in diabetics [65]. Future blood sample sensors will be needle free, intelligent and wearable. They will read all the blood parameters, such as white blood cells (WBCs) and red blood cells (RBCs) and will be connected to the 6G Internet. A blood sample will be periodically sent to the testing center for test results, either automatically or with the patient's permission. In addition, such a sensor can easily monitor the spread of a deadly virus in real time. Therefore, BSR sensors will be highly sought-after medical devices in the future. Intelligent wearable devices connected to the Internet will transmit and monitor heart rate, blood pressure, blood tests, the health status of the patient and their body weight and diet. IVDs will also learn from the patient's personal history to offer advice for a specific action, such as advice on walking or running or on diet [65].

By applying such technologies, the detection of minor physical problems will reduce the frequency of hospital visits, while hospitals will focus on more complex diseases. In addition, the IVD will read blood samples and enable early detection of cancer, improving health conditions and thereby extending people's life expectancy. Also, services for older people who need intensive care will be improved. Future IVDs will combine multiple functions in one device, and over time, such devices will become affordable for the most of the population. Ambulances are currently only for the function of transporting patients with the priority of giving oxygen in order to revive the natural functions of the body and to transfer the patient from a certain location to the hospital. They does not have the possibility to offer genuine emergency assistance to the patient, due to the absence of quality intelligence. So, emergency services do not fundamentally affect our lives. Any normal car can also serve the same purpose if it is equipped with an oxygen cylinder and has an emergency signal [63–65].

Thus, a new type of emergency care is needed to improve lifestyles. In the future, it will be on the way from home to hospital, and transportation will be provided with intelligent vehicles that will be fully powered by AI [66].

18.7 TELESURGERY, EPIDEMICS AND PANDEMICS AND PRECISION MEDICINE

Telesurgery requires robots, nurses and remote physician intermediaries, as well as very high data transfer speeds. For this kind of support, 6G technology is necessary, which enables real-time communication [67]. Finally, thanks to 6G networks, it is possible to provide interactive verbal guidance with the support of holographic communication, during which the doctor can be present in the office for the necessary verbal instructions while solving a medical problem. Also, by applying such technologies, a specific operational area is presented visually. It is crucial to show the operation at a distance, using telestration by video. In intelligent healthcare, AR and VR will also be used for telestration. In addition, physician(s) will also use tactile/haptic technology. With all that in mind, it is believed that all the requirements of telesurgery will be able to be fully met by 6G communication technology, paving the way for more frequent remote operations [67].

Communication technology will play an important role pandemics, bearing in mind that in such situations, medical personnel are exposed to great risk. Recently, COVID-19 has claimed thousands of lives, including medical personnel. Outbreaks of pandemics like COVID-19 can be easily stopped with the IIoMT by analyzing blood samples using a BSR sensor at home. A blood sample will be taken using intelligent portable technology (BSR sensor) and transported to testing centers. Thus, the human chain of disease transmission can be easily stopped and the epidemic can be monitored in real time. In addition, precision medicine is developing treatments for better patient care [42], which will greatly benefit from 6G technology. For better treatment, the health data of people undergoing clinical trials is needed [68].

6G networks will significantly improve business, redefining existing hospital business models. Currently, the cost of treatment is paid by the patient directly to the hospital or through the health insurance policy. The health insurance policy will be managed by a company, forming a network of hospitals. Such hospitals will enable cashless treatment. Since today, most insurances do not cover many diseases and health services for the elderly, because this business model defines the hospital and insurance as separate entities during treatment, this will be a significant improvement. Today, the insurance company usually pays the hospital for the service. Sometimes these are enormous amounts, which is why hospital services are often very inaccessible for patients. In other words, neither the hospital nor the insurance company is responsible for our treatment from birth to death. Unlike existing models, the new business model is expected to abolish health insurance, and hospitals will play the role of health insurance companies [67, 68].

Such insurance will be hospital health insurance. HIH will form a network of hospitals and remove the middleman (health insurance). The annual or monthly insurance premium will be paid directly to the hospital, so the hospital will use the insurance money to care for patients and their health from birth to death. It is enough for the patient to call the H2H service to arrive at the hospital, where they will verify their HIH identification and then be admitted to any partner hospital for priority treatment. After discharge from the hospital, the patient will not have to pay any medical bill. Such services will include IVD connection and monitoring, H2H services, telesurgery, surgery, pregnancy and delivery, vaccines, intensive care services for the elderly, personalization and appropriate therapy. HIH will cover all types of illnesses and accidents, including cancer, influenza, cardiovascular and neurological problems. There will be no limit on the number of treatments per patient [67, 68].

In addition, 6G communication technology promises the highest level of security, using artificial intelligence, quantum machine learning, quantum computing and THz communication, which is resistant to eavesdropping and jamming [56]. Today, as healthcare requires a high level of security for data transmission over the network, any change in health data may be unsafe for the patient, so the key question has become how to protect health data from attackers. In addition, 6G communication technology will focus on the secrecy of the most sensitive data, which will be protected from being viewed by anyone other than the data owner.

Also, administrators will not be allowed to see this sensitive data, such as family history. In addition, 6G will also focus on privacy, which is a crucial healthcare parameter, relying on edge technology, where edge nodes are located closer to intelligent devices. Such data will be analyzed in those nodes. Since edge nodes have limited memory, different data will be concentrated in different locations. Another essential point is data filtering using edge nodes. That is, edge nodes will filter data and transmit only necessary information to the cloud. This will result in less user information being stored in the cloud. In the current scenario, blockchain provides a high degree of privacy for health data [56, 68].

18.8 THE METAVERSE AND HOLOGRAPHIC SIMULATION

Many tools, digital and analog, have been used to ensure anti-aging mechanisms. Such tools often include food tracking applications, which allow users to quantify their food intake in terms of the number of calories or macronutrient balance. Most wearable devices (fitness trackers, smart watches) are tools for monitoring and improving health by monitoring physical activity and estimation of calories burned, essential information for fitness management and user nutrition goals. In addition, entertainment apps help users maintain good mental health, thus increasing the chances of a long life. The new generation of Internet, named the Metaverse, which represents the network of 3D virtual worlds focused on creating social networks, as a hypothetical iteration of the Internet of a single universal virtual world facilitated by the use of virtual or augmented reality headsets, is also very important in the future development of intelligent healthcare, because it provides a unique virtual environment that offers more interactivity when used in combination with new technologies (artificial intelligence, blockchain, Internet of Things), which helps create more effective anti-aging strategies and solutions that mitigate the aging process itself and create conditions for a better quality of life [5, 20, 69].

The Metaverse can also assist medical professionals while performing surgeries. Medical professionals can also use the Metaverse platform for learning and training purposes. The success of this practice will lead many medical institutions to move from the traditional way of learning to virtual reality, mixed reality and artificial intelligence–supported systems to train their employees and students as effectively as possible [5], since the Metaverse itself is a virtual space that includes a mix of different technologies, such as mixed reality, virtual reality, blockchain and artificial intelligence, to enable virtual communication between users with a high degree of immersive experience, which imitates scenarios from real life [5, 20, 69].

Although the Metaverse was primarily developed for social communication and entertainment, it certainly affects various fields of social activity, including digital anti-aging in healthcare. Metaverse enables virtual healthcare, thereby helping elderly people cope with their health problems more easily. It provides a virtual environment in which patients can communicate with healthcare professionals and receive medical assistance during treatment in their own home, particularly useful for older people who have mobility or transportation problems [70, 71]. Also, this technology helps develop virtual fitness programs, which provide a personalized exercise regimen adapted to the user's age, fitness level and health status while providing a platform for socialization and building a good social environment for older adults. By providing a virtual space for social interaction, the Metaverse helps combat social isolation and promotes overall well-being [5, 20, 69–71]. Major chronic diseases include heart disease and stroke, cancer, diabetes, Alzheimer's disease, Parkinson's disease, arthritis, chronic obstructive pulmonary disease (COPD) and obesity.

The stage immediately preceding a holographic simulation is holographic construction, during which a static geometric model of the virtual world is formed, consisting of virtual hospitals, medical personnel and medical tools. All objects in the environment are classified into three categories: scenes, events and people. The second step is a holographic simulation, in which the real environment is implemented in a virtual world, which includes numerous technologies that connect medical information with existing data systems, as well as devices for recording movements in real time [5, 20, 69–71].

The next stage after the holographic simulation stage is the fusion of virtual and real, where it is crucial that the virtual world look as authentic as possible, which is achieved by using mixed reality, which overcomes the boundaries between the virtual medical world and the real world. Finally, there is the fourth stage of connecting the virtual and real worlds, by combining artificial intelligence, IoT and brain–computer interfaces (BCI), to create intelligent medical equipment and improve methods of simulating the process of transformation of virtual events into real ones and vice versa. The four given phases create the possibility of implementing medical solutions in the Metaverse. As entertainment becomes more important as we age, entertainment programs increasingly include puzzles, card games, coffee and playing games, as these all help reduce stress [5, 20, 69–71]. The Metaverse environment, combined with other digital technologies such as AI, BC and IoT entertainment programs, not only does not limit the user to games but also provides a new social environment that makes the user's life much more interesting. In the Metaverse it is possible to meet and collaborate with others; socialize and make new friends; buy real and virtual products; play virtual games; and attend events such as concerts, fairs and learning events. The Metaverse, through the use of VR gaming technologies, plays an essential role in human well-being. The use of VR devices has been proven to help stimulate brain activity, especially in individuals with dementia [37]; as such, patients can use the Metaverse to connect to other environments and thus simulate memories and connect with friends and family [5, 20, 69–71].

Mental health is among the crucial sectors of healthcare for the elderly because it directly affects the quality of their aging process. A healthy mental state leads to a lower risk of a shortened lifespan.

The Metaverse provides the possibility of improving a person's mental state, serving as a rehabilitation medium for patients with mental illnesses. The Metaverse is used in training hospitals but also for remote consultations. VR, AR and mixed reality are the crucial technologies that enable this type of treatment, as well as mental health diagnostics. Some applications of mental health disorders created within the Metaverse include diseases such as attention deficit hyperactivity disorder, eating disorders, anxiety, phobias and post-traumatic stress disorders, autism and Alzheimer's disease. Various software and hardware applications are used to create 3D virtual data, creating a 3D virtual environment [5, 20, 69–71].

18.9 CONCLUSION

One of the most significant new technologies is holography, which has many applications in medicine, military, weather forecasting, virtual reality, digital art and security. This technology has extraordinary importance in the industry and medicine development, improving the efficiency of existing products and services in various technological fields, such as architecture, 3D modeling, mechatronics, robotics and health and medical engineering. 3D holography uses digital image inputs and provides extensive data visualization for training physicians, surgeons and students.

It converts information about the body into a digital format and has the potential to inform, promote and entertain medical students and doctors. Holographic 3D images have a considerable depth of field, so a doctor can zoom in on them for better medical imaging of body parts. This technology quickly detects problems in different organs, such as the brain, heart, liver or kidneys, thus allowing doctors to see organs from more angles and with better precision.

Digital holography has also advanced tremendously in recent times due to advances in experimental and algorithmic techniques. The introduction of machine learning and deep learning has significantly improved pattern recognition and prediction procedures related to data stored in visual images. The combination of DH and ML/DL has also shown significant potential not only in biomedical microscopy, including the identification and classification of cellular and subcellular structures, but also in the detection of pathogenic microbes. Additionally, the convergence of artificial intelligence, blockchain, the Internet of Things, immersive technologies and digital twins in the metaverse environment presents new opportunities for future smart/intelligent healthcare development.

Knowing that the tactile Internet [2, 3] enables a new type of human–machine interaction characterized by extremely low latency and short transit, high availability, high reliability and an exceptional level of security when creating systems with real-time interactive actions with the advent of the 6G network [1–3], the integration of mobile edge cloud and augmented reality for sensory and haptic controls will be enabled. In this way, future smart/intelligent health systems will have a response time of less than 1 millisecond while simultaneously offering tactile physical experiences at a distance.

REFERENCES

1. V. Jokanović, S. Živković, Controversies related to real protection against SARS-CoV-2 virus of the most frequently used face masks, Zastita Materijala 63(3) (2022), 221–229.
2. V. Jokanović, M. Živković, S. Živković, Artificial intelligence as a powerful tool in overcoming substantial health problems of the COVID-19 pandemic, Stomatološku glasnik Srbije 68 (2021), 143–152.
3. V. Jokanović, The wondrous challenges of the exotic worlds of nanomachines and bio-inspired artificial intelligence, In Technological Prospects and Social Applications of Society 5.0, Taylor and Francis, Boca Raton, London, New York (2022).
4. J. Hopkins, Performs its first augmented reality surgeries in patients. Available online: www.hopkinsmedicine.org/news/articles/johns-hopkins-performs-its-first-augmented-reality-surgeries-in-patients/ (accessed on 16 February 2021).
5. C. W. Lee, Application of metaverse service to healthcare industry: A strategic perspective, Int. J. Environ. Res. Public Health 19 (2022), 13038.

6. Y. Xie, L. Lu, F. Gao, S.-J. He, H.-J. Zhao, Y. Fang, J.-M. Yang, Y. An, Z.-W. Ye, Z. Dong, Integration of artificial intelligence, blockchain, and wearable technology for chronic disease management: A new paradigm in smart healthcare, Curr. Med. Sci. 41 (2021), 1123–1133.
7. O. T. Picot, R. Alcalá, C. Sánchez, M. Dai, N. F. Hughes-Brittain, D. J. Broer, C. W. Bastiaansen, Manufacturing of surface relief structures in moving substrates using photo embossing and pulsed-interference holography, Macromol. Mater. Eng. 298(1) (2013), 33–37.
8. M. Fratz, T. Seyler, A. Bertz, D. Carl, Digital holography in production: An overview, Light Adv. Manuf. 2(2) (2021), 134–146.
9. R. Ashima, A. Haleem, S. Bahl, M. Javaid, S. K. Mahla, S. Singh, Automation and manufacturing of smart materials in Additive Manufacturing technologies using the Internet of Things towards the adoption of Industry 4.0, Mater. Today Proc. 45 (2021), 5081–5088.
10. A. Lonnqvist, J. Ala-Laurinaho, J. Hakli, T. Koskinen, V. Viikari, J. Saily, A. V. Raisanen, Manufacturing of large-sized amplitude holograms for a submm-wave CATR (IEEE Cat. No. 02CH37313), IEEE Antennas Propag. Soc. Int. Symp. 4 (2002), 394–397.
11. H. I. Bjelkhagen, D. Brotherton-Ratcliffe, Ultrarealistic imaging: The future of display holography, Opt. Eng. 53(11) (2014), 112310.
12. E. Marino, L. Barbieri, B. Colacino, A. K. Fleri, F. Bruno, An augmented reality inspection tool to support workers in Industry 4.0 environments, Comput. Ind. 127 (2021), 103412.
13. D. Vather, I. Naydenova, D. Cody, M. Zawadzka, S. Martin, E. Mihaylova, V. Toal, Serialized holography for brand protection and authentication, Appl. Opt. 57(22) (2018), E131–E137.
14. L. N. Hoon, S. S. Shaharuddin, Learning effectiveness of 3D hologram animation on primary school learners, J. Vis. Art Des. 1(2) (2019), 93–104.
15. J. Butt, A strategic roadmap for the manufacturing industry to implement industry 4.0, Design 4(2) (2020), 11–42.
16. G. Valiño, J. C. Rico, P. Fernández, B. J. Alvarez, Y. Fernandez, Capability of colonoscopic holography for digitizing and measuring of layer thickness on PLA parts built by FFF, Procedia Manuf. 41 (2019), 129–136.
17. B. Bordbar, M. M. Hussain, P. P. Banerjee, Application of complex field imaging sensor to additive manufacturing, In Ultra-High-Definition Imaging Systems III, 11305, International Society for Optics and Photonics, San Francisco, CA (2020), 113050G.
18. Y. Yang, K. Siau, W. Xie, Y. Sun, Smart health intelligent healthcare systems in the metaverse, artificial intelligence, and data science era, J. Organ. End User Comput. (JOEUC) 34 (2022), 1–14.
19. M. A. Mozumder, T. P. T. Armand, S. M. Imtiyaj Uddin, A. Athar, R. I. Umon, R. I. A. Hussain, H.-C. Kim, Metaverse for digital anti-aging healthcare: An overview of potential use cases based on artificial intelligence, blockchain, IoT technologies, its challenges, and future directions, Appl. Sci. 13 (2023), 5127–5146.
20. M. N. Ahmed, A. S. Toor, K. O'Neil, D. Friedland, Cognitive computing and the future of health care cognitive computing and the future of healthcare: The cognitive power of IBM Watson has the potential to transform global personalized medicine, IEEE Pulse 8 (2017), 4–9.
21. X. Zhang, Y. Chen, L. Hu, Y. Wang, The metaverse in education: Definition, framework, features, potential applications, challenges, and future research topics, Front. Psychol. 13 (2022), 1016300.
22. P. K. Padhi, F. Charrua-Santos, 6G enabled tactile internet and cognitive internet of healthcare everything: Towards a theoretical framework, Appl. Syst. Innov. 4 (2021), 66–86.
23. J. Lin, W. M. Chen, Y. Lin, J. Cohn, C. Gan, S. Han, MCUNet: Tiny deep learning on IoT devices. arXiv 1 (2020), 10319.
24. H.-N. Dai, Z. Zheng, Z. Y. Zhang, Blockchain for Internet of Things: A survey. IEEE Internet Things J. 2019, 8076–8094.
25. P. Padma, Unlocking the power of tactile internet via 5G network, Internet of Things latest news. 2020. Available online: www.analyticsinsight.net/unlocking-the-power-of-tactile-internet-via-5g-network/ (accessed on 19 April 2021).
26. G. Cisotto, E. Casarin, S. Tomasin, Performance requirements of advanced healthcare services over future cellular systems, arXiv 2019.
27. P. G. Polson, C. Lewis, J. Rieman, C. Wharton, Cognitive walkthroughs: A method for theory-based evaluation of user interfaces, Int. J. Man-Mach. Stud. 36 (1992), 741–773.
28. C. H. Tsai, Theory, social cognitive theory, and the technology acceptance model to explore a behavioral model of telehealth systems, Int. J. Environ. Res. Public Health 11 (2014), 4905–4925.
29. V. Jokanović, Smart healthcare in smart cities, In L. Sharna (ed.) Towards Smart World: Homes to Cities Using Internet of Things, 1st edition, Chapter 4, Taylor and Francis Group, New York (2020).

30. V. Jokanović, B. Jokanović, Brain-computer interface: State of art, challenges and future, In Artificial Intelligence Technologies, Applications, and Challenges (paper in printing), Chapter 27, Taylor and Francis Group, New York (2021).
31. V. Jokanović, Synthetic biology and artificial intelligence, In Computer Vision and Internet of Things: Technology and Applications (paper in printing), Taylor and Francis Group, New York (2021).
32. V. Jokanović, S. Živković, M. Živković, State of the art of artificial intelligence in dentistry and its expected future, In Computer Vision and Internet of Things: Technology and Applications (paper in printing), Taylor and Francis Group (2021).
33. V. Jokanović, Bridge Between Nanophysics and Alternative Medicine: A New Energetic Approach to the Human Cell Treatment and Their Healing, Lap Lambert Academic Publishing, New York (2016).
34. V. Jokanović, Nanomedicine, the Greatest Challenge of 21th Century, Monograph (830 pages), Data Status, Beograd (2012).
35. V. Jokanović, How Died and Lives Our Cells, Monograph (530 pages), Institute of Nuclear Science Vinča, Beograd (2013).
36. S. A. Frank, The price equation program: Simple invariances unify population dynamics, thermodynamics, probability, information, and inference, Entropy 20 (2018), 978.
37. M. Lohstroh, E. A. Lee, An interface theory for the Internet of Things, In SEFM 2015 Collocated Workshops, Springer, Cham, (2015), 20–34.
38. V. Jokanović, Instrumental Methods, a Key for Understanding Nanotechnology and Nanomedicine, Institute of Nuclear Sciences and Serbian Engineering Academy, Belgrade (2014).
39. U. Schnars, W. P. O. Juptner, Digital recording and numerical reconstruction of holograms, Meas. Sci. Technol. 13 (2002), R85.
40. W. Xu, M. H. Jericho, I. A. Meinertzhagen, H. J. Kreuzer, Digital in-line holography for biological applications, Proc. Natl. Acad. Sci. U.S.A. 98 (2002), 11301.
41. T. Nguyen, V. Bui, V. Lam, C. B. Raub, L.-C. Chang, G. Nehmetallah, Automatic phase aberration compensation for digital holographic microscopy based on deep learning background detection, Opt. Express 25 (2017), 15043.
42. A. U. Dar, A. B. Ahanger, M. Rasool, M. Singh, A. Assad, M. A. Macha, S. W. Aalam, A. N. Ahanger, Applications of artificial intelligence and digital holography in biomedical microscopy, Authorea 21 (2023), 1–28.
43. W. Jeon, W. Jeong, K. Son, H. Yang, Speckle noise reduction for digital holographic images using multi-scale convolutional neural networks, Opt. Lett. 43 (2018), 4240.
44. M. Tahon, S. Montresor, P. Picart, Towards reduced CNNs for de-noising phase images corrupted with speckle noise, Photonics 8 (2021), 255.
45. D.-Y. Park and J.-H. Park, Hologram conversion for speckle free reconstruction using light field extraction and deep learning, Opt. Express 28 (2020), 5393.
46. A. Elmorshidy, Holographic projection technology: The world is changing, arXiv 2(2) (2010), 104–112.
47. M. Paturzo, P. Memmolo, A. Finizio, R. Näsänen, T. J. Naughton, P. Ferraro, Synthesis and display of dynamic holographic 3D scenes with real-world objects, Opt. Express 18(9) (2010), 8806–8815.
48. W. Zheng, L. Cao, H. Zhang, D. Kong, S. Zong, G. Jin, Three-dimensional display based on angular multiplexing of computer-generated holograms, In Digital Holography and Three-Dimensional Imaging, Optica Publishing Group, Heidelberg, Germany (2016), DT4D-1.
49. C. P. Goncalves, Quantum cybernetics and complex quantum systems science—a quantum connectionist exploration, In Conference on Quantum Biology, Guilford (2014).
50. G. Brassard, S. Gamb, E. Aimeur, Machine learning in a quantum world, In Advances in Artificial Intelligence, Springer, Quebec (2010), 431–442.
51. A. Haleem, M. Javaid, I. H. Khan, Holography applications toward medical field: An overview, Indian J. Radiol. Imaging 30(3) (2020), 354–361.
52. S. Mishra, Hologram the future of medicine—from star wars to clinical imaging, Indian Heart J. 69 (2017): 566–567.
53. A. Haleem, M. Javaid, R. Vaishya, Holography applications for orthopaedics, Indian J. Radiol. Imaging 29 (2019), 477–479.
54. W. Kreider, P. V. Yuldashev, O. A. Sapozhnikov, N. Farr, A. Partanen, M. R. Bailey, V. Khokhlova, Characterization of a multi-element clinical HIFU system using acoustic holography and nonlinear modeling, IEEE Trans. Ultrason. Ferroelectr. Freq. Control 60 (2913), 1683–1698.
55. M. Khaleghi, J. Guignard, C. Furlong, J. J. Rosowski, Simultaneous full-field 3-D vibrometry of the human eardrum using spatial-bandwidth multiplexed holography, J Biomed. Opt. 20 (2015), 111202.

56. A. A. Aarnisalo, I. T. Cheng, M. E. Ravicz, N. Hulli, E. J. Harrington, M. S. Hernandez-Montes, C. Furlong, S. N. Merchant, J. J. Rosowski, Middle ear mechanics of cartilage tympanoplasty evaluated by laser holography and vibrometry, Otol. Neurotol. 30 (2009), 1209–1214.
57. D. Pathania, A. Im, H. Kilcoyne, A. E. Sohani, L. Fexon, M. Pivovarov, J. S. Abramson, T. C. Randall, B. A. Chabner, R. Weissleder, H. Lee, C. M. Castro, Holographic assessment of lymphoma tissue (HALT) for global oncology field applications, Theranostics 6 (2016), 1603–1610.
58. M. Bernhardt, J. D. Nicolas, M. Osterhoff, H. Mittelstädt, M. Reuss, B. Harke, et al., Correlative microscopy approach for biology using X-ray holography, X-ray scanning diffraction and STED microscopy, Nat. Commun. 9 (2018), 3641.
59. S. O. Isikman, W. Bishara, O. Mudanyali, I. Sencan, T. W. Su, D. Tseng, O. Yaglidere, U. Sikora, A. Ozcan, Lensfree on-chip microscopy and tomography for bio-medical applications, IEEE J. Sel. Top Quantum Electron. 18 (2011), 1059–1072.
60. W. T. Lin, C. Y. Lin, V. R. Singh, Y. Luo, Speckle illumination holographic non-scanning fluorescence endoscopy, J. Biophotonics 11 (2018), e201800010.
61. O. A. Sapozhnikov, S. A. Tsysar, V. A. Khokhlova, W. Kreider, Acoustic holography as a metrological tool for characterizing medical ultrasound sources and fields, J. Acoust. Soc. Am. 138 (2015), 1515–1532.
62. M. Guillon, B. C. Forget, A. J. Foust, V. De Sars, N. Ritsch-Marte, V. Emiliani, Vortex-free phase profiles for uniform patterning with computer-generated holography, Opt. Express 25 (2017), 12640–12652.
63. M. Bedrossian, C. Barr, C. A. Lindensmith, K. Nealson, J. L. Nadeau, Quantifying microorganisms at low concentrations using digital holographic microscopy (DHM), J. Vis. Exp. (2017), e56343.
64. G. L. Rodríguez, J. Weber, J. S. Sandhu, M. A. Anastasio, Feasibility study of complex wavefield retrieval in off-axis acoustic holography employing an acousto-optic sensor, Ultrasonics 51 (2011), 847–852.
65. Y. Jo, S. Park, J. Jung, J. Yoon, H. Joo, M. H. Kim, S.-J. Kang, M. C. Choi, S. Y. Lee, Y. K. Park, Holographic deep learning for rapid optical screening of anthrax spores, Sci Adv. 3 (2017), e1700606.
66. M. Krenkel, M. Toepperwien, F. Alves, T. Salditt, Three-dimensional single-cell imaging with X-ray waveguides in the holographic regime, Acta Crystallogr. A Found Adv. 73 (2017), 282–292.
67. H. Bocanegra Evans, S. Gorumlu, B. Aksak, L. Castillo, J. Sheng, Holographic microscopy and microfluidics platform for measuring wall stress and 3D flow over surfaces textured by micro-pillars, Sci. Rep. 6 (2016), 28753.
68. F. Merola, P. Memmolo, L. Miccio, R. Savoia, M. Mugnano, A. Fontana, G. D'Ippolito, A. Sardo, A. Iolascon, A. Gambale, P. Ferraro, Tomographic flow cytometry by digital holography, Light Sci. Appl. 6 (2017), e16241.
69. J. Thomason, MetaHealth-how will the metaverse change health care? J. Metaverse 1 (2021), 13–16.
70. M. Damar, What the literature on medicine, nursing, public health, midwifery, and dentistry reveals: An overview of the rapidly approaching metaverse, J. Metaverse 2 (2022), 62–70.
71. A. Garavand, N. Aslani, Metaverse phenomenon and its impact on health: A scoping review, Inform. Med. Unlocked 32 (2022), 101029.

19 Tracking of Disease—A Review of the State of the Art of Technology for Next Generation Healthcare

Sanjay Ghosh and Vipasha Sharma

19.1 INTRODUCTION

In the rapidly changing landscape of healthcare, tracking disease plays a crucial role in identifying, monitoring, and controlling the spread of various illnesses [1–3]. Accurate and timely tracking of disease helps healthcare providers, public health agencies, and policymakers in efficient decision making, allocation of resources, and implementing intervention strategies [2]. Tracking disease has evolved with advancements in technology, laboratory techniques, and surveillance systems, with organisations like World Health Organization (WHO) coordinating global efforts for diseases like dengue, malaria, smallpox, polio, and measles [4, 5]. In the 21st century, disease tracking has gained significance due to emergence of infectious diseases like dengue, malaria, typhoid, cholera, zika virus, Ebola, and COVID-19. Technological advancements, such as real-time data collection and digital epidemiology, have revolutionised tracking of disease, as observed during the COVID-19 pandemic using contact tracing apps [6]. However, ambiguity is often reported when using the terms "tracking of disease" and "surveillance of disease"; therefore, a comparison between these terms is shown in Table 19.1.

In 2015, United Nations outlined 17 Sustainable Development Goals (SDGs) to end poverty and protect the planet. Tracking disease is critical for global health security and aligns with the Sustainable Development Goals. SDG 3: Good Health and Well-Being highlights the role of tracking of disease in providing real-time information, detecting outbreaks, and guiding response strategies. SDG 9: Industry, Innovation, and Infrastructure promotes investment in innovation and technology for tracking of disease, while SDG 17: Partnerships for the Goals highlights the importance of collaboration in addressing infectious diseases [7]. Effective tracking of disease contributes to achieving specific SDGs and overall development goals by reducing illness burden, preventing deaths, and improving population well-being. It supports evidence-based decision-making, resource allocation, and targeted interventions, improving health outcomes [4, 8].

In healthcare, tracking disease is an important aspect and should not be underestimated. Overall, it serves as a crucial tool for surveillance, enabling the detection and monitoring of disease patterns and trends. By tracking diseases, healthcare professionals may identify shifts in disease prevalence, changes in transmission patterns, and emerging infectious agents [9, 10]. This information allows for implementing proactive measures to prevent and control the spread of diseases. This may include actions such as tracing of contact, quarantine protocols, and targeted vaccination campaigns [6, 11]. Rapid response to outbreaks is crucial for restricting the spread of disease and minimising its impact on individuals and communities. Further, tracking of disease facilitates the generation of accurate epidemiological data, which forms the foundation for evidence-based decision-making in healthcare [12]. By collecting and analysing data on incidence of disease, prevalence, and mortality, researchers and

DOI: 10.1201/9781003451846-19

TABLE 19.1
Comparison of "Tracking of Disease" and "Surveillance of Disease"

Aspect	Tracking of disease	Surveillance of disease
Definition	The process of monitoring and recording the progression of a disease over time, focusing on individual cases and their characteristics.	The systematic and continuous collection of data, its analysis, and interpretation for public health actions.
Scope	Emphasises individual-level data and follows specific cases or outbreaks.	Focuses on population-level data and covers a broader range of health indicators.
Purpose	Provides detailed information about the characteristics and patterns of individual cases or outbreaks.	Aims to detect, monitor, and respond to changes in health status, identify trends, and guide public health interventions.
Focus	Centres on specific diseases or outbreaks of interest.	Includes a wide range of health conditions and events, including infectious and non-infectious diseases.
Data Collection	Involves detailed case investigations and data collection from individual patients and affected areas.	Relies on various data sources, such as healthcare facilities, laboratories, and other health systems, to collect population-level data.
Data Analysis	Analyses individual case data, including symptoms, demographics, associated risk factors, and outcomes.	Analyses aggregated data to identify trends, patterns of spread, and changes in disease occurrence and distribution.
Response	Often used for immediate response to outbreaks or individual cases, guiding targeted interventions.	Used for long-term surveillance and monitoring, guiding prevention, control, and policy planning.
Timeframe	Focuses on the short-term tracking of specific cases or outbreaks.	Emphasises continuous, long-term monitoring and surveillance of diseases.

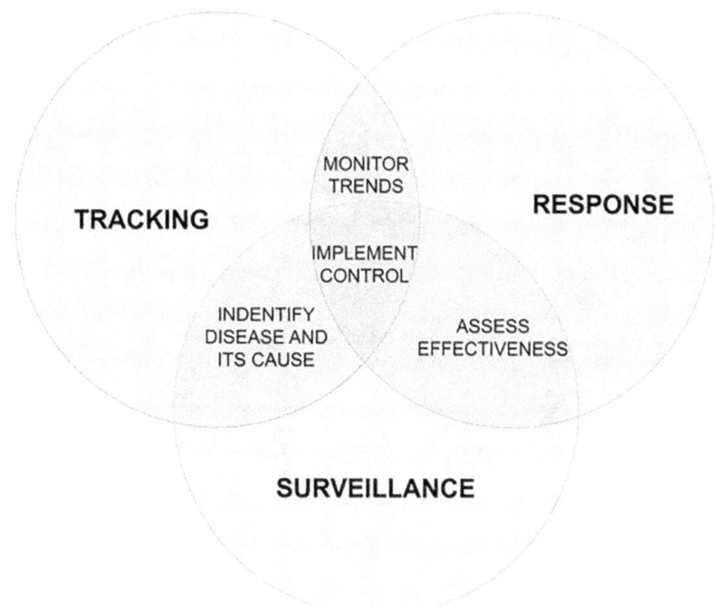

FIGURE 19.1 Principles of disease tracking, surveillance, and response.

policymakers may have better understanding of the pattern of diseases, risk factors, and effectiveness of interventions. This knowledge contributes to developing targeted prevention strategies, improved treatment protocols, and better resource allocation [13]. By understanding disease burden and distribution, healthcare providers and policymakers may allocate resources, such as medical supplies, personnel, and funding, as required. This targeted approach ensures that healthcare systems effectively respond to disease outbreaks and provide timely and appropriate care to affected individuals. Integrating advanced technologies like the Internet of Things (IoT) and deep learning further enhances disease-tracking capabilities, opening new avenues for proactive and personalised healthcare solutions.

19.2 APPROACHES FOR TRACKING OF DISEASE

Traditionally, conventional methods of tracking disease have relied upon monitoring and controlling the spread of infectious diseases [14]. Such practices have evolved over time, along with different infectious disease outbreaks around the world. However, as societies strive to achieve sustainable development goals, there is a growing need to adopt innovative and sustainable approaches to track disease [15]. This section explores conventional and sustainable tracking of disease, highlighting the benefits and implications of each. In addition, this section also discusses the different methods used in tracking infectious disease.

19.2.1 Conventional Tracking of Disease

Conventional or traditional methods of tracking disease refers to the approaches used for surveillance and response to infectious diseases. This approach typically relies on passive surveillance, where healthcare providers and laboratories report cases to public health agencies based on predefined protocols [16, 17]. Conventional tracking of disease often focuses on well-known diseases with established surveillance systems, such as influenza or tuberculosis [18]. The data collection and analysis in conventional tracking systems may be fragmented and lack real-time capabilities, leading to delayed reporting and limited situational awareness [9, 19]. Decision-making in conventional tracking of disease is typically hierarchical, with public health authorities leading in disseminating information and guiding response efforts [12, 16], as shown in Figure 19.2.

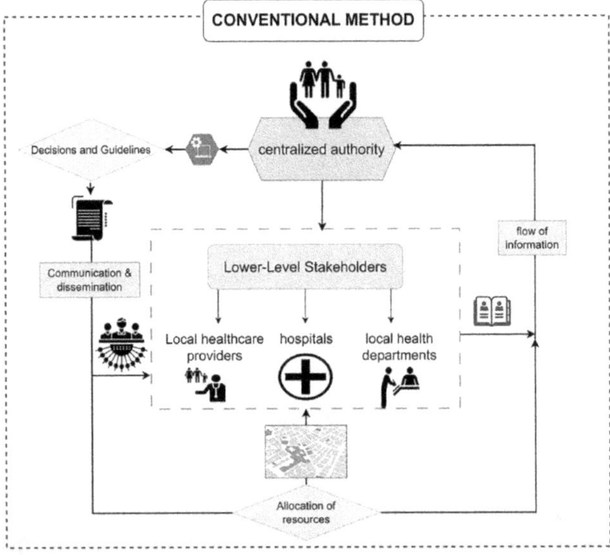

FIGURE 19.2 Sequential steps in the traditional disease tracking process highlight the conventional method's workflow.

The centralised authority, such as national or regional public health agencies, control surveillance of disease, coordination of response, and allocation of resources. The central authority is the hub for receiving, aggregating, and analysing the collected data. They establish guidelines, protocols, and standards for tracking of disease. The lower-level stakeholders, including healthcare providers, local health departments, and laboratories, are the primary sources of disease data and reports. They are crucial in identifying and reporting cases to the central authority. For example, a primary care physician in a local clinic encounters patients with respiratory symptoms and reports suspected cases to the local health department. Further, they follow the guidelines and protocols set by the central authority, collect and report case information, and conduct initial investigations. The local health department collects relevant case information, including demographics, symptoms, and laboratory results, and compiles it into a standardised report. This report is then transmitted vertically to the national public health agency for analysis, validation, and decision-making. These decisions are then communicated back down the hierarchy through the ring structure. The central authority disseminates information, guidance, and directives to lower-level stakeholders, ensuring consistency and coordination in tracking of disease and response efforts. The central authority assesses the resource needs based on the severity of the outbreak and allocates resources accordingly. Allocation of resources includes deploying additional healthcare personnel, providing medical supplies, and allocating funding to support local response activities. The resources are distributed down the hierarchy to assist in managing the outbreak at the local level.

While conventional tracking of disease has effectively monitored and controlled certain diseases, it may face challenges in detecting and reacting to emerging or re-emerging infectious diseases on time [16, 17]. For example, for infectious disease like dengue, malaria, cholera, typhoid, jaundice and COVID-19, many conventional applications are not adequate to monitor an ongoing outbreak and its spread [16, 17, 20]. Also, in case of active outbreak, such surveillance may slow down the response due to slower flow of information [18]. Although the hierarchical approach in conventional tracking of disease provides a transparent chain of command, standardised protocols, and centralised decision-making, it may also face challenges such as delayed information flow, limited local autonomy, and potential bottlenecks in decision-making. Conventional systems often suffer from limited data integration, with information stored across different agencies and organisations [16]. Such an approach may hinder the timely sharing of critical data and stakeholder collaboration. These limitations have led to exploring alternative methods, such as sustainable tracking of disease, emphasising more decentralised, community-driven, and flexible strategies.

19.2.2 Sustainable Tracking of Disease

As the world continuously faces never-ending health challenges, adopting sustainable disease-tracking practices becomes vital for a resilient and healthier future. Sustainable tracking of disease signifies a shift towards more advanced and holistic approaches to surveillance of disease. While conventional disease-tracking methods have been the foundation of public health surveillance for decades, sustainable disease tracking offers a more comprehensive and progressive approach. Sustainable tracking of disease represents a modern and comprehensive approach to surveillance and response, leveraging advanced technologies and community engagement to enhance effectiveness and timeliness [21–23].

This approach emphasises active and real-time surveillance methods, such as syndromic, digital, and participatory surveillance, enabling proactive monitoring and early detection of disease outbreaks. Sustainable tracking of disease also integrates data from multiple sources, including clinical records, laboratory data, environmental monitoring, and social media platforms, enabling comprehensive analysis and forecasting of disease trends [22, 24, 25]. Furthermore, the establishment of sustainable disease tracking methods actively engages communities and individuals through initiatives in public health, mobile health applications, and community-led reporting. This empowers them to contribute valuable data and participate in early warning systems [26, 27]. By embracing innovation and technology, sustainable disease-tracking methods have the capability to revolutionise the health surveillance and response to known and emerging infectious diseases.

The process of sustainable tracking of disease highlights the importance of engaging communities, leveraging technology, promoting interdisciplinary collaboration, and empowering local stakeholders to achieve effective and sustainable tracking of disease outcomes, as shown in Figure 19.3. The method of sustainable tracking of disease is an ongoing and iterative one. It requires continuous monitoring, learning, and adaptation to emerging infectious diseases, changing environmental factors, technological advancements, and community needs. Active engagement with communities and stakeholders is established to ensure their involvement, collaboration, and ownership in disease-tracking efforts. Active engagement involves conducting community consultations, building relationships, and involving community members in data collection and decision-making processes. Innovative technologies and tools are utilised to enhance disease-tracking capabilities. This includes the use of digital surveillance systems, real-time data collection methods, mobile health applications, and advanced analytics for data processing and analysis. Collaboration among various disciplines, such as healthcare professionals, epidemiologists, environmental scientists, social scientists, policymakers, and other stakeholders, is facilitated.

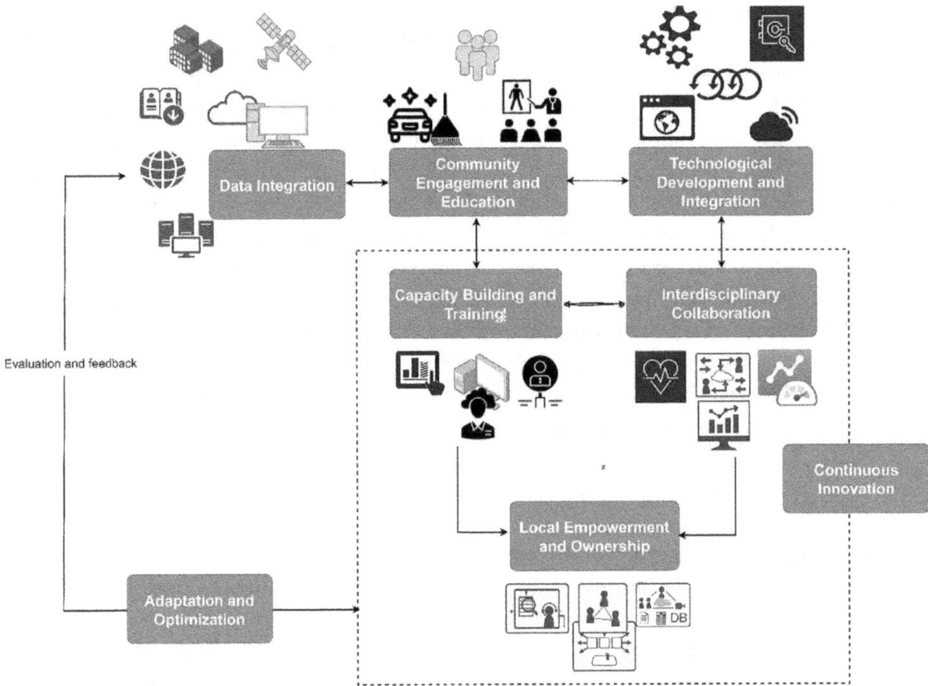

FIGURE 19.3 A sustainable framework for disease tracking, highlighting community engagement, and continuous engagement.

This interdisciplinary approach ensures a holistic understanding of disease dynamics and facilitates comprehensive response strategies. Local communities, healthcare providers, and public health agencies are empowered and provided with resources, training, and decision-making authority. Ongoing research and adoption of innovative approaches, methods and technologies are encouraged to enhance the effectiveness and efficiency of disease-tracking efforts. The disease-tracking process is regularly evaluated to assess its efficacy and gather feedback from stakeholders and communities. This evaluation helps identify areas for improvement, address challenges, and guide future enhancements. Based on the assessment and feedback received, necessary adjustments, optimisations, and refinements are made to improve the overall efficiency and impact of sustainable disease-tracking efforts. This involves adapting to emerging challenges, incorporating lessons learned, and optimising processes and technologies to meet the needs of the communities.

Table 19.2 highlights the key differences between approaches of conventional and sustainable tracking of disease in terms of surveillance, data collection, decision-making, community involvement, technology adoption, data integration, timeliness, and flexibility. Sustainable tracking of disease emphasises real-time surveillance, comprehensive data integration, collaborative decision-making, community engagement, and innovative technologies to enhance disease monitoring and response capabilities [15].

TABLE 19.2
Comparison of Conventional and Sustainable Tracking of Disease Approaches

Parameter	Conventional Tracking of Disease	Sustainable Tracking of Disease
Surveillance Approach	Passive surveillance	Active surveillance
Data Collection	Fragmented and delayed	Comprehensive and real time
Focus	Well-known diseases with established surveillance	Known and emerging diseases
Decision-Making	Hierarchical	Collaborative and community driven
Technology	Relies on traditional methods	Embraces innovation and advanced technologies
Community Involvement	Limited community involvement	Actively involves communities and citizen participation
Data Integration	Limited integration of data sources	Integrates data from multiple sources for comprehensive analysis
Timeliness	May experience delays in reporting and response	Enables proactive monitoring and early detection
Flexibility	Less adaptable to emerging or re-emerging diseases	Flexible and adaptable to changing disease landscapes

19.2.3 Methods of Tracking of Disease

Methods of tracking disease encompasses various strategies and techniques used to detect, monitor, and control the spread of infectious diseases. According to WHO, such methods may be classified as (Figure 19.4) [19]:

1. surveillance,
2. laboratory testing, and
3. digital methods

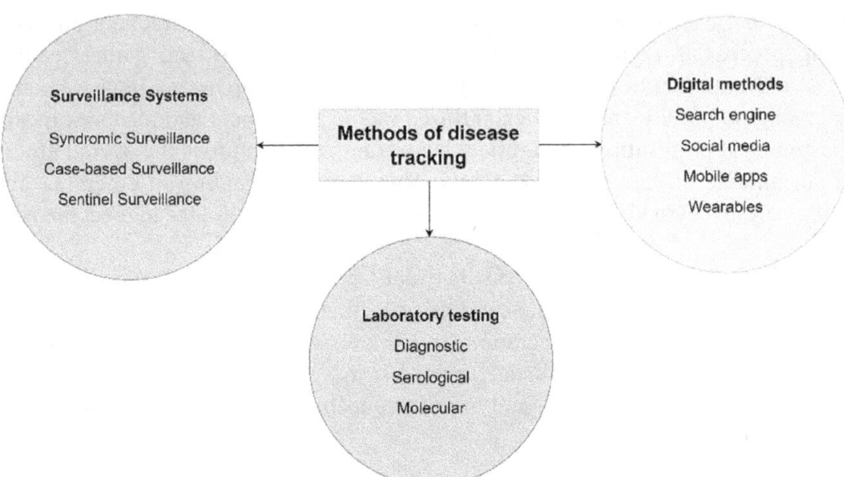

FIGURE 19.4 An overview of different methods utilised for effective disease tracking.

19.2.3.1 Surveillance Systems

It involves systematic collection, analysis, and interpretation of data related to health to monitor and track the occurrence and spread of diseases [21]. These may help to identify disease trends, detect outbreaks, and inform public health interventions. The surveillance systems are further classified as syndromic, case-based, and sentinel surveillance. The syndromic surveillance method involves monitoring and analysing non-specific symptoms or syndromes, such as fever or respiratory distress, to detect potential outbreaks or changes in disease patterns [22]. On the other hand, case-based surveillance focuses on tracking individual cases of specific diseases. It involves reporting and monitoring diagnosed cases through healthcare providers, laboratories, or other reporting mechanisms [18]. Sentinel surveillance involves monitoring a selected network of healthcare providers or institutions to gather data on specific diseases or conditions [23]. These sentinel sites provide representative data on disease occurrence and trends.

19.2.3.2 Laboratory Testing

It is a critical component of tracking of disease, involving the analysis of clinical specimens to detect the presence of infectious agents [24]. It confirms clinical diagnoses, identifies the causative agents of outbreaks, and tracks the spread of disease. Advances in laboratory testing technologies, such as rapid diagnostic tests, involve the analysis of biological samples to detect the presence of pathogens or specific markers [15, 25]. Diagnostic testing aims to identify the specific pathogen causing disease in an individual. It involves techniques like polymerase chain reaction (PCR), culture, or antigen tests. Serological testing examines the presence of antibodies in blood samples to determine if an individual has been exposed to a particular disease or has developed immunity. Molecular testing involves using advanced techniques, such as DNA sequencing or genotyping, to characterise the genetic makeup of pathogens and track their evolution and transmission patterns.

19.2.3.3 Digital Methods

In addition to these traditional methods, advancements in technology have led to the development of digital disease-tracking tools. These tools, including online symptom checkers, social media monitoring, and mobile health apps, enable real-time data collection and analysis [6, 26]. Digital methods leverage technology and digital platforms to gather data and insights for tracking of disease. They offer real-time information and may complement traditional surveillance systems. Search engines, like Google, may provide access to vast information. Analysis of search queries related to diseases may offer insights into public concerns, disease spread, and emerging health threats. Social media interfaces, such as Twitter, Facebook, and LinkedIn, provide near–real-time data on public discussions, behaviours, and sentiments related to diseases [14, 27]. Monitoring social media may help identify outbreaks, track disease trends, and detect misinformation. Mobile applications, or apps, may enable individuals to report symptoms, access health information, or participate in contact tracing. Mobile apps may enhance tracking of disease by providing data on disease symptoms, geographical locations, and behavioural patterns.

These methods of tracking of disease work together, providing a comprehensive and multidimensional approach to monitoring and understanding the occurrence, spread, and impact of diseases [18, 19, 28, 29]. Each technique brings unique advantages and contributes to the overall surveillance and response efforts in public health. Wearable technology, mobile health (mHealth) apps, and the One Health approach that considers human, animal, and environmental health will also improve disease-tracking efforts [26, 30]. The broad applications of digital technologies in tracking of disease are summarised in Figure 19.5.

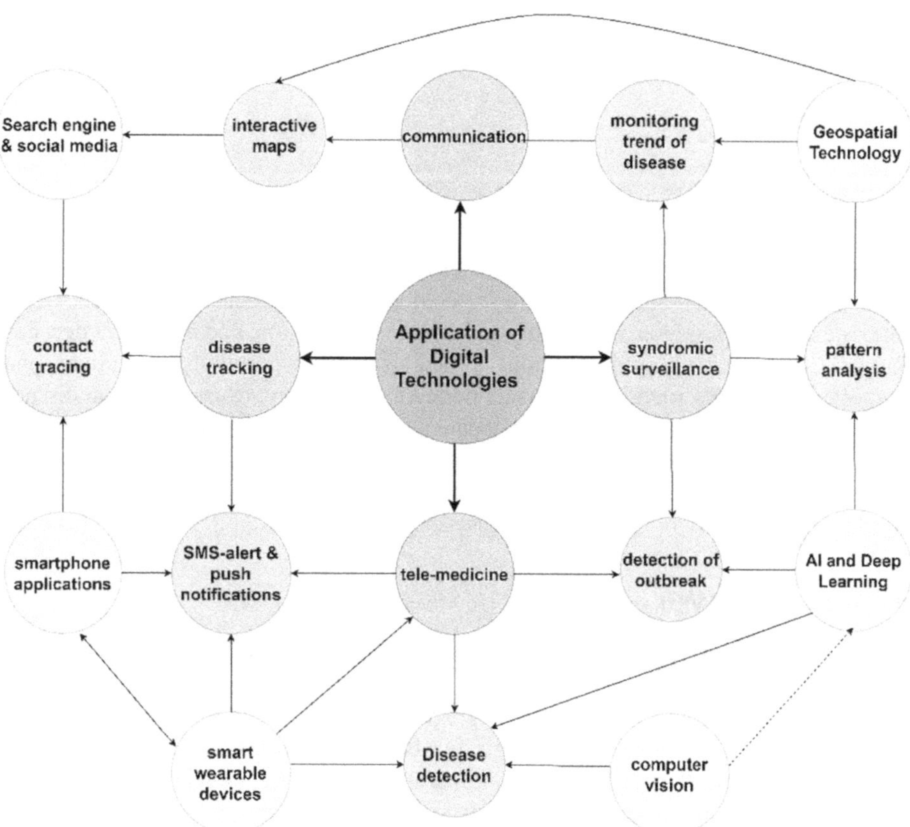

FIGURE 19.5 Comprehensive diagram highlighting the extensive applications of digital technologies in the tracking of disease.

19.3 ROLE OF THE IoT IN TRACKING OF DISEASE

The Internet of Things (IoT) is based on the interconnection of physical devices and sensors via internet to collect and exchange data. This extends the capabilities of traditional computing devices by incorporating everyday objects into a networked ecosystem [31]. The IoT-enabled healthcare system consists of multiple layers. The sensing layer incorporates various sensors, including wearable sensors like ECG, smart wearables, and RFID for identification. The network layer facilitates secure data transmission using communication protocols such as ZigBee, NB-IOT, and LoRa. The data processing layer employs learning-based approaches to extract valuable knowledge from sensor data. Finally, intelligent services and applications like diagnosis of disease, recognition of behaviour, and smart assistance are delivered based on the insights derived from the preceding layers (Figure 19.6).

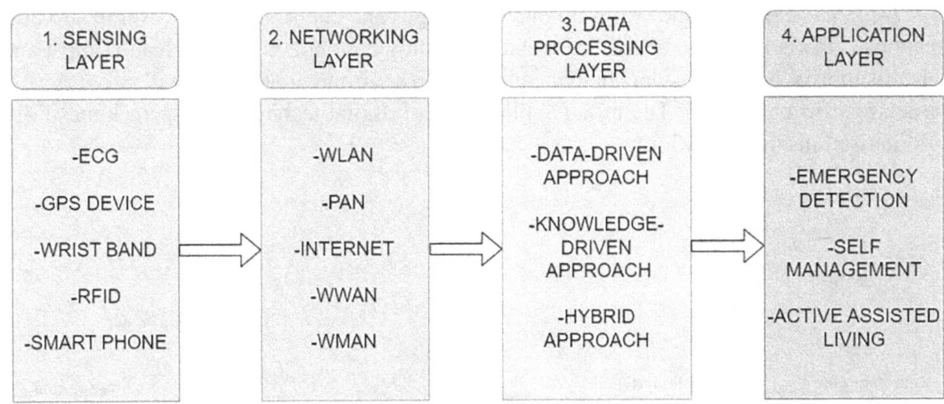

FIGURE 19.6 A framework of integrating IoT technologies for personalised healthcare [32].

The core concept of the IoT is to enhance efficiency, convenience, and productivity by enabling seamless connectivity and communication between objects and systems. This connectivity enables real-time data collection, remote monitoring and control, automation, and intelligent decision-making. The IoT has wide-ranging applications in healthcare, transportation, agriculture, and other domains, offering benefits such as improved operational efficiency, resource utilisation, and decision-making. The IoT has revolutionised healthcare by transforming tracking of disease and surveillance [17, 32, 33]. By interconnecting devices and sensors, the IoT enables continuous monitoring of various health parameters, providing valuable real-time data for tracking of disease. This section explores the role of the IoT in tracking of disease and highlights its applications and benefits.

19.3.1 IoT-Enabled Wearable Devices for Health Monitoring

The IoT plays a important role in tracking of disease by efficient collection and analysis of large volumes of health data [34]. IoT devices seamlessly capture and transmit data to centralised databases or cloud platforms, enabling real-time data aggregation and analysis. This data may include vital signs, symptoms, medication adherence, and lifestyle behaviours. Integrating IoT-generated data with advanced analytics approaches, such as machine learning and deep learning, enhances disease-tracking capabilities. By leveraging these techniques, healthcare providers may extract valuable insights from the collected data, including disease trends, risk factors, and early warning signs. This knowledge may inform preventive strategies, support accurate diagnosis, and improve disease management.

One of the significant contributions of the IoT towards tracking of disease is the development of wearable devices that collect and transmit health data [35]. They have the capability to continuously track vital signs, symptoms, and other health parameters of individuals. This allows healthcare professionals to remotely monitor patients even in non-clinical settings to detect any abnormal changes and identify potential signs of disease onset or progression [29]. This remote monitoring capability is vital in managing infectious diseases, such as COVID-19, dengue, or jaundice, where regular monitoring is essential [31, 33]. These devices provide relevant health indicators, provide health-care professionals insights into the health status of patients, detect early warning signs, and track disease progression. Further, wearable devices may facilitate early detection of infectious diseases and assist in contact tracing efforts [36]. IoT-based products, such as Bluetooth-enabled devices or smartphone applications, aid in contact tracing efforts during infectious disease outbreaks [36, 37]. These devices have the capability to detect and record interactions between individuals and provide alerts if they have been in close proximity to someone infected with a particular disease. Additionally, wearable devices track movements of individuals and interactions, aiding in contact tracing and identifying potential disease transmission pathways. This provides an advantage, as it aids active outbreak management, which significantly reduces action time as compared to those provided by retrospective studies.

19.3.2 IoT in Environmental Monitoring for Prediction of Disease Outbreak

IoT technologies also play a crucial role in environmental monitoring for disease outbreak prediction. By deploying IoT sensors in environmental settings, such as water sources, air quality monitoring stations, and vector surveillance systems, healthcare professionals may collect real-time data on environmental factors that influence disease transmission [34, 38].

IoT devices enable the collection of large volumes of real-time data, which may be analysed using advanced analytics techniques. IoT facilitates data-driven disease surveillance by integrating data from multiple sources, such as wearable devices, health records, social media, remote sensing, routine investigation data being saved in the cloud, and environmental sensors. Patterns and trends in the data identify disease hotspots, track disease spread, and predict future outbreaks. IoT sensors may be deployed to monitor environmental factors contributing to the spread of diseases, such as air quality, humidity, temperature, or the presence of specific pathogens. Real-time data from these sensors helps identify high-risk areas or detect early warning signs of disease outbreaks.

For example, IoT sensors monitor water quality in areas prone to waterborne diseases, providing early warnings of potential outbreaks. Figure 19.7 represents a cloud-based system that utilises sensors to monitor and control water contamination. The IoT devices are equipped with AI and machine learning capabilities, enabling them to detect and determine the level of contamination in the water body. This operation requires collection of data from various sensors, such as an aqua sensor, which is then transferred to the cloud for analysis using IoT-based techniques. Through this analysis, the system performs quality checks on the water to identify any contamination. Thus, the integration of IoT devices, sensors, and cloud-based analysis provides an efficient and intelligent approach for monitoring and controlling water quality [39]. Similarly, air quality monitoring stations equipped with IoT sensors may detect pollutants or pathogens in the air, helping identify regions at risk of respiratory diseases or airborne infections [40]. Integrating this environmental data with surveillance of disease systems allows healthcare providers to predict and prevent disease outbreaks more effectively.

Remote sensing technologies, using satellite imagery and aerial photography, may help identify environmental factors such as land use; vegetation cover; urban/rural areas; and hydro-meteorological parameters like temperature, precipitation, humidity, and wind speed contributing to disease transmission [4]. For example, remote sensing data may reveal patterns of water stagnation, vegetation density, or urban development associated with mosquito-borne diseases like malaria or dengue fever. By analysing these spatial variables, healthcare professionals may effectively target vector control efforts and implement preventive measures. GPS technology allows for precise location tracking, invaluable in surveillance of disease and contact tracing [3, 6]. By tracking the movements and interactions of people, healthcare providers may identify potential disease transmission pathways and promptly notify individuals who may have been exposed to infectious diseases. GPS data may also help monitor compliance with quarantine protocols and assess the effectiveness of social distancing measures.

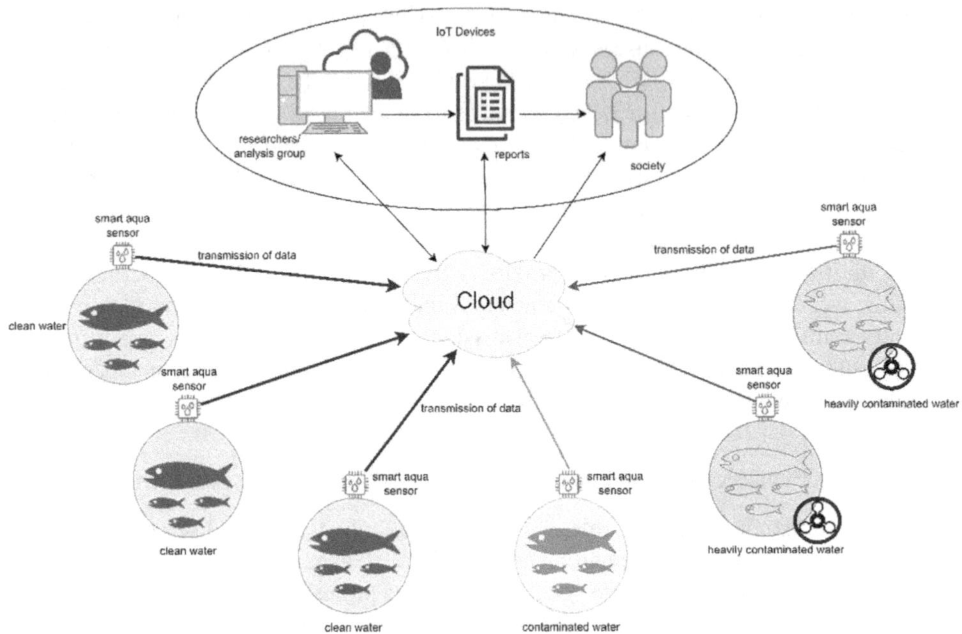

FIGURE 19.7 Use of cloud technology to connect IoT devices and sensors for real-time monitoring of water bodies.

19.3.3 IoT-Based Predictive Analysis for Tracking of Disease

Additionally, IoT-based data collection and analysis enable the implementation of predictive analytics models in tracking of disease [32, 36]. By combining historical and real-time IoT-generated data, predictive models may forecast disease trends, identify high-risk populations, and guide resource allocation. This proactive approach allows healthcare systems to allocate resources efficiently, implement preventive interventions, and improve public health outcomes. GIS plays a vital role in tracking of disease by integrating spatial data and providing valuable insights into disease patterns, transmission dynamics, and risk factors [28, 41–43]. It contributes to the understanding and visualisation of spread of disease, aids in early detection and response, supports resource allocation and planning, and facilitates targeted interventions. These technologies enable integrating location-specific data such as GPS with disease surveillance systems, providing valuable spatial insights into disease patterns, transmission pathways, and high-risk areas. GIS combines spatial data with various layers of information, such as demographic data, health facility locations, and disease incidence rates, to create detailed disease mapping and visualisation tools. These tools enable healthcare professionals to identify disease hotspots, assess the impact of socioeconomic factors on disease prevalence, and plan targeted interventions [43, 44]. GIS-based disease mapping enhances situational awareness, supports resource allocation decisions, and enables effective communication with stakeholders. It plays a vital role in tracking disease by enabling spatial analysis and visualisation of disease patterns. GIS technology allows for mapping and geospatial analysis of disease cases, identifying high-risk areas, and guiding targeted interventions and resource allocation.

By combining IoT data with advanced algorithms, predictive analytics may be applied to forecast disease outbreaks, identify populations at risk, and optimise resource allocation for prevention and control measures. This approach allows for timely interventions and more efficient disease tracking. This may be further used to create real-time alerts and notifications to individuals, healthcare providers, or public health authorities when certain disease-related conditions or thresholds are met. This helps in rapid response and timely intervention, minimising the spread of diseases.

In summary, the IoT complements the tracking of disease by providing spatial context to disease data. These technologies enable the integration of location-specific information, aiding in identifying disease patterns, transmission pathways, and high-risk areas. By leveraging geospatial data, healthcare professionals may develop targeted interventions, improve resource allocation, and enhance surveillance of disease and control efforts. The utilisation of IoT for disease detection and tracking offers several advantages, including early detection, near–real-time surveillance, data-driven decision-making, and improved resource allocation. However, the challenges related to data privacy, security, standardisation, and scalability need to be addressed to ensure the widespread adoption of IoT-based disease tracking solutions.

19.4 DEEP LEARNING TECHNIQUES FOR TRACKING OF DISEASE

Deep learning has emerged as a dominant tool in the tracking of disease and surveillance for analysing complex medical data, enabling accurate classification, early detection, and prediction of diseases [45]. Deep learning techniques have revolutionised the tracking of disease and surveillance by leveraging complex neural networks to analyse large volumes of medical data and extract valuable insights. Deep learning algorithms have shown remarkable capabilities in disease classification. By training on huge datasets of medical imagery like X-rays, CT scans, or pathology slides, deep learning models may learn intricate patterns and features associated with specific diseases [46, 47]. These models may then accurately classify images and aid in identifying various conditions, including cancers, cardiovascular diseases, and infectious diseases.

This section explores the application of deep learning algorithms in the tracking and detection of disease, highlighting their effectiveness in various healthcare applications. By leveraging deep neural networks, these algorithms may uncover intricate patterns and relationships within data, improving disease-tracking capabilities and more informed decision-making in healthcare [48–50].

19.4.1 Deep Learning Algorithms Used in Tracking of Disease

This section explores the specific deep learning algorithms employed in tracking of disease and detection tasks. Further, their unique characteristics, architectures, and applications in different areas of healthcare are discussed. By understanding the capabilities and limitations of these algorithms, insights regarding their contribution towards advancing tracking of disease and detection, ultimately leading to improved patient outcomes and public health, may be explored. Several deep learning algorithms have proven effective in tracking of disease and detection and classification tasks. The key deep learning algorithms used in healthcare applications are as follows.

19.4.1.1 Convolutional Neural Networks

CNNs are particularly effective in image-based learning tasks due to their automatic mechanism of feature extraction. A CNN operates by passing the input image through multiple layers, containing convolutional layers, activation functions, and pooling layers (Figure 19.8). In the convolution layer, the image is filtered by observing a specific area, either 3 × 3 pixels or 5 × 5 pixels in size [51]. The observed area of the image is subjected to a dot product operation with predefined weights in the layer, which is known as convolution. The results of the dot product are then summed, resulting in a single number that represents the observed image area. The convolutional layer produces a smaller matrix compared to the original image. This output is then passed through the activation layer, which introduces non-linearity to the input received from the convolutional layer. The inclusion of non-linearity enables the network to learn and train effectively using the backpropagation algorithm.

In the pooling layer, the matrix obtained from the activation layer is further reduced in size by applying a pooling operation, such as max pooling or min pooling. This operation selects the maximum or minimum value from each group of values, respectively. By reducing the size of the matrix, the pooling layer helps to speed up the training process by reducing the computational complexity and retaining the most relevant information for subsequent layers.

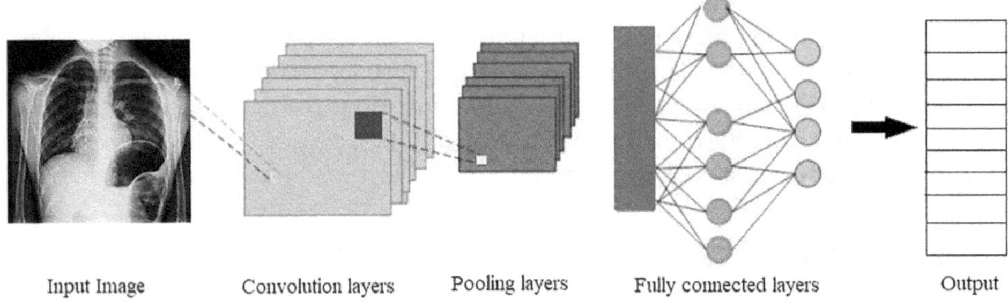

FIGURE 19.8 Diagram outlining the architecture of a convolutional neural network (CNN) for image processing in healthcare.

These layers work together to extract meaningful features from the image while reducing its spatial dimensions. The learned features are then moved through fully connected layers, which perform classification or regression tasks. The network is trained using labelled data, adjusting the biases and weights to minimise the difference between predicted outputs and ground truth labels. Such a process allows the CNN to learn recognising and differentiating various patterns and features in the input images, enabling it to make predictions on unseen data. Overall, the hierarchical and data-driven architecture of CNNs enables them to automatically extract relevant information from images and make predictions.

CNNs are thus well suited for processing visual data, making them valuable for tracking infectious diseases through medical image analysis or spatial data processing [52, 53]. CNNs are widely employed in disease tracking and detection tasks, particularly in medical imaging analysis [16, 37, 52]. These studies highlight the diverse applications of CNNs in medical domains, ranging from electroencephalography (EEG) analysis and radiology to endoscopic ultrasound (EUS) imaging, diagnosis of disease, and analysis of structured medical records and speech data [16, 53, 54]. CNNs are capable of learning intricate features and patterns from images, enabling classification and detection of diseases. They have been successfully used for tasks such as detecting tumours in medical scans, identifying abnormalities in radiology images, and classifying skin lesions. CNN-based models like CheXNet have outperformed human experts in classifying chest ailments [52]. Furthermore, CNNs have demonstrated their dominance in the detection of COVID-19 using chest X-rays/CT scans [54, 55].

19.4.1.2 Recurrent Neural Networks

RNNs are mainly used in speech processing and NLP environments [56]. RNNs have a cyclic connection in the hidden layer, enabling them to process sequential data. The hidden units in the RNN perform cyclic calculations to process input data in sequence [51]. Each hidden unit stores a state vector that holds information from previous inputs (Figure 19.9). These state vectors are used to compute the output. RNNs calculate new outputs by considering both the current input and the previous inputs. This allows them to capture dependencies and patterns in sequential data. However, RNNs face challenges during backpropagation, specifically with gradient calculation. By multiplication of many partial derivatives, gradients can become very small (vanishing gradient) or very large (exploding gradient), making it difficult for RNNs to learn long-distance dependencies. To address this problem, long short-term memory (LSTM) networks were introduced.

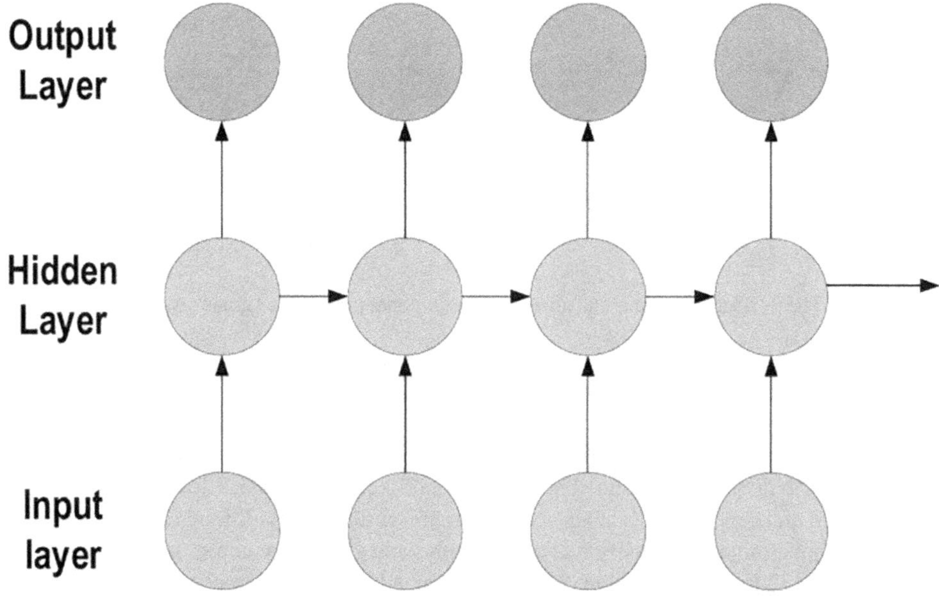

FIGURE 19.9 A typical structure of a recurrent neural network (RNN) for sequential data processing.

LSTM networks utilise a gating mechanism and incorporate three main gates, the input gate, forget gate, and output gate. The input gate controls the amount of information or input to be integrated into the cell state. It controls the flow of information into the current cell. The forget gate controls the information from the previous time step that should be forgotten or discarded. It helps the model selectively retain or discard relevant information. The output gate determines the information that to be output. It thus controls the flow of information in the system. By using these gates, LSTM networks can store and retain information over long sequences, allowing them to capture long-term dependencies and solve the gradient vanishing problem. A gated recurrent unit (GRU) is a simplified form of LSTM that aims to reduce the complexity of the gating mechanism.

A GRU replaces the three gates of LSTM with two gates, the update gate and the reset gate. The update gate in a GRU combines the roles of the forget gate and input gate in LSTM. It determines the importance or weight given to the past and present information. The reset gate controls the effect of the previous hidden layer state (representing past information) on the current word or input. It helps decide which parts of the past information should be used in the current computation. A GRU simplifies the structure of LSTM and reduces the number of matrix operations involved, resulting in faster computation. Despite the simplifications, a GRU still retains the ability to identify long-term dependencies and perform well in tasks involving sequential data, especially when there is a large amount of training data. RNNs are beneficial in tracking of disease and detection scenarios where sequential data plays a vital role [57]. They excel at capturing temporal dependencies and are well suited for analysing time-series data. RNNs may be applied to modelling of disease progression, monitoring vital signs of patients, and predicting disease outbreaks [58, 59].

19.4.1.3 Generative Adversarial Network

GANs assist in tracking of infectious disease by generating synthetic data that aids in training models, simulation of disease spread, or generating realistic patient data [60]. GANs have demonstrated potential in tracking of disease and detection tasks, particularly in generating synthetic data to augment limited datasets. They consist of a generator network which generates realistic data samples and a discriminator network that differentiates real and synthetic samples (Figure 19.10) [60, 61].

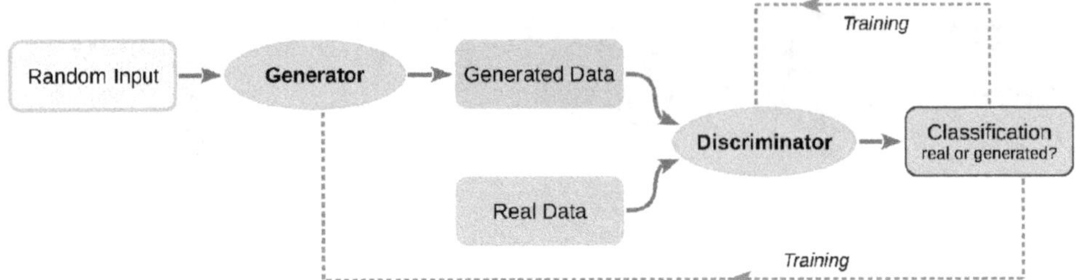

FIGURE 19.10 The intricate structure and adversarial components within a Generative Adversarial Network architecture [59].

The generator network takes random noise as an input to generate synthetic data samples. It consists of multiple layers, such as convolutional layers, to transform the random noise into meaningful data representations that are indistinguishable from real data samples. The discriminator network acts as a binary classifier which distinguishes between real and generated data. It takes input data (either real or generated) and generates a probability score representing the likelihood of the input to be real. The discriminator is trained to classify real data samples and generated data samples as real and fake, respectively. The training process of a GAN involves an adversarial interaction of the generator and the discriminator. This process continues until an equilibrium is reached, that is, when the generator produces indistinguishable data from real data, which cannot be differentiated by the discriminator.

19.4.1.4 Deep Belief Networks

DBNs have been widely used in various applications in healthcare. Like deep learning models, a DBN consists of multiple layers of interconnected units or nodes, similar to other deep neural network architectures [62]. DBN are composed of stacked restricted Boltzmann machines (RBMs) or their variants, such as deep Boltzmann machines (DBMs) (Figure 19.11). RBMs are generative stochastic neural networks that learn to represent the underlying dissemination of the input data. The structure of a DBN typically includes input layer, multiple hidden layers, and an output layer. Each layer is trained in unsupervised manner, one layer at a time, using a contrastive divergence algorithm or other training methods specific to RBMs. This unsupervised pre-training allows each layer to progressively learn complex representations of the input data. Once the RBMs are pre-trained, the DBN may be fine-tuned using supervised learning methods such as backpropagation or gradient descent. During fine-tuning, the whole network is trained to optimise the weights and biases for a specific task, such as classification or regression.

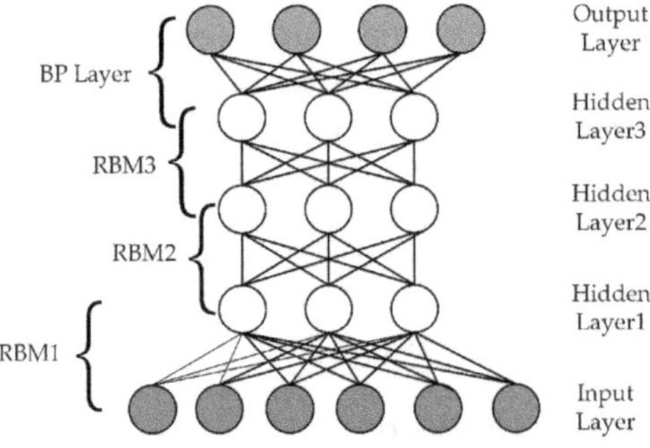

FIGURE 19.11 A graphical depiction of the basic building blocks and connections in the structure of a Deep Belief Network [60].

19.4.1.5 Capsule Networks

Capsule networks aim to overcome some limitations of CNNs, particularly in handling spatial hierarchies and viewpoint invariance [53, 63]. The architecture of a capsule network (CapsNet) includes multiple layers of capsules, which are the fundamental building blocks of the network (Figure 19.12). Each capsule represents a vector denoting the probability of entity existence and orientation, capturing its various characteristics such as position, size, texture, velocity, and albedo. A CapsNet uses a squashing function at the capsule level, which restricts the capsule length under 1 and enables easy classification of different capsules. The hierarchical arrangement of capsules is similar to the layers in a basic neural network. Lower-level capsules have a larger number and smaller dimensionality, representing smaller input areas and capturing spatial relationships effectively, and vice-versa. As the network moves from lower-level to higher-level capsules, the dimensionality increases. The conversion of lower-level to higher-level capsules is facilitated by dynamic routing, where higher-level capsules are denoted as a weighted summation of lower-level capsules. This routing-by-agreement method helps strengthen the support of capsules that align most with the parent output, enhancing the learning process. In summary, the overall architecture of a CapsNet typically consists of a convolution layer followed by a layer of primary capsules, which are the resized output of the convolutional layer. The connection between capsules in different layers allows information flow and aggregation across the network. It's important to note that a CapsNet differs from conventional CNN architectures by replacing max-pooling layers with convolutional layers with larger strides for dimension reduction and by using the routing-by-agreement mechanism for dynamic routing between capsules [54]. They have shown promise in tracking of disease and detection tasks, such as classifying lung nodules in CT scans and detecting diabetic retinopathy in retinal images [54, 63, 64]. Capsule networks are designed to capture hierarchical relationships between image components and may provide more robust and interpretable representations.

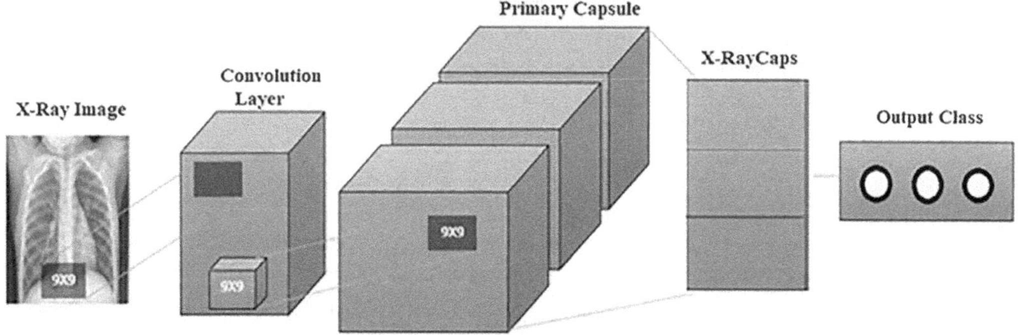

FIGURE 19.12 An example of the architecture of the capsule network used for detection of COVID-19 [64].

These deep learning algorithms have significantly advanced tracking of disease and detection capabilities. The applications, along with advantages and disadvantages, are summarised in Table 19.3. They have facilitated accurate disease classification, early detection of abnormalities, and improved prediction accuracy. By leveraging the power of these algorithms, healthcare professionals may enhance their tracking of disease and detection efforts, leading to more effective interventions, personalised treatment strategies, and improved patient outcomes.

TABLE 19.3
Comparison of Deep Learning Algorithms for Tracking of Disease

Algorithm	Applications	Advantages	Disadvantages	Algorithms Used
CNN (convolutional neural network)	Image-based disease diagnosis, medical image analysis, pathology detection.	• Effective in capturing local features and spatial relationships in images. • Can handle large datasets. • Robust to variations in image scale, rotation, and translation.	• Limited ability for capturing long-range dependencies in sequential data. • Computationally expensive for large models. • Requires large amount of labelled training data.	CheXNet, ResNet, DenseNet
RNN (recurrent neural network)	Time series analysis, disease progression modelling, outbreak prediction.	• Ability to model temporal dependencies and capture long-range dependencies in sequential data. • Can handle variable-length input sequences. • Efficient for online learning.	• Prone to vanishing/exploding gradients. • Limited memory for capturing very long-term dependencies. • Difficulty in parallelising computations.	LSTM, GRU, EpidemicRNN
GAN (generative adversarial network)	Synthetic data generation for disease simulation, data augmentation, anomaly detection.	• Ability to generate realistic synthetic data. • Can learn complex data distributions. • Useful for data augmentation and anomaly detection tasks.	• Training instability and mode collapse. • Difficulty in evaluating the quality of created samples. • Sensitive to hyper-parameter settings.	MedGAN, DCGAN, InfoGAN
DBN (deep belief networks)	Disease diagnosis, risk prediction, gene expression analysis.	• Ability to learn complex hierarchical representations of data. • Unsupervised feature learning. • Ability to handle high-dimensional data. • Robust to missing data.	• Computationally expensive training process. • Requires large amounts of training data. • Sensitive to hyper-parameter settings.	Deep belief networks
Capsule networks	Disease classification, medical image segmentation, anomaly detection in medical images.	• Ability to model hierarchical relationships between features. • Robust to small variations in object pose and viewpoint. • Efficient in parameter usage.	• Limited interpretability of capsule networks. • Require large amounts of training data. • Computationally expensive for large-scale models.	CapsNet, MedCaps

19.4.2 Applications of Deep Learning in Tracking of Disease

This section explores the broad applications of deep learning algorithms discussed in Section 19.4.1. The applications are broadly classified into classification, diagnosis of disease, and predictive analytics.

19.4.2.1 Deep Learning Models for Disease Classification

Deep learning algorithms have shown remarkable capabilities in classification of disease. By training on huge datasets consisting of medical images, like as X-rays, CT scans, or pathology slides, deep learning models may learn intricate patterns and features associated with specific diseases [53, 54]. These models may then accurately classify images and aid in identifying various conditions, including cancers, cardiovascular diseases, and infectious diseases. For example, CNNs have shown promising results in detecting various types of cancer, heart ailments, infections like COVID-19, and asthma [52, 54]. These models may assist radiologists in identifying disease markers and anomalies, enabling early detection and timely intervention. Deep learning algorithms process and analyse large volumes of electronic health records, extracting valuable insights for disease tracking. By analysing structured and unstructured data from electronic health records (EHRs), such as patient demographics, medical histories, laboratory results, and clinical notes, deep learning models may identify disease patterns, predict disease progression, and assess treatment outcomes.

This information may help healthcare administrators to make the required decisions and improve patient care. These techniques may be applied to genomic data analysis, contributing to personalised medicine and disease tracking. By examining DNA sequences, gene expression patterns, and genetic variations, deep learning models may identify disease-related genetic markers, predict disease risks, and enable precision medicine approaches. These models may thus, aid in the understanding of complex genetic interactions and facilitate targeted interventions. The use of deep learning in disease classification offers several advantages. It may help reduce diagnostic errors and variability, as the algorithms may consistently analyse medical images with high precision [53]. Moreover, deep learning models have capability to handle complex and diverse data, allowing for detecting subtle abnormalities or early-stage diseases that may be challenging for human interpretation [55]. By improving diagnostic accuracy and efficiency, deep learning contributes to timely treatment and improved patient outcomes.

19.4.2.2 Deep Learning Models for Diagnosis of Disease

Deep learning techniques also play a major role in predictive analytics for tracking of disease. Deep learning models may identify patterns and risk factors associated with disease development by analysing large datasets containing medical records, genetic profiles, lifestyle data, and environmental factors [54]. These models may then predict the likelihood of an individual developing a particular disease or estimate disease progression. Early disease detection is crucial to tracking of disease, enabling proactive interventions and timely treatment.

Deep learning models have shown great potential in disease diagnosis by analysing medical images. These models may learn intricate patterns and features associated with specific diseases, enabling accurate classification and identification. Deep learning models, like CNN, RNN, and GAN, have shown remarkable effectiveness in identification of disease from medical imaging data. These models are used to extract meaningful features and patterns from complex and high-dimensional medical images, enabling accurate disease diagnosis and classification.

CNNs are particularly well suited for image-based tasks and have achieved remarkable success in medical imaging analysis. Such models are designed to learn hierarchical representations of images automatically by employing multiple layers of convolutional and pooling operations [41]. These layers enable the network to capture local features and gradually build up to more abstract representations. In the context of identification of disease, CNN may effectively learn and discriminate between subtle visual patterns associated with specific diseases. By training on large datasets of labelled medical images, CNN may accurately identify disease-specific features and make precise predictions.

RNNs are another type of deep learning model effective in disease identification from medical imaging data. Unlike CNNs, which primarily focus on spatial information, RNNs are designed to capture temporal dependencies in sequential data. In medical imaging, RNNs may be used to analyse dynamic image sequences, such as time-series data from medical scans or video recordings [54]. RNNs may effectively model the temporal evolution of disease-related changes, allowing for more accurate disease identification and monitoring over time.

The effectiveness of these deep learning models in identification of diseases from medical imaging data arises from their ability to learn and extract relevant features from raw image data automatically. These models may capture subtle visual patterns and complex relationships that may not be readily noticeable to humans. By training on large datasets, deep learning models generalise their learned representations to identify diseases in unseen images accurately. Such techniques have significant implications for clinical practice, as deep learning models may assist healthcare professionals in making more accurate and timely diagnoses and more efficient healthcare delivery.

The performance and effectiveness of deep learning models in identification of disease depend on several factors, including availability of high-quality labelled datasets, appropriate model architecture, hyper-parameter tuning, and careful validation and evaluation [54]. Additionally, ongoing research and development efforts are continuously improving these models and advancing their capabilities in medical imaging analysis. The use of deep learning in diagnosis of disease offers several advantages. First of all, it reduces diagnostic errors and variability, as the algorithms may consistently analyse medical images with high precision [44]. Moreover, deep learning models have the capability to handle complex and diverse data, allowing for detecting subtle abnormalities or early-stage of a disease, which otherwise may be challenging for human interpretation. Deep learning significantly impacts patient outcomes and treatment decisions by improving diagnostic accuracy and efficiency.

19.4.2.3 Deep Learning for Predictive Analytics in Tracking of Disease

Deep learning techniques are instrumental in predictive analytics for tracking of disease, enabling the identification of patterns and risk factors associated with disease development. By analysing large datasets of medical records, genetic profiles, lifestyle data, and environmental factors, deep learning models may predict the likelihood of an individual developing a particular disease or estimate disease progression. Early disease detection is critical to tracking of disease, as it enables proactive interventions and timely treatment. Deep learning models may analyse diverse data sources and identify early warning signs, such as biomarkers or subtle changes in health parameters, that may indicate the onset of a disease [44]. This early detection may lead to personalised preventive measures, early interventions, and improved health outcomes for individuals.

Furthermore, deep learning algorithms support population-level disease prediction and outbreak forecasting [48, 56]. By integrating data from various sources, including surveillance of disease systems, environmental data, and socio-demographic information, deep learning models may forecast disease trends and identify regions at risk of outbreaks [48, 56]. This information empowers healthcare providers and policymakers to allocate resources efficiently, implement targeted interventions, and prevent the spread of diseases. Deep learning techniques analyse social media feeds, online forums, and text data to track disease-related discussions and sentiments. By mining social media data, deep learning models may identify disease outbreaks, track disease spread, and analyse public perceptions and behaviours related to health. This information may support public health agencies in implementing targeted interventions and communication strategies.

Deep learning models leverage historical disease data to make predictions and forecasts about disease trends [41, 48, 49, 51]. By considering various factors such as environmental conditions, population demographics, and disease surveillance data, these models have capability to estimate disease prevalence, identify high-risk areas, and forecast disease outbreaks. This information aids in resource allocation, planning public health strategies, and implementing preventive measures.

In summary, deep learning techniques are crucial in tracking of disease by enabling accurate diagnosis of disease, predicting disease development, and optimising treatment strategies. Deep learning models excel at analysing complex medical data and extracting valuable insights. By leveraging these insights, healthcare professionals may improve surveillance of disease, enhance early detection, and develop personalised interventions. The applications of deep learning in tracking of disease have the potential to significantly improve healthcare and contribute to the advancement of next-generation healthcare systems.

19.5 INTEGRATION OF IoT AND DEEP LEARNING IN TRACKING OF DISEASE

IoT and deep learning technologies have revolutionised tracking of disease and surveillance, enabling real-time monitoring, predictive analytics, and enhanced data analysis. This section explores the synergistic relationship between the IoT and deep learning in tracking of disease and highlights the benefits of this integration.

19.5.1 Leveraging IoT Data for Deep Learning Models

IoT devices, equipped with sensors and connected to the internet, generate vast amounts of real-time data that may be leveraged for tracking of disease. Deep learning models effectively analyse the data and extract valuable insights to improve surveillance of disease and its management. By integrating IoT data into deep learning models, healthcare professionals may enhance disease prediction and diagnosis accuracy and reliability. For example, wearable devices like smart watches collect continuous health data, including vital signs, physical activity levels, and sleep patterns [16, 33, 65]. This data may be fed into deep learning algorithms, allowing for personalised disease risk assessment and early detection of abnormalities.

Moreover, IoT-enabled devices in healthcare settings, such as hospital monitoring systems or remote patient monitoring devices, generate rich and diverse data streams. Deep learning models further process this data to identify patterns, detect anomalies, and provide real-time alerts for potential disease outbreaks or adverse events. Integrating IoT data into deep learning algorithms strengthens disease-tracking capabilities and facilitates proactive interventions.

19.5.2 Real-Time Tracking of Disease and Early Warning Systems

The combination of IoT and deep learning enables real-time tracking of disease and the development of early warning systems. IoT devices provide continuous data streams that may be analysed in real time by deep learning models, allowing for prompt detection of disease-related anomalies or trends [34]. For instance, IoT devices may capture various parameters such as body temperature, heart rate, or respiratory patterns in the context of infectious diseases. Deep learning algorithms have the capability to monitor these data streams, detect abnormal patterns indicative of infections, and trigger early warnings. This real-time monitoring and alert system facilitates timely testing, contact tracing, and implementation of preventive measures to control disease spread.

Additionally, integrating IoT and deep learning facilitates the deployment of intelligent surveillance systems. By combining IoT-generated data, such as environmental conditions, population density, and social interactions, with deep learning algorithms, healthcare providers may develop advanced surveillance models. These models have the capability to monitor disease patterns, identify high-risk areas or populations, and enable timely interventions to prevent outbreaks.

19.5.3 Data Fusion and Integration for Enhanced Tracking of Disease

IoT devices generate data from diverse sources, including medical devices, wearables, environmental sensors, and social media platforms. Deep learning techniques may effectively integrate and fuse these heterogeneous data sources, enabling a comprehensive view of tracking of disease.

Data fusion and integration enhance tracking of disease by combining information from multiple domains. For example, by integrating medical records, genetic profiles, IoT sensor data, and environmental information, deep learning models may provide a holistic understanding of disease risk factors, progression, and transmission dynamics. This integrated approach enables healthcare professionals to make informed decisions, implement targeted interventions, and optimise resource allocation. Further, integrating geospatial technologies, such as remote sensing, GPS, and GIS, with IoT and deep learning adds another layer of valuable information for tracking of disease. Geospatial data, including environmental factors, population distribution, and healthcare facility locations, can be integrated with IoT-generated data to create detailed disease mapping and visualisation tools. These tools facilitate spatial analysis, identify disease hotspots, and support targeted interventions to control disease outbreaks.

Thus, integrating IoT and deep learning in tracking of disease enables the leverage of real-time data, facilitates early warning systems, and enhances data fusion and integration for comprehensive surveillance of disease. This synergistic approach improves disease prediction, diagnosis, and management, leading to more effective healthcare interventions and better health outcomes. Integrating geospatial technologies enhances disease-tracking capabilities, enabling spatial analysis and targeted interventions. The combination of IoT and deep learning represents a dominant paradigm for next-generation tracking of disease and surveillance systems.

19.6 CHALLENGES AND FUTURE DIRECTIONS

This section discusses the challenges and future directions in integrating IoT and deep learning for tracking of disease. Some of the challenges are:

1. Ethical considerations
2. Scalability and interoperability challenges
3. Newly emerging diseases
4. Emerging trends and future directions in tracking of disease

19.6.1 Ethical Considerations

Tracking of disease plays a crucial role in safeguarding public health; however, it raises ethical concerns regarding individual rights and privacy. One of the foremost ethical considerations associated with tracking of disease involves the potential for privacy breaches [6, 28]. The collection of health data necessitates trust, and individuals must have assurance that their data is secure and protected.

Another ethical challenge in tracking of disease is balancing public health needs and individual rights [66]. Tracking of disease involves gathering personal health information, which may be sensitive and private. Ensuring that this data is collected and utilised with due consideration for individual autonomy and privacy is crucial. Additionally, disease-tracking efforts must address the potential for stigmatisation of certain individuals or groups. For instance, during the COVID-19 pandemic, there were instances of stigmatisation towards Asian individuals due to the association of the virus with China [67, 68]. Tracking of disease should prevent data collection and usage practices from contributing to discrimination or stigmatisation, proactively addressing unintended consequences. Using location data or social media data for tracking disease outbreaks may raise concerns regarding surveillance and privacy. It is vital to ensure that the application of such technologies is balanced with respect for individual rights and privacy [18].

To address these ethical challenges, governments and health organisations must develop explicit policies and guidelines for tracking of disease that prioritise individual rights and privacy while protecting public health. These policies should be informed by transparency, accountability, and respect for personal autonomy [18, 66, 69].

19.6.2 Scalability and Interoperability Challenges

As disease-tracking systems expand in scope and coverage, scalability and interoperability become significant challenges. Scaling up the infrastructure to handle large volumes of data generated by IoT devices and deep learning algorithms requires robust computational resources and efficient data processing techniques [26, 45]. Interoperability issues arise when integrating data from various sources and platforms, such as IoT devices, electronic health records, and public health databases. Standardisation of data formats, interoperability protocols, and integration frameworks is essential to ensure seamless data exchange and collaboration among different stakeholders in the disease-tracking ecosystem [70]. Collaborative partnerships between governments, international organisations, and non-governmental organisations may support capacity-building efforts and knowledge exchange.

19.6.3 Newly Emerging Diseases

Another challenge is the difficulty in tracking certain diseases, such as those with long incubation periods or asymptomatic cases [19, 29, 71, 72]. For example, tracking the transmission of diseases like tuberculosis, which may remain dormant in the body for years, maybe challenging [24]. Similarly, tracking asymptomatic cases, such as COVID-19, may be difficult, as individuals may not present with symptoms or seek healthcare [24]. Newly emerging diseases present unique challenges in tracking of disease, as they often catch healthcare systems off guard and require rapid response to prevent their spread. The challenges may be, but are not limited to:

1. Identification and Diagnosis: One of the primary challenges is the timely identification and diagnosis of newly emerging diseases [6]. These diseases may have unfamiliar clinical presentations and may initially be mistaken for other, more common illnesses. It may be challenging to accurately identify and confirm cases without a specific diagnostic test or clear understanding of the disease. This delays the implementation of targeted control measures and hampers disease-tracking efforts.
2. Surveillance and Reporting: Establishing effective surveillance systems for newly emerging diseases may be difficult. Often, no infrastructure or protocols may be in place to track and report these diseases [71, 73]. Developing surveillance networks, training healthcare workers, and creating data collection and reporting mechanisms are crucial but may take time and resources. Delays in surveillance and reporting may impede early detection and response, allowing the disease to spread undetected.

19.6.4 Emerging Trends and Future Directions in Tracking of Disease

The field of tracking of disease is constantly evolving, and several emerging trends and future directions hold great promise. These include:

1. Edge Computing: Adopting edge computing techniques may alleviate the computational burden of transmitting and processing large volumes of data in centralised cloud systems. Edge devices may perform data processing and analysis locally, reducing latency and improving real-time disease-tracking capabilities.
2. Federated Learning: Federated learning allows collaborative training of models on decentralised data sources without sharing raw data. This approach may address privacy concerns by keeping data localised while leveraging collective intelligence for disease-tracking model development.
3. Explainable AI: As deep learning models become more complex, there is a necessity for transparency and interpretability. Explainable AI techniques provide insights into the

decision-making process of deep learning models, enabling healthcare professionals to understand and trust the generated predictions or recommendations.

4. Integration of Social Determinants of Health: Incorporating social factors associated with health, such as socioeconomic factors, environmental conditions, and behavioural data, into tracking of disease models may provide a more holistic understanding of disease spread and its underlying factors. This integration may help develop targeted interventions and policies to address health disparities.
5. One Health Approach: The One Health approach highlights the interlinkage of human, animal, and environmental health. Integrating the IoT and deep learning in tracking of disease across these domains may enhance the early detection of zoonotic diseases, track environmental factors influencing disease spread, and support interdisciplinary collaborations.

By addressing the challenges and leveraging emerging trends, the future of tracking of disease holds great potential for improving public health surveillance, enabling early detection of outbreaks, and guiding effective interventions.

19.7 CONCLUSION

The overall integration of the IoT and deep learning technologies holds great potential to revolutionise tracking of disease and enhance public health surveillance. IoT devices play a critical role in tracking of disease by enabling real-time data collection of vital health parameters, environmental factors, and behavioural data. Such continuous monitoring allows for early detection of disease outbreaks, providing a valuable opportunity for prompt response and containment measures. Deep learning algorithms further enhance tracking of disease by leveraging advanced pattern recognition and predictive analytics capabilities. These algorithms may detect disease patterns, facilitate accurate diagnosis, and enable personalised disease management strategies. Integrating the IoT and deep learning also brings the advantage of data fusion and analysis from diverse sources. Tracking of disease systems may achieve greater accuracy and comprehensiveness in their insights by combining data from different channels, such as IoT devices, electronic health records, and public health databases.

The impact of IoT and deep learning on tracking of disease is substantial. These technologies have the capabilities to transform public health surveillance by enabling early detection and rapid response to disease outbreaks, thereby minimising the spread of infectious diseases and alleviating the burden on healthcare systems. Additionally, they empower individuals with personalised disease management strategies, leading to improved health outcomes and better quality of life. Real-time monitoring and surveillance facilitated by IoT and deep learning allow healthcare authorities to allocate resources more efficiently and implement targeted interventions for optimal effectiveness.

REFERENCES

[1] D. F. Attaway, K. H. Jacobsen, A. Falconer, G. Manca, and N. M. Waters, "Risk analysis for dengue suitability in Africa using the ArcGIS predictive analysis tools (PA tools)," *Acta Trop.*, vol. 158, pp. 248–257, 2016, doi: 10.1016/j.actatropica.2016.02.018.

[2] L. C. Backer *et al.*, "Environmental public health surveillance: Possible estuary-associated syndrome," *Environ. Health Perspect.*, vol. 109, no. Suppl. 5, pp. 797–801, 2001, doi: 10.1289/ehp.01109s5797.

[3] M. N. Kamel Boulos and E. M. Geraghty, "Geographical tracking and mapping of coronavirus disease COVID-19/severe acute respiratory syndrome coronavirus 2 (SARS-CoV-2) epidemic and associated events around the world: How 21st century GIS technologies are supporting the global fight against outbr," *Int. J. Health Geogr.*, vol. 19, no. 1, pp. 1–12, 2020, doi: 10.1186/s12942-020-00202-8.

[4] P. Ceccato, B. Ramirez, T. Manyangadze, P. Gwakisa, and M. C. Thomson, "Data and tools to integrate climate and environmental information into public health," *Infect. Dis. Poverty*, vol. 7, no. 1, pp. 1–11, 2018, doi: 10.1186/s40249-018-0501-9.

[5] P. A. Villarreal, "International law and digital disease surveillance in pandemics: On the margins of regulation," *Ger. Law J.*, vol. 24, no. 3, pp. 603–617, 2023, doi: 10.1017/glj.2023.26.
[6] J. Budd *et al.*, "Digital technologies in the public-health response to COVID-19," *Nat. Med.*, vol. 26, no. 8, pp. 1183–1192, 2020, doi: 10.1038/s41591-020-1011-4.
[7] WHO, *Ending the Neglect to Attain the Sustainable Development Goals: A Sustainability Framework for Action Against Neglected Tropical Diseases 2021–2030.* World Health Organization, 2021.
[8] C. Coussens and E. Rusch, *Public Health Linkages with Sustainability*, 2013, doi: 10.17226/18375.
[9] E. Viennet, S. A. Ritchie, H. M. Faddy, C. R. Williams, and D. Harley, "Epidemiology of dengue in a high-income country: A case study in Queensland, Australia," *Parasit. Vectors*, vol. 7, no. 1, pp. 1–16, 2014, doi: 10.1186/1756-3305-7-379.
[10] H. A. Hatherell, H. Simpson, R. F. Baggaley, T. D. Hollingsworth, and R. L. Pullan, "Sustainable surveillance of neglected tropical diseases for the post-elimination era," *Clin. Infect. Dis.*, vol. 72, no. Suppl. 3, pp. S210–S216, 2021, doi: 10.1093/cid/ciab211.
[11] M. A. Viray *et al.*, "Public health investigation and response to a hepatitis A outbreak from imported scallops consumed raw-Hawaii, 2016," *Epidemiol. Infect.*, vol. 147, 2019, doi: 10.1017/S0950268818002844.
[12] V. J. Jayaraj, R. Avoi, N. Gopalakrishnan, D. B. Raja, and Y. Umasa, "Developing a dengue prediction model based on climate in Tawau, Malaysia," *Acta Trop.*, vol. 197, p. 105055, 2019, doi: 10.1016/j.actatropica.2019.105055.
[13] S. Doi, H. Ide, S. Ogawa, K. Takabayashi, S. Fujita, and S. Koike, "Probabilistic model to analyze patient accessibility to medical facilities using geographic information systems," *Procedia Comput. Sci.*, vol. 60, no. 1, pp. 1631–1639, 2015, doi: 10.1016/j.procs.2015.08.273.
[14] E. Rees *et al.*, "Risk assessment strategies for early detection and prediction of infectious disease outbreaks associated with climate change," *Canada Commun. Dis. Rep.*, vol. 45, no. 5, pp. 119–126, 2019, doi: 10.14745/ccdr.v45i05a02.
[15] N. K. Lee, M. A. Stewart, J. S. Dymond, and S. L. Lewis, "An implementation strategy to develop sustainable surveillance activities through adoption of a target operating model," *Front. Public Heal.*, vol. 10, pp. 1–7, 2022, doi: 10.3389/fpubh.2022.871114.
[16] W. N. Ismail, M. M. Hassan, H. A. Alsalamah, and G. Fortino, "CNN-based health model for regular health factors analysis in internet-of-medical things environment," *IEEE Access*, vol. 8, pp. 52541–52549, 2020, doi: 10.1109/ACCESS.2020.2980938.
[17] M. H. Kashani, M. Madanipour, M. Nikravan, P. Asghari, and E. Mahdipour, "A systematic review of IoT in healthcare: Applications, techniques, and trends," *J. Netw. Comput. Appl.*, vol. 192, p. 103164, 2021, doi: 10.1016/j.jnca.2021.103164.
[18] H. A. Lee *et al.*, "Global infectious disease surveillance and case tracking system for COVID-19: Development study," *JMIR Med. Inform.*, vol. 8, no. 12, pp. 1–17, 2020, doi: 10.2196/20567.
[19] WHO, *Strengthening the Global Architecture for Health Emergency Preparedness, Response and Resilience. Part 2. The Five Cs of Health Emergency Prevention, Preparedness, Response, and Resilience*, pp. 11–14. World Health Organization, 2022.
[20] D. Kaul, H. Raju, and B. K. Tripathy, Deep learning in healthcare. In: D. P. Acharjya, A. Mitra, and N. Zaman (eds) *Deep Learning in Data Analytics: Studies in Big Data*, vol. 91. Springer, 2022, doi: 10.1007/978-3-030-75855-4_6.
[21] T. Wuhib, T. L. Chorba, V. Davidiants, W. R. Mac Kenzie, and S. J. N. McNabb, "Assessment of the infectious diseases surveillance system of the Republic of Armenia: An example of surveillance in the republics of the former Soviet Union," *BMC Public Health*, vol. 2, pp. 1–8, 2002, doi: 10.1186/1471-2458-2-3.
[22] N. M. M'ikanatha, R. Lynfield, C. A. Van Beneden, and H. de Valk, "Infectious Disease Surveillance: A Cornerstone for Prevention and Control, Emerging Infectious Diseases," *Clinical Microbiology and Infection, Elsevier*, p. 560. 2007, doi: 10.3201/eid1604.090584.
[23] A. Wilder-Smith and D. J. Gubler, "Geographic expansion of dengue: The impact of international travel," *Med. Clin. North Am.*, vol. 92, no. 6, pp. 1377–1390, 2008, doi: 10.1016/j.mcna.2008.07.002.
[24] N. K. Tran *et al.*, "Evolving applications of artificial intelligence and machine learning in infectious diseases testing," *Clin. Chem.*, vol. 68, no. 1, pp. 125–133, 2022, doi: 10.1093/clinchem/hvab239.
[25] M. U. G. Kraemer *et al.*, "Reconstruction and prediction of viral disease epidemics," *Epidemiol. Infect.*, vol. 147, pp. 1–7, 2019, doi: 10.1017/S0950268818002881.
[26] A. E. Aiello, A. Renson, and P. Zivich, "Social media- and internet-based disease surveillance for public health," *Annu. Rev. Public Health*, vol. 41, no. 26, pp. 101–118, 2020, doi: 10.1146/annurev-publhealth-040119-094402.Social.

[27] L. E. Charles-Smith *et al.*, "Using social media for actionable disease surveillance and outbreak management: A systematic literature review," *PLoS One*, vol. 10, no. 10, pp. 1–20, 2015, doi: 10.1371/journal.pone.0139701.
[28] H. Luan and J. Law, "Web GIS-based public health surveillance systems: A systematic review," *ISPRS Int. J. GeoInf.*, vol. 3, no. 2, pp. 481–506, 2014, doi: 10.3390/ijgi3020481.
[29] J. Choi, Y. Cho, E. Shim, and H. Woo, "Web-based infectious disease surveillance systems and public health perspectives: A systematic review," *BMC Public Health*, vol. 16, no. 1, pp. 1–10, 2016, doi: 10.1186/s12889-016-3893-0.
[30] S. E. Roche, M. G. Garner, R. L. Sanson, C. Cook, and C. Birch, "Evaluating vaccination strategies to control foot-and-mouth disease: A model comparison study," *Epidemiol Infect.*, vol. 146, pp. 1256–1275, 2015, doi: 10.1017/S0950268814001927.
[31] J. Calvillo-Arbizu, I. Román-Martínez, and J. Reina-Tosina, "Computer methods and programs in biomedicine Internet of Things in health: Requirements, issues, and gaps," *Comput. Methods Programs Biomed.*, vol. 208, p. 106231, 2021, doi: 10.1016/j.cmpb.2021.106231.
[32] V. Bhardwaj, R. Joshi, and A. Mli, "IoT – based smart health monitoring system for COVID-19," *SN Comput. Sci.*, vol. 3, no. 2, pp. 1–11, 2022, doi: 10.1007/s42979-022-01015-1.
[33] M. Javaid and I. Haleem, "Internet of Things (IoT) enabled healthcare helps to take the challenges of COVID-19 pandemic," *J. Oral Biol. Craniofacial Res.*, vol. 11, no. 2, pp. 209–214, 2021, doi: 10.1016/j.jobcr.2021.01.015.
[34] K. S. Sahu, S. E. Majowicz, and J. A. Dubin, "NextGen public health surveillance and the Internet of Things (IoT)," *Front. Public Heal.*, vol. 9, pp. 1–9, 2021, doi: 10.3389/fpubh.2021.756675.
[35] M. R. Ullah, M. A. R. Bhuiyan, and A. K. Das, "IHEMHA: Interactive healthcare system design with emotion computing and medical history analysis," *2017 6th Int. Conf. Informatics, Electron. Vis. 2017 7th Int. Symp. Comput. Med. Heal. Technol. ICIEV-ISCMHT 2017*, vol. 2018, pp. 1–8, 2018, doi: 10.1109/ICIEV.2017.8338606.
[36] S. Jaya and S. Rajasekar, "An enhanced IoT based tracing and tracking model for COVID-19 cases," *SN Comput. Sci.*, vol. 2, no. 1, pp. 1–4, 2021, doi: 10.1007/s42979-020-00400-y.
[37] A. A. Malibari, "An efficient IoT-artificial intelligence-based disease prediction using lightweight CNN in healthcare system," *Meas. Sensors*, vol. 26, p. 100695, 2023, doi: 10.1016/j.measen.2023.100695.
[38] M. Islam, A. Rahaman, and R. Islam, "Development of smart healthcare monitoring system in IoT environment," *SN Comput. Sci.*, vol. 1, no. 3, pp. 1–11, 2020, doi: 10.1007/s42979-020-00195-y.
[39] S. L. Ullo and G. R. Sinha, "Advances in smart environment monitoring systems using iot and sensors," *Sensors (Switzerland)*, vol. 20, no. 11, 2020, doi: 10.3390/s20113113.
[40] S. Selvaraj and S. Sundaravaradhan, "Challenges and opportunities in IoT healthcare systems: A systematic review," *SN Appl. Sci.*, vol. 2, no. 1, pp. 1–8, 2020, doi: 10.1007/s42452-019-1925-y.
[41] E. Chanda, V. M. Mukonka, D. Mthembu, M. Kamuliwo, S. Coetzer, and C. J. Shinondo, "Using a geographical-information-system-based decision support to enhance malaria vector control in Zambia," *J. Trop. Med.*, vol. 2012, 2012, doi: 10.1155/2012/363520.
[42] L. Eisen and R. J. Eisen, "Using geographic information systems and decision support systems for the prediction, prevention, and control of vector-borne diseases," *Annu. Rev. Entomol.*, vol. 56, pp. 41–61, 2011, doi: 10.1146/annurev-ento-120709-144847.
[43] V. Sharma, S. K. Ghosh, and S. Khare, "A proposed framework for surveillance of dengue disease and prediction," *Int. Arch. Photogramm. Remote Sens. Spat. Inf. Sci. ISPRS Arch.*, vol. 48, no. M-1-2023, pp. 317–323, 2023, doi: 10.5194/isprs-archives-XLVIII-M-1-2023-317-2023.
[44] A. Diptyanusa, L. Lazuardi, and R. H. Jatmiko, "Implementation of geographical information systems for the study of diseases caused by vector-borne arboviruses in Southeast Asia: A review based on the publication record," *Geospat. Health*, vol. 15, no. 1, 2020, doi: 10.4081/gh.2020.862.
[45] D. Zeng, Z. Cao, and D. B. Neill, *Artificial Intelligence–Enabled Public Health Surveillance—From Local Detection to Global Epidemic Monitoring and Control.* INC, 2021, doi: 10.1016/b978-0-12-821259-2.00022-3.
[46] X. Chen *et al.*, "Recent advances and clinical applications of deep learning in medical image analysis," *Med. Image Anal.*, vol. 79, p. 102444, 2022, doi: 10.1016/j.media.2022.102444.
[47] S. Gao and D. Lima, "A review of the application of deep learning in the detection of Alzheimer's disease," *Int. J. Cogn. Comput. Eng.*, vol. 3, pp. 1–8, 2022, doi: 10.1016/j.ijcce.2021.12.002.
[48] A. Esteva *et al.*, "A guide to deep learning in healthcare," *Nat. Med.*, vol. 25, 2019, doi: 10.1038/s41591-018-0316-z.

[49] D. Kaul, H. Raju, and B. K. Tripathy, "Deep learning in healthcare," January 2022, doi: 10.1007/978-3-030-75855-4.

[50] D. Bordoloi, V. Singh, S. Sanober, S. M. Buhari, J. A. Ujjan, and R. Boddu, "Deep learning in healthcare system for quality of service," *J. Healthc. Eng.*, vol. 2022, p. 11, 2022, doi: 10.1155/2022/8169203.

[51] Z. Yu, K. Wang, Z. Wan, S. Xie, and Z. Lv, "Popular deep learning algorithms for disease prediction: A review," *Cluster Comput.*, vol. 26, no. 2, pp. 1231–1251, 2023, doi: 10.1007/s10586-022-03707-y.

[52] D. R. Sarvamangala and R. V. Kulkarni, "Convolutional neural networks in medical image understanding: A survey," *Evol. Intell.*, vol. 15, no. 1, pp. 1–22, 2022, doi: 10.1007/s12065-020-00540-3.

[53] Y. Jiao, H. Qi, and J. Wu, "Capsule network assisted electrocardiogram classification model for smart healthcare," *Biocybern. Biomed. Eng.*, vol. 42, no. 2, pp. 543–555, 2022, doi: 10.1016/j.bbe.2022.03.006.

[54] S. Tiwari and A. Jain, "Convolutional capsule network for COVID-19 detection using radiography images," *Int. J. Imaging Syst. Technol.*, vol. 31, no. 2, pp. 525–539, 2021, doi: 10.1002/ima.22566.

[55] F. Khozeimeh *et al.*, "Combining a convolutional neural network with autoencoders to predict the survival chance of COVID-19 patients," *Sci. Rep.*, vol. 11, no. 1, pp. 1–18, 2021, doi: 10.1038/s41598-021-93543-8.

[56] L. Alzubaidi *et al.*, *Review of deep learning: Concepts, CNN architectures, challenges, applications, future directions*, vol. 8, no. 1. Springer International Publishing, 2021. doi: 10.1186/s40537-021-00444-8.

[57] J. Xu *et al.*, "Forecast of dengue cases in 20 Chinese cities based on the deep learning method," *Int. J. Environ. Res. Public Health*, vol. 17, no. 2, 2020, doi: 10.3390/ijerph17020453.

[58] E. Choi, A. Schuetz, W. F. Stewart, and J. Sun, "Using recurrent neural network models for early detection of heart failure onset," *J. Am. Med. Inform. Assoc.*, vol. 24, no. 2, pp. 361–370, 2017, doi: 10.1093/jamia/ocw112.

[59] L. Rasmy *et al.*, "Recurrent neural network models (CovRNN) for predicting outcomes of patients with COVID-19 on admission to hospital: Model development and validation using electronic health record data," *Lancet Digit. Heal.*, vol. 4, no. 6, pp. e415–e425, 2022, doi: 10.1016/S2589-7500(22)00049-8.

[60] Y. Zhang, Q. Zhang, Y. Zhao, Y. Deng, and H. Zheng, "Urban spatial risk prediction and optimization analysis of POI based on deep learning from the perspective of an epidemic," *Int. J. Appl. Earth Obs. Geoinf.*, vol. 112, p. 102942, 2022, doi: 10.1016/j.jag.2022.102942.

[61] M. Abedi, L. Hempel, S. Sadeghi, and T. Kirsten, "GAN-based approaches for generating structured data in the medical domain," *Appl. Sci.*, vol. 12, no. 14, 2022, doi: 10.3390/app12147075.

[62] X. M. Chen *et al.*, "Design and analysis for early warning of rotor UAV based on data-driven DBN," *Electron.*, vol. 8, no. 11, pp. 1–22, 2019, doi: 10.3390/electronics8111350.

[63] P. Sharma, R. Arya, R. Verma, and B. Verma, "Conv-CapsNet: Capsule based network for COVID-19 detection through X-Ray scans," *Multimed. Tools Appl.*, 2023, doi: 10.1007/s11042-023-14353-w.

[64] S. Suganyadevi, V. Seethalakshmi, and K. Balasamy, "A review on deep learning in medical image analysis," *Int. J. Multimed. Inf. Retr.*, vol. 11, no. 1, pp. 19–38, 2022, doi: 10.1007/s13735-021-00218-1.

[65] Á. V. Espinosa, L. Luis, and F. M. Mata, "Application of IoT in healthcare: Keys to implementation of the sustainable development goals," *Sensors (Basel)*, vol. 21, no. 7, p. 2330, 2021, doi: 10.3390/s21072330.

[66] M. Raviglione and D. Maher, "Ending infectious diseases in the era of the sustainable development goals," *Porto Biomed. J.*, vol. 2, no. 5, pp. 140–142, 2017, doi: 10.1016/j.pbj.2017.08.001.

[67] M. Kim, S. Liu, Y. Lee, C. Hee, and S. Mariano, "COVID-19 related racial discrimination in small Asian communities: A cross sectional study," *J. Immigr. Minor. Heal.*, vol. 24, no. 1, pp. 38–47, 2022, doi: 10.1007/s10903-021-01295-4.

[68] S. Misra, P. T. D. Le, E. Goldmann, and L. H. Yang, "Psychological impact of anti-asian stigma due to the COVID-19 pandemic: A call for research, practice, and policy responses," *Psychol Trauma.*, vol. 12, no. 5, pp. 461–464, 2020, doi: 10.1037/tra0000821.Psychological.

[69] C. Degeling *et al.*, "Implementing a one health approach to emerging infectious disease: Reflections on the socio-political, ethical and legal dimensions," *BMC Public Health*, vol. 15, no. 1, pp. 1–11, 2015, doi: 10.1186/s12889-015-2617-1.

[70] W. Hoyos, J. Aguilar, and M. Toro, "Dengue models based on machine learning techniques: A systematic literature review," *Artif. Intell. Med.*, vol. 119, p. 102157, 2021, doi: 10.1016/j.artmed.2021.102157.

[71] F. M. Burkle, "Declining public health protections within autocratic regimes: Impact on global public health security, infectious disease outbreaks, epidemics, and pandemics," *Prehosp. Disaster Med.*, vol. 35, no. 3, pp. 237–246, 2020, doi: 10.1017/S1049023X20000424.

[72] C. Qi *et al.*, "Epidemiological characteristics and spatial-temporal analysis of COVID-19 in Shandong Province, China," *Epidemiol. Infect.*, vol. 148, pp. 1–8, 2020, doi: 10.1017/S095026882000151X.

[73] L. Gibson and D. Rush, "Novel coronavirus in Cape Town informal settlements: Feasibility of using informal dwelling outlines to identify high risk areas for COVID-19 transmission from a social distancing perspective," *JMIR Public Heal. Surveill.*, vol. 6, no. 2, 2020, doi: 10.2196/18844.

[74] Sharma, L., & Garg, P.K. (Eds.). (2023). *Technological Prospects and Social Applications of Society* 5.0 (1st ed.). Chapman and Hall/CRC. https://doi.org/10.1201/9781003324720.

[75] Sharma, L. (Ed.). (2020). *Towards Smart World: Homes to Cities Using Internet of Things* (1st ed.). Chapman and Hall/CRC. https://doi.org/10.1201/9781003056751.

20 Disease Detection Using TensorFlow Methodology

Shipra Verma

20.1 INTRODUCTION

Japanese encephalitis (JE) is a major public health problem worldwide and mainly affects children and young adults (Mutheneni *et al.*, 2014). Disease health sector are required carefully designed and implemented system which concerns individual patient care (Stansfield *et al.*, 2006). In real time, detection and prevention of disease is very difficult as it required perfect algorithms, and accurate analysis (Solomon *et al.*, 2000). The disease incidence is estimated at about 50,000 cases and 10,000 deaths over 3 billion people who live in JE endemic regions annually (Fischer *et al.*, 2008; Van den Hurk *et al.*, 2009). JEV originated in the Malay Archipelago (Bista, 2005) and was isolated from human cases in 1934 and 1938 (Mitamura *et al.*, 1936, 1938; Grossman *et al.*, 1973). According to the WHO, encephalitis cases are defined as: "a person of any age, at any time of the year, with the acute onset of fever and a change in mental status or new onset seizures (excluding simple febrile seizures)" (WHO, 2006, 2007; Keiser *et al.*, 2005). Due to scarce medical facilities, the JE disease data collection is higher (Peiris *et al.*, 1992; Tsai, 2000). Much research has been conducted on the disease (Bunnel *et al.*, 2005; Kalluri *et al.*, 2007; Verma and Gupta, 2014), but it is expensive and time consuming.

Machine learning is an advanced computational technique and provides strong support in the field of disease outbreaks (Ahsan *et al.*, 2020). It is a self-improving process and entered health sector in the 1970s. Many different approaches are adopted using ML techniques, such as support vector machine (SVM), naïve Bayes, and artificial neural networks (Kononenko, 2001). TensorFlow is an interface for implementing and expressing such algorithms (Arvind and Culler, 1986). It is a subset of artificial intelligence and uses data as an input function (Stafford *et al.*, 2022).

Machine learning algorithms are used to carry out the work. Different algorithms are used to optimize and generate the input data at the fittest point. It also obtains a precise and validated data along with justification (Thakkar and Lohiya, 2021). Today, machine learning has come to predict information using past data (Mitchell, 1997). The use of the Internet on computers and laptops and frequent use of mobile devices are influenced by the surroundings. It is needed to perform best algorithm for particular diseases. Handling and understanding health datasets in ML are the most important and dynamic factor (Massaro *et al.*, 2018). TensorFlow, an open-source framework, is used with multiple sets of health data under the Keras environment. It is the most widely used deep learning library for pre-processing, building, and training machine learning models. It helps load highly scalable data using common input values and provides a tool to transform and validate large sets of data (Anshik, 2021).

20.2 OBJECTIVE

The objective of the present chapter is to examine the features related to JE such as age, location, gender, month of detection, and outcome to predict the disease from the history of the disease data using a machine learning model. A good data feature enhances the accuracy of

DOI: 10.1201/9781003451846-20

the model and identifies feature importance in the data. Machine learning algorithms can solve JE health issues efficiently and allow us to build models to quickly clean and process data and deliver results faster. In this work, the Pandas libraries can be used to compare the performance of multiple ML approaches to diagnosing a disease for a given dataset with a couple of lines of code.

This technique helps in building mathematical models and creating information using health-related historical data. ML algorithm development usually has two phases: 1) training and 2) testing. To improve the accuracy of large data, the existing work will be done on unstructured or textual data. For the prediction of diseases, will be done on Tensor Flow (TF) using a neural network (NN) algorithm. This will decrease the probability of inaccurate diagnosis, which is a significant consideration when dealing with the health of people.

20.3 DATA, ALGORITHMS, AND METHODS

The important feature of data is block, age, gender, month of detection, and outcome, that is, the target outcome of the data. The data set has four attributes and one class variable named Outcome. The attributes of location in terms of blocks in a district which has highly number of diseases, particular age in which disease detected, months of disease detection and the gender wise distribution of disease. A dataset table consists of columns that contains attributes and class variables which are used to build ML model for disease diagnosis. Here, the class variables indicated disease to be positively diagnosed under disease consideration. It predicts the class values, where 1 means positively diagnosed and 0 means negatively diagnosed. At present study, ML model for disease diagnosing has 18 possible outcomes with value in between 0 and 1.

A deep neural network model (NLP) with the Keras function is used for training and testing data with input, hidden, and output layers. These values are compiled and provide the output value in a binary label encoder. Model is trained and turned into validation to find accuracy.

20.4 METHODOLOGY

Pandas is used for data processing work. The Keras framework is used for training the model. For visualization, Matplotlib was used. These packages are used for the development of Pandas, Tensor Flow, Numpy, and Matplotlib (Massaro *et al.*, 2018). ML algorithms offer efficient and refined multi-dimensional disease data, although the accuracy of diagnosing diseases is still a major concern. Different health datasets need to use different ML approaches and find indications to apply and adjust the algorithms on the matching dataset (Quest, 2022). ML functions perform on the kaggle platform and require efficient time with minimal lines of code. It supports searching for the best ML method and to diagnose a particular disease problem for a given set of data with optimal lines of code. This method delineates the predicted inaccurate diagnosis and will decrease the probability of inaccurate diagnoses and provide an effective approach for the patients and communicate their health.

20.4.1 Data Processing System

The collection of health data and information for the Gorakhpur district enables the machine learning platform using the TensorFlow framework.

The functions using Keras models can predict disease on the basis of their training, testing, and validation data (Figure 20.1). The disease data is processed in such a way to transform specific information and help compile and analyze the data. The developed model can easily predict the chance of infection using different functions. The prediction value is in binary form between 0 and 1. It helps monitor patient health using recorded data.

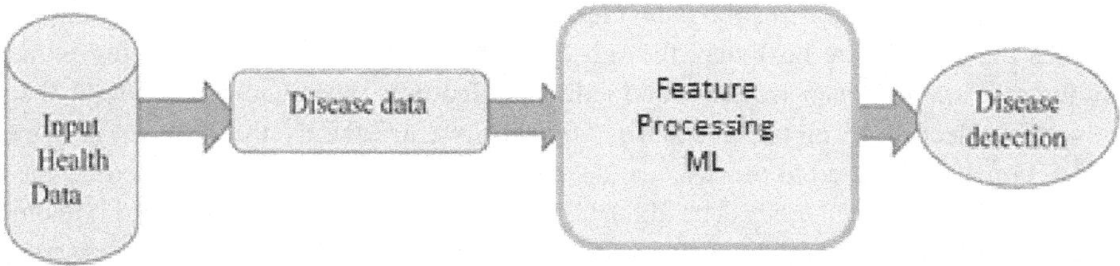

FIGURE 20.1 Data processing system.

20.4.2 Data Architecture Using Machine Learning Techniques

The health dataset of JE disease was collected from the district from 2009 to 2020. The first step of data architecture is data acquisition. This involves data collection and preparation.

Figure 20.2 shows the steps. The collection of JE disease data is segregated on the basis of feature selection, which is involved with decision making. Feature engineering helps identify the features that hold the most relevant information to the predicted target (Ramalingam *et al.*, 2018). The development of model is in three phases. First the dataset is trained for the appropriate task, then, at the time of training, the training data is evaluated and continuously validates the trained data. After training, the model is tested and deployed.

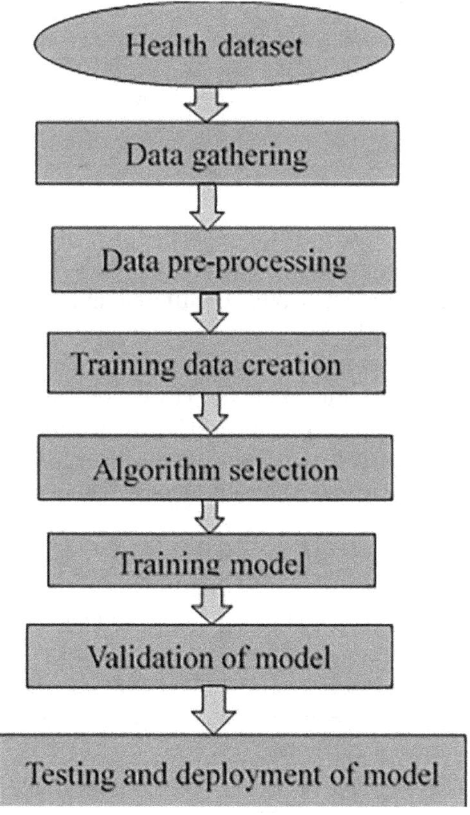

FIGURE 20.2 Block diagram of decision flow architecture of ML-based disease model.

The processing unit normalizes the data, cleans the data, and does a step-by-step transformation and encodes the data. In the next step, the subset of feature selection is involved for extraction of relevant features and removes irrelevant and redundant features. The architecture adopts the system to involve the selection of algorithm, that is, TensorFlow, to identify the problem (Figure 20.2). The Keras framework is used to process the disease data. The trained model proceeds to the testing phase and reduces the dependency. The algorithm extracts and predicts the required outcomes, and the further refined solution is ready to make decisions (Shvets *et al.*, 2018). The output model allows one to directly make decisions.

20.4.3 Calculating Feature Importance

It calculates a performance evaluation matrix in terms of binary methods and expresses positive/negative (Figure 20.3) in between all features.

```
['block', 'age', 'gender', 'month_of_detection']
Epoch 1/10
8/8 [==============================] - 1s 31ms/step - loss: 0.7637 - accuracy: 0.5350 - val_loss: 0.7266 - val_accuracy: 0.4262
Epoch 2/10
8/8 [==============================] - 0s 6ms/step - loss: 0.6877 - accuracy: 0.5473 - val_loss: 0.6606 - val_accuracy: 0.4426
Epoch 3/10
8/8 [==============================] - 0s 6ms/step - loss: 0.6159 - accuracy: 0.7407 - val_loss: 0.5819 - val_accuracy: 0.8033
Epoch 4/10
8/8 [==============================] - 0s 6ms/step - loss: 0.5713 - accuracy: 0.9053 - val_loss: 0.5669 - val_accuracy: 0.9836
Epoch 5/10
8/8 [==============================] - 0s 6ms/step - loss: 0.5342 - accuracy: 0.8807 - val_loss: 0.5194 - val_accuracy: 0.9836
Epoch 6/10
8/8 [==============================] - 0s 6ms/step - loss: 0.4838 - accuracy: 0.9712 - val_loss: 0.4635 - val_accuracy: 1.0000
Epoch 7/10
8/8 [==============================] - 0s 6ms/step - loss: 0.4290 - accuracy: 1.0000 - val_loss: 0.4213 - val_accuracy: 1.0000
Epoch 8/10
8/8 [==============================] - 0s 7ms/step - loss: 0.3675 - accuracy: 1.0000 - val_loss: 0.3428 - val_accuracy: 1.0000
Epoch 9/10
8/8 [==============================] - 0s 6ms/step - loss: 0.3029 - accuracy: 1.0000 - val_loss: 0.2809 - val_accuracy: 1.0000
Epoch 10/10
8/8 [==============================] - 0s 7ms/step - loss: 0.2426 - accuracy: 1.0000 - val_loss: 0.2362 - val_accuracy: 1.0000
```

FIGURE 20.3 Feature importance.

Identifying the features and feature importance can help to find potential issues and diagnose behavior of models and their interpretability. Feature importance is set for a specific dataset and particular model. It may assign different scores for different models to the same features. Feature importance is generated by the model and shows the scores about important features in the prediction of disease. The four measurements values: recall, precision, accuracy, and F1, measure the performance of binary class. A true positive (TP) denotes the number of results correctly predicted, true negative (TN) denotes the number of correctly classified which are not required means negative class, false positive (FP) the number of results incorrectly classified in reference to positive, false negative (FN) (the number of results incorrectly classified as negative) respectively (Powers, 2011).

The accuracy of correctly classified samples and the total number of samples in the evaluation dataset are shown, respectively (Figures 20.4 and 20.5).

A lower loss means the model is better at fitting. In the training data, accuracy is increased, loss is decreased, and the model is trained. The data frame model is encoded with categorical data, then passes the test data into the model. It will give a prediction. It's an evaluation metric used after training to measure how well the model generalizes to new, unseen data. A higher accuracy indicates that the model is making more correct predictions.

The mean of the model loss is a training metric used to guide optimization, while accuracy is an evaluation metric used to assess the model's performance on new data. Both metrics are essential in

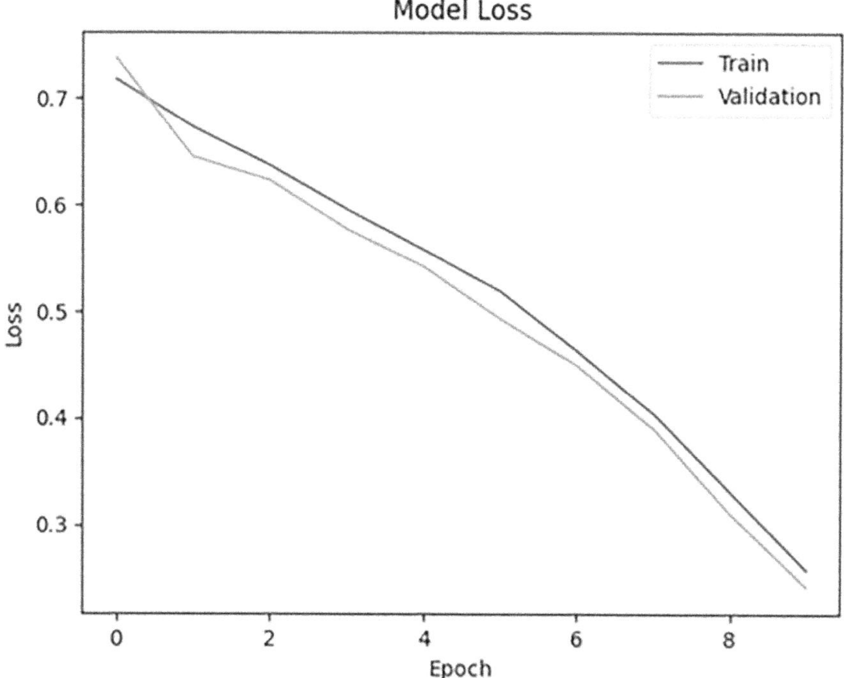

FIGURE 20.4 Model loss.

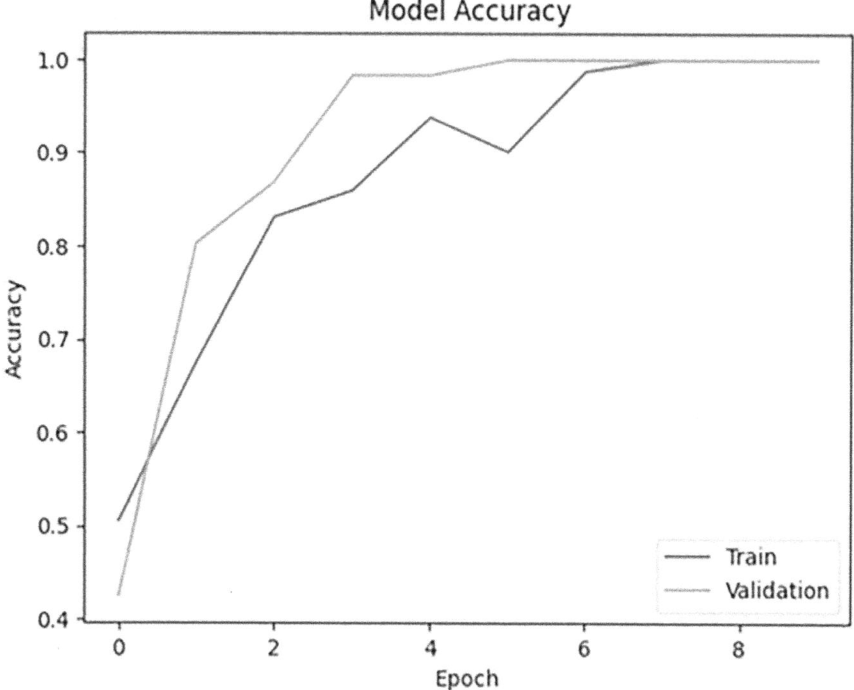

FIGURE 20.5 Model accuracy.

the machine learning workflow, but they serve different purposes. As a binary set model imbalanced outcome class, the F1 score is often used to balanced and predict performance in a single numerical value in terms of positives or negatives (Eq. 20.1):

$$F1 - Score = \frac{2 * precision * recall}{Precision + recall} \qquad 20.1$$

where *precision* measures the accuracy of true positive prediction, that is, the ratio of true positive predictions to the total positive predictions made by the model (Eq. 20.2).

$$Precision = \frac{TruePositive}{TruePositive + FalsePositive} \qquad 20.2$$

and *recall* is the ratio of correctly identified positive instances (true positives) from all the actual positive samples in the dataset. It is the ratio of true positive predictions and to the actual positive instances in the dataset (Eq. 20.3).

$$Recall = \frac{TruePositive}{TruePositive + FalseNegative} \qquad 20.3$$

Here the feature score shows (Figure 20.6) that the age highly affects the prediction of JE disease, with a value of 3.1385. The gender and blocks, 2.089 and 1.214, also have important features, while the month of detection, at 0.4583, is less important. The F1 score ranges from 0 to 1. One set of test data is used for testing the model and receives the probability of detection (Figure 20.7). The test is on block Sahjanwa, age of detection 1 to 5, "gender" mainly male, and month "April to October". The chance of infection is 0.845, which is near 1 and would show the person is affected.

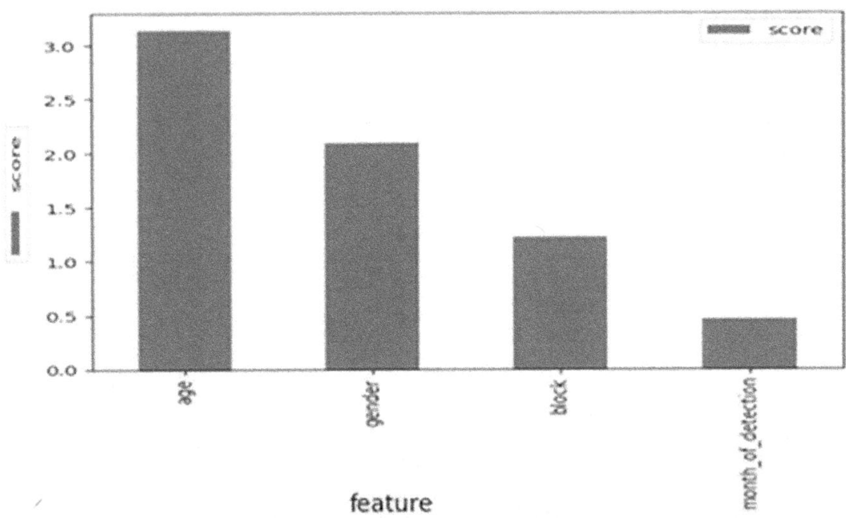

FIGURE 20.6 Feature score.

```
        block       age gender month_of_detection
0  SAHJANWA  1 to 5       M         April to Oct
   block  age  gender  month_of_detection
0     15    1       1                   0
1/1 [==============================] - 0s 17ms/step
[[0.845477]]
Probability / Chance  of Infection:  0.845477
The person is infected: 1
```

FIGURE 20.7 Test data: top of form.

20.4.4 Training and Validation Loss Curves

The validation curve balances the metric distribution between precision and recall and maintains values with poor generalization. It helps to distribute classes evenly and make decisions about threshold selection and model improvement.

$$Validate = \frac{TruePositive}{TruePositive + False\,Negative} \qquad 20.4$$

Here, validation loss has decreased greatly, along with training loss. Hence, the model is neither overfitted nor underfitted (Figure 20.8). It is a perfect fit model, providing decent accuracy, so we can see that the model is getting trained perfectly with each increasing epoch.

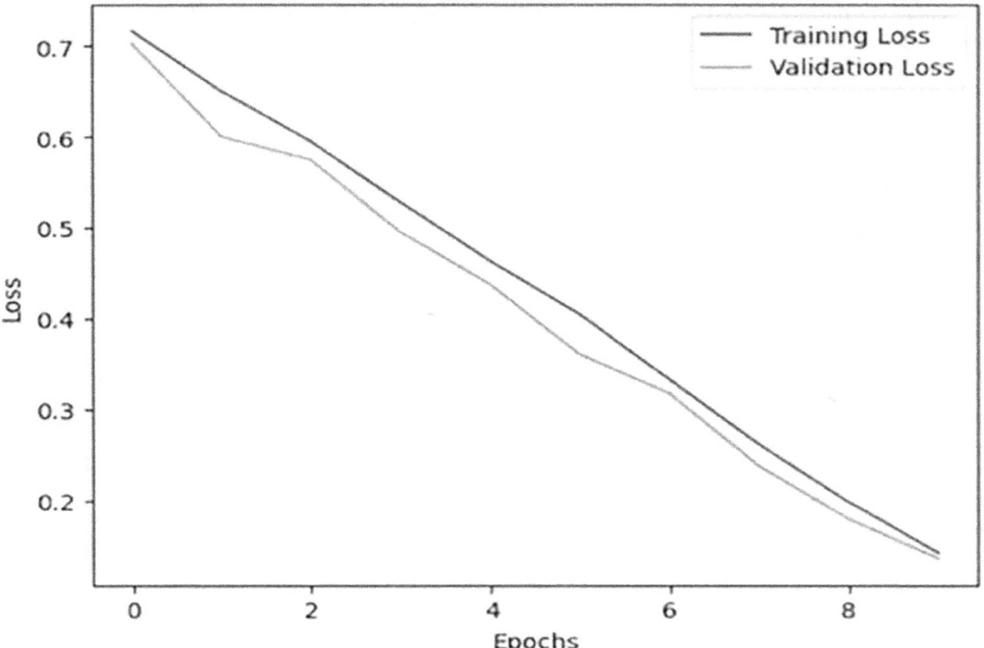

FIGURE 20.8 Training and validation loss.

20.5 CONCLUSION

In healthcare diagnosis and disease detection, machine learning algorithms are highly applicable. In the present work, Panda libraries help in performing and finding the best ML approaches for determining a disease with minimal lines of code. In the present study, different features of disease are predicted that are responsible for disease. Based on their performance, "age" corresponds to a high impact on disease detection with respect to "gender", "block", and "month of detection". This shows that in a very simple and optimal number of lines of code, we diagnosed which data features are high impact and how we can predict the disease in a particular area. The proposed model predicts the chance of occurrence of disease, and it also alerts the system to effective algorithms for numerous occurrences of disease in common populations. This model helps to predict the waiting time for affected persons so that additional healthcare practice can be involved and recommend an effective remedy in an appropriate manner. This prediction model helps doctors to make good decisions related to patient diagnoses, and according to that, good treatment will be given to the patient, which increases improvement in healthcare services.

Machine learning can be helpful in analyzing past hidden data and provide an interface with reference to a model with automated response and can create predictions for the future. The improvement in the performance of present models in future with health dataset features. More feature dataset should have more features. We could train the model and help to relate the feature to each other. It provides highly correlated features. This will make it easier to control disease occurrence and provide patient care.

REFERENCES

Ahsan, M. M., Gupta, K. D., Islam, M. M., Sen, S., Rahman, M., and Shakhawat Hossain, M. (2020). COVID-19 symptoms detection based on nasnetmobile with explainable AI using various imaging modalities. Mach. Learn. Knowl. Extr. 2, 490–504.

Anshik (2021). Predicting hospital readmission by analyzing patient HER records. In: AI for Healthcare with Keras and TensorFlow 2.0. Apress, Berkeley, CA. https://doi.org/10.1007/978-1-4842-7086-8_3.

Bista, M. B., and Shrestha, J. M. (2005). Epidemiological situation of Japanese encephalitis in Nepal. J. Nepal Med. Assoc. 44(158), 51–56.

Bunnel, E. J., Karlsen, W. A., Finkelman, B. R., and Shield, M. T. (2005). GIS in Human Health Studies, Essentials of Medical Geology. Elsevier, Amsterdam, 633–644.

Fischer, M., Hills, S., Staples, E., Johnson, B., Yaich, M., and Solomon, T. (2008). Japanese encephalitis prevention and control: advances, challenges, and new initiatives. In: Scheld, W. M., Hammer, S. M., Hughes, J. M., eds. Emerging Infections 8. ASM Press, Washington, DC, 93–124.

Grossman, R. A., Edelman, R., Chiewanich, P., Voodhikul, P., and Siriwan, C. (1973). Study of Japanese encephalitis virus in Chiangmai Valley, Thailand. II. Human clinical infections. Am. J. Epidemiol. 98(2): 121–132.

Kalluri, S., Gilruth, P., Rogers, D., and Szczur, M. (2007). Surveillance of arthropod vector-borne infectious diseases using remote sensing techniques: a review. PLoS Pathog. (3), 1361–1371.

Keiser, J., Maltese, M. F., Erlanger, T. E., Bos, R., Tanner, M., Singer, B. H., and Utzinger, J. (2005). Effect of irrigated rice agriculture on Japanese encephalitis, including challenges and opportunities for integrated vector management. Acta Trop. 95(1), 40–57.

Kononenko, I. (2001). Machine learning for medical diagnosis: history, state of the art and perspective. Artif. Intell. Med. 23(1), 89–109. doi:10.1016/S0933-3657(01)00077-X.

Massaro, A., Maritati, V., Savino, N., and Galiano, A. (2018). Neural networks for automated smart health platforms oriented on heart predictive diagnostic big data systems. In Proceedings of the 2018 AEIT International Annual Conference, Bari, 3–5 October.

Mitamura, T., Kitaoka, M., Mori, K., and Okuba, K. (1938). Isolation of the virus of Japanese epidemic encephalitis from mosquitoes caught in nature. Tokyo Iji Shinshi 62, 820–824.

Mitamura, T., Kitaoka, M., Watanabe, M., Okuba, K., Tenjin, S., Yamada, S., Mori, K., and Asada, J. (1936). Study on Japanese encephalitis virus. Animal experiments and mosquito transmission experiments. Kansai Iji 1, 260–261.

Mitchell, T. M. (1997). Machine Learning. McGraw-Hill, New York.

Mutheneni, R. S., Upadhyayula, M. S., and Natarajan, A. (2014). Prevalence of Japanese encephalitis and its modulation by weather variables. J. Public Health Epidemiol. 6(1), 52–59.

Peiris, J. S., Amerasinghe, F. P., Amerasinghe, P. H., Ratnayake, C. B., Karunaratne, S. H., and Tsai, T. F. (1992). Japanese encephalitis in Sri Lanka–The study of an epidemic: vector incrimination, porcine infection and human disease. Trans. R. Soc. Trop. Med. Hyg. 86: 307–313.

Powers, D. M.W. (2011). Evaluation: from precision, recall and F-measure to ROC, informedness, markedness & correlation. J. Mach. Learn. Technol. 2(1), 37–63.

Quest, D. (2022). Demystifying AI in Healthcare: historical perspectives and current considerations. www.physicianleaders.org/articles/demystifying-ai-healthcare-historical-perspectives-and-current-considerations.

Ramalingam, V., Dandapath, A., and Raja, M. K. (2018). Heart disease prediction using machine learning techniques: A survey. Int. J. Eng. Technol. 7(2), 684–687.

Sharma, L. (Ed.). (2020). Towards Smart World: *Homes to Cities Using Internet of Things* (1st ed.). Chapman and Hall/CRC. https://doi.org/10.1201/9781003056751

Sharma, L., & Garg, P.K. (Eds.). (2019). *From Visual Surveillance to Internet of Things: Technology and Applications* (1st ed.). Chapman and Hall/CRC. https://doi.org/10.1201/9780429297922

Shvets, A., Rakhlin, A., Kalinin, A. A., and Iglovikov, V. (2018). Automatic instrument segmentation in robot-assisted surgery using deep learning. https://arxiv.org/abs/1803.01207.

Solomon, T., Dung, N. M., Kneen, R., Gainsborough, M., Vaughn, D. W., and Khanh, V. T. (2000). Japanese encephalitis. J. Neurol. Neurosurg. Psychiatry 68, 405–415.

Stafford, I., Kellermann, M., Mossotto, E., Beattie, R., MacArthur, B., and Ennis, S. (2022). A systematic review of the applications of artificial intelligence and machine learning in autoimmune diseases. NPJ Digit. Med. 3, 1–11.

Thakkar, A., and Lohiya, R. (2021). Attack classification using feature selection techniques: a comparative study. J. Ambient Intell. Humaniz. Comput. 12(1), 1249–1266.

Tsai, T. F. (2000). New initiatives for the control of Japanese encephalitis by vaccination: minutes of a WHO/CVI Meeting, Bangkok, Thailand, 13–15 Oct. 1998. Vaccine. 18(Suppl 2), 1–25.

Van den Hurk, A. F., Ritchie, S. A., and Meckenzie, J. S. (2009). Ecological and geographical expansion of Japanese encephalitis virus. Annu. Rev. Entomol. 54, 17–35.

Verma, S., and Gupta, R. D. (2014). Spatial and temporal variation of Japanese encephalitis disease and detection of disease hotspots: a case study of Gorakhpur District, Uttar Pradesh, India. ISPRS Ann. Photogramm. Remote Sens. Spat. Inf. Sci. II-8.

World Health Organization. (2006). Japanese encephalitis surveillance standards. www.path.org/files/WHO_surveillance_standards_JE.pdf. Accessed 15 August 2014.

World Health Organization. (2007). Third bi-regional meeting on control of Japanese encephalitis. Meeting Report. World Health Organization, Ho Chi Minh City; Regional Office for the Western Pacific, Manila.

21 AI and Deep Learning
Applications in Healthcare

Rashmi Kandwal

21.1 INTRODUCTION

In the past decade, if someone were to pinpoint the most ubiquitous topic that has been discussed in healthcare, it's undoubtedly COVID-19. However, during those challenging times, a close second contender emerged, artificial intelligence (AI), accompanied by its power siblings machine learning (ML) and deep learning (DL). Technology experts refer to it as the foremost disruptive technology reshaping industries [1]. It has shown unparalleled potential, defying all prior expectations. While the concept of AI dates back to the 1950s, the past decade has witnessed leaps and bounds in ML and DL realms [2–4]. The generative and predictive powers of AI and its ability to detect patterns make it a phenomenon that is here to stay. Among the industries poised to be most disrupted by AI, healthcare is in the top few [5–7]. As Rebitzer et al. [8] note, "It has a potential to improve every aspect of healthcare". This potential comes primarily from the data-rich health industry and spans improving medical advice for patients and decreasing paperwork. While there are innumerable benefits of AI in the medical world, it also brings with it a set of ethical, legal, and privacy challenges, including concerns about data security and bias [9]. When it comes to the well-being of individuals, these are issues that cannot be simply ignored. As a result, any conversation regarding AI's role in healthcare requires a concurrent consideration of these critical challenges.

This chapter focuses on the scope and significance of these technological advancements in the healthcare domain. It then delves into a comprehensive exploration of several common applications of AI in the medical sphere, including but not limited to disease diagnosis, drug discovery, treatment options, remote monitoring and telehealth, and fraud detection. Through these applications, the chapter underscores the benefits of integrating DL, ML, and AI technology into healthcare practices and the challenges that come with it.

The chapter wraps up with a forward-looking discussion on the future trends and challenges in this dynamic landscape of AI-driven healthcare.

21.2 UNDERSTANDING AI, MACHINE LEARNING, AND DEEP LEARNING IN HEALTHCARE

Let's start with understanding what AI is. In simplistic terms, AI means computer systems that are similar to the human mind and capable of cognitive functions such as perceiving, reasoning, learning, interacting with an environment, and problem solving [1, 2]. To offer a more formal definition, the AI watch group at the European Commission's Science and Knowledge Services conducted an extensive analysis of 55 documents focusing on policy, research, and industry. They defined AI as follows:

> Artificial intelligence (AI) systems are software (and possibly also hardware) systems designed by humans that, given a complex goal, act in the physical or digital dimension by perceiving their environment through data acquisition, interpreting the collected structured or unstructured data, reasoning on

DOI: 10.1201/9781003451846-21

> the knowledge, or processing the information, derived from this data and deciding the best action(s) to take to achieve the given goal. AI systems can either use symbolic rules or learn a numeric model, and they can also adapt their behavior by analyzing how the environment is affected by their previous actions [10].
>
> AI's primary goal is to build an intelligent machine. The second goal is to find out about the nature of intelligence [11].

To discuss AI in healthcare, it is important to understand the distinction between generative AI and predictive AI. The recent attention fueled by entities like ChatGPT has been more about generative AI, which, though powerful, has limited use in medicine [7]. As the McKinsey report [2, 12] states, "Generative artificial intelligence (AI) describes algorithms (such as ChatGPT) that can be used to create new content, including audio, code, images, text, simulations, and videos". Predictive AI, as the name suggests, uses statistical, ML, and deep learning techniques to make predictions based on historical data and make informed future decisions [2, 12–15].

Applications of predictive AI discussed in this chapter draw from various AI sub-fields such as ML, DL, and neural networks. AI is the big umbrella encompassing the technology of ML and deep learning (Figure 21.1). ML, a subset of AI, refers to the study of algorithms that allow computer programs to automatically improve through experience, fostering optimization [2, 14, 16]. It further branches into supervised learning, unsupervised learning, reinforced learning, and deep learning [17]. DL, a subset of machine learning, automates most of the feature extraction piece of the process, requiring minimal user input, and boasts the ability to handle much larger and complex datasets, hence earning the moniker "scalable machine leaning" [1, 14, 17, 16]. Neural networks, on the other hand, are also subsets of machine learning and form the elementary bricks of deep learning. The areas of image processing and speech recognition in healthcare have significantly benefitted from neural deep learning [2, 16, 18]

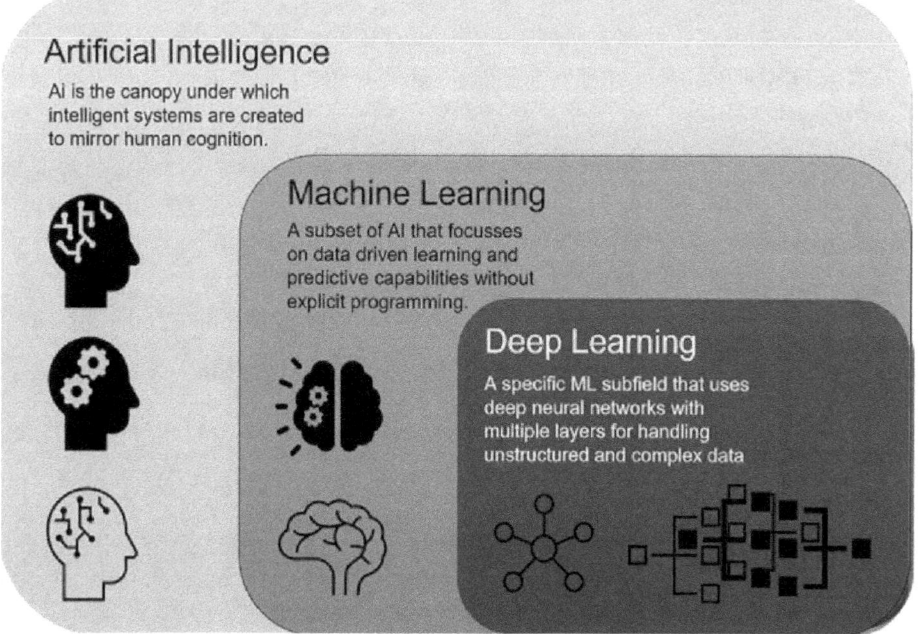

FIGURE 21.1 Relationship of AI, machine learning, and deep learning.

21.2.1 Scopes of Applying AI in Healthcare

The scope of AI and DL in healthcare is limitless and offers a wide array of benefits to various stakeholders, including providers, patients, payers, pharmaceuticals, the medical device industry, and hospital and health systems.

For healthcare providers, the technology holds the promise of enhancing patient outcomes, assisting physicians by collating patient and medical information from various sources, reducing diagnostics and therapeutic errors and improving overall patient care, informing social determinants of health (SDOH) studies, and mitigating health disparities. Patients, on the other hand, benefit from increased healthcare efficiency, cost savings, personalized treatment plans, better access to services like telemedicine, and more precise medical image analysis leading to more accurate diagnoses [7, 16–21]. In the pharmaceutical industry, AI revolutionizes both preclinical studies and clinical trials, expediting and streamlining drug development pipelines, resulting in shorter timeframes and cost reductions [22, 23]. Payers leverage AI for fraud detection, machine-assisted claims review, reducing administrative burdens, and safeguarding electronic health records (EHRs) against data breaches, potentially saving billions [21]. Health systems find advantages in managing administrative and operational costs, achieving greater efficiencies, and enhancing patient outcomes, including improved hospital census data, optimized operating room efficiency, and appointment scheduling improvements [12, 24, 25]. For device manufacturers, the potential lies in the realm of wearables that have already harnessed the power of AI. These wearable health devices enable continuous monitoring of the important body vitals [26, 27]. Their applications extend to both self-monitoring by individuals and clinical use in medical settings. Figure 21.2, adopted from Kalis, Collier, and Fu [21], depicts the top ten applications in healthcare ranked on the likelihood of their adoption and the potential in annual savings. It estimates up to $150 billion in annual savings for U.S. healthcare by 2026 [21]

This section elaborates on the many use cases and applications of AI and DL in healthcare. We will individually dive into areas of disease diagnosis and prediction, drug discovery, healthcare operations, fraud detection, remote monitoring, and public health.

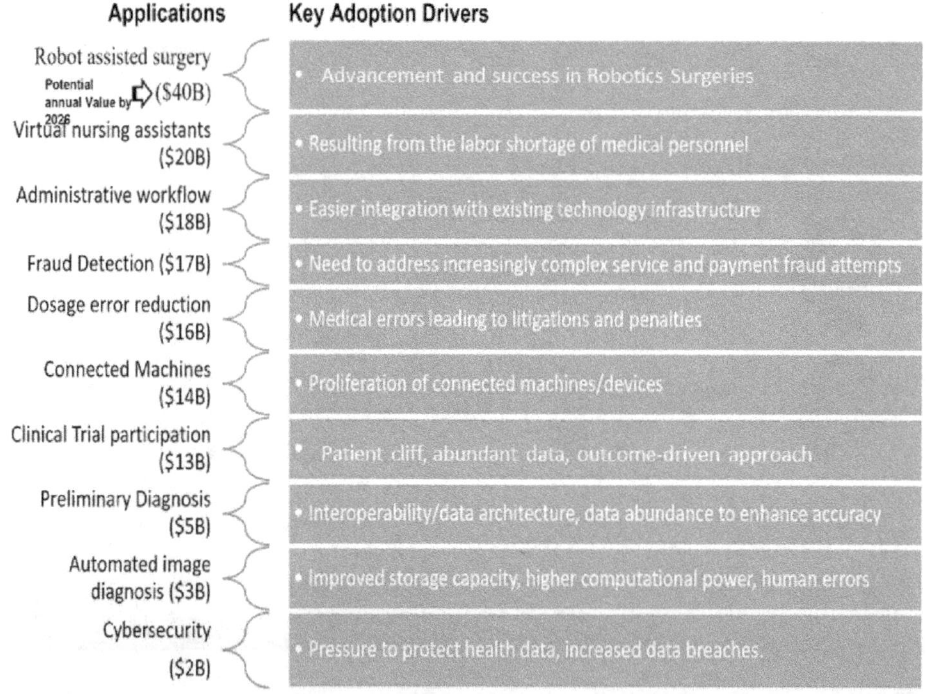

FIGURE 21.2 Applications of AI and DL in healthcare.

- **Drug development and discovery**
  As stated, in the pharmaceutical industry, AI revolutionizes both preclinical studies and clinical trials, expediting and streamlining drug development pipelines by analyzing massive datasets and predicting potential drug candidates. DL is one of the most extensively utilized methods in these applications. DL algorithms are used for various stages of drug development and discovery, including drug-target interactions, drug–drug similarity interactions, drug sensitivity and responsiveness, and drug side effect predictions. Several DL algorithms are used to accelerate these processes in the drug design pipeline and improve its efficiency. Some notable ones are convolutional neural networks (CNNs), recurrent neural networks (RNNs) long short-term memory (LSTM) network autoencoders, graph neural networks (GNNs), and transformer models. A combination of these techniques has resulted in shorter timeframes of new drug development and reduced costs to bring new drugs to the market and optimize clinical trial designs [22, 23, 28, 29].
- **Robotic surgery**
  According to an HBR article [21], robot-assisted-surgery is among the top ten applications of AI in healthcare. AI not only helps in guiding the surgeon's instrument in real-time surgery but also uses data from past surgeries to inform new surgical techniques. DL techniques in robotic surgery have been used for workflow analysis, for example, collecting data from predicting surgical tool usage and determining surgery duration. In future it is expected that DL methods will be trained to predict estimated survival after certain life-threatening surgeries or predict secondary side effects like incisional hernia post-surgery [30–33].
- **Medical image analysis**
  Medical images like X-rays, MRIs, CT scans, and pathology slides are prone to human errors. DL models, such as CNNs, RNNs, LSTM networks, U-Net, ResNets, and 3D convolutional neural networks excel at interpreting such data. These models, trained on large amounts of previously analyzed scans and reports by doctors, help clinicians and radiologists detect anomalies and tumors and other conditions with a high degree of accuracy [21, 28, 30, 34]. Radiomics is another emerging field within medical imaging that aims to convert medical images into high-dimensional data that can then be analyzed using ML and DL techniques. Radiomics has shown promise in earlier detection and diagnosis of diseases like cancer and in predicting disease outcomes and prognosis [35].
- **Disease diagnosis and prediction**
  AI's ability to accurately analyze medical images helps in diagnosing diseases like diabetic retinopathy, cancer, and pulmonary and skin diseases with a high degree of accuracy. DL models can predict cardiovascular diseases, rare diseases, and neurodegenerative diseases by analyzing a combination of medical records, genetic data, scans, and clinical symptoms. AI models can also analyze genomic data to identify genetic markers and predict potential disease risks. Timely interventions designed for such cases improve patient outcomes [21, 34].
- **Clinical decision support systems**
  AI-powered decision tools feeding on patient data, medical records, and the latest medical advancements can help providers curate targeted treatment plans and diagnostic tests. This approach enhances treatment effectiveness and minimizes adverse effects. They can also predict future outcomes based on genetics and lifestyle choices. These systems are often powered with Chatbots and virtual assistants that can provide patients support on medication reminders, personalized treatment advice, and education and answer health-related queries [21, 24, 25, 28, 34, 36]
- **Healthcare operations and management**
  Hospitals and health systems significantly benefit from AI-powered systems in managing administrative and operational costs, enhancing efficiency and patient outcomes.

Hospital and clinic operations are supported through efficient staff scheduling, resource allocation, and a streamlined patient flow. Additionally, hospitals benefit from the predictive analytics that help in reducing readmission rates and timely disease diagnosis, and predictions help improve patient outcomes [24, 25, 28, 30, 34]. Predictive analytics can also effectively assess the demand and supply of critical health equipment and supplies [37].

- **Remote monitoring and telehealth**
  The infinite potential of sensor-enabled smartphones and wearables in healthcare market is already underway. These wearable health devices enable continuous monitoring of vital health data like blood pressure, oxygen level, heart rate, and blood glucose levels, allowing the patients to monitor their health and updating the providers with real-time data, thus enabling remote patient care [26, 27]. On the other hand, virtual health assistants and AI-enabled chatbots provide continuous and personalized access to care by answering health-related queries and giving medication reminders and personalized lifestyle plans. Telehealth services also address access issues, especially in remote or underserved areas. AI-driven chatbots and apps are also being used to provide mental health support, offering therapy, monitoring, and crisis intervention [26, 27, 30, 34].
- **Integration with electronic health records**
  DL models, such as RNNs and LSTMs in combination with natural language processing (NLP), can be applied to EHRs that encompass structured elements like patient demographics, diagnosis, medications, and lab tests and unstructured elements like free-text clinical notes. Utilizing NLP algorithms, valuable information can be extracted from unstructured clinical notes, making it easier for healthcare providers to access and utilize patient data. The insights from EHRs help in identifying disease patterns, crafting personalized patient plans, predicting outbreaks, and improving hospital operations and management [34, 38].
- **Fraud detection and claims processing**
  AI algorithms can comb through massive claims datasets and use pattern detection techniques to identify irregular patterns and identify data anomalies that might indicate fraudulent activities. These might include anomalies like overbilling for certain procedures or unnecessary procedures performed. In claims processing, AI algorithms can automate the data entry process, thus speeding up the claims processing cycle, reducing human error, and lowering costs by reducing administrative burdens [21, 24].

21.2.2 Real-Time Case Studies

The industry is witnessing a high number of use cases of successful implementation of AI and deep learning in healthcare [28, 30]. For instance, a collaborative effort involving researchers from Google, Stanford Medicine, University of Chicago, and UC San Francisco used deep learning to address some challenging issues that hospitals face on a routine basis. The team combined data across two hospitals containing 46 billion data points, including free text clinical notes from more than 216,000 EHRs. The model that they developed achieved high accuracy in predicting inpatient mortality, unexpected readmissions, and prolonged length of stay [28, 36, 38]. Though the researchers admitted to some limitations in the study, it showcases the potential of deep learning in transforming healthcare delivery.

In another example, the US-based Mayo Clinic, ranked as one of the best hospitals in the world, is already working on almost 184 predictive AI models, including both clinical and research stages. At the Mayo Clinic, applications of AI are already in practice in many diagnostic procedures and process management. Remote diagnostics, EHR integration, disease prediction, and radiology labs are other areas harnessing AI technology in this large health system. As part of a streamlined approach to save time for healthcare providers, the institution employs generative AI to summarize clinical visits, leverage speech and text analytics to improve the summaries, and automate the creation of message drafts for patient's benefit [12, 36, 39].

In a 2017 study published in *Nature* [40], a group of scientists from Stanford University developed a deep learning algorithm that studied skin cancer from 130,000 images of skin lesions that represented over 2,000 different skin diseases and was tested against 21 board-certified dermatologists. The algorithm matched the performance of the skin specialists.

Meanwhile, Da Vinci, a surgical robot, has become a widely adopted robotic modality since its FDA approval in the US in 2011. It aids surgeons by enhancing precision, facilitating access to hard-to reach anatomical areas, and mitigating hand tremors during intricate surgical processes [32].

These use cases highlight the potential of deep learning and AI in healthcare to enhance efficiency, reduce costs, and improve outcomes.

21.3 CHALLENGES AND OPPORTUNITIES

The benefits of AI and deep learning in healthcare are everywhere. We have already discussed its potential in reducing costs and improving patient outcomes, generating widespread optimism. However, it is imperative to delve into the accompanying challenges that come with it. Companies and hospitals are in a rush to deploy AI solutions, yet we must pause to contemplate the wisdom in Ginni Rometty's words:

> Be very careful right now because it's really your brand and trust that are at stake, what we have on our hands is not a technology issue. It's going to be a trust and people issue, particularly as we tackle problems of importance and personal impact. I'm completely convinced of it.

AI adoption fundamentally is a people issue, with data privacy and security translating into matters of trust. Maintaining data privacy and ensuing compliance with regulations is paramount. The data volume needed to train models, especially in the fields of new drug discovery, disease prediction, and image analysis, brings forth a data storage challenge. Data quality stemming from unstructured, incomplete, and non-standardized data adds another layer of complexity to these challenges [25, 34, 41]. Interoperability, the ability of different systems, applications, and devices to exchange information and seamlessly work together, is a big challenge in technology applications. In healthcare where data originates from multiple sources, this challenge is amplified, especially given the critical importance of patient data security [9, 25, 34, 36].

Outside of the data realm, there are challenges stemming from the socioeconomic implications of people losing their jobs and technology adoption in the workforce needing new education and training. Existing disparities in healthcare might be exacerbated in the absence of AI technology being readily available to everyone. Last, there are challenges of ethical dilemmas, assigning responsibility when AI makes a mistake [9, 41].

All these challenges present several opportunities for all stakeholders in healthcare to collaborate and ensure the seamless and regulated integration of deep learning in healthcare in the future. This includes developing improved ethical frameworks and guidelines for responsible AI use driving transparency, fairness, and accountability. Relevant data regulations and guidelines are needed to safeguard patient rights [41]. As Tesla and SpaceX founder Elon Musk aptly stated: "I'm increasingly inclined to think that there should be some regulatory oversight, maybe at the national and international level, just to make sure that we don't do something very foolish. I mean with the artificial intelligence we are summoning the demon" [9].

21.4 FUTURE TRENDS

There is no doubt that deep learning in healthcare will play a vital role in providing the best-quality care to consumers. The trends that have already started, such as AI-assisted surgery, remote monitoring, AI-powered genomics, and personalized medicine will get more sophisticated as the models improve with the growing amount of data getting integrated in the algorithms [30–32]. As suggested by Miotto et al. [34], deep learning has the potential to lead to a new healthcare system with unified patient representation, including EHRs, genomics, environmental factors, wearables, and social interactions to create a comprehensive individual health profile. Deep learning models can then be integrated into a hospital's EHR system and can be continuously updated with shifts in the patient population. With everyone taking note, strong investment from major players in the industry, and governments getting involved, it is believed that in the future, AI will have more transparency and regulatory frameworks to ensure ethical AI use. The debate is already on [28, 41, 42].

21.5 CONCLUSION

We talked about the transformative potential of AI in healthcare, and we explored the numerous applications of AI and deep learning in healthcare—including disease and drug discovery, precision medicine, fraud detection, and electronic health records. From the many examples we saw of machine learning's potential in enhancing patient outcomes and improving operations for healthcare delivery, we also saw the potential of deep learning in disrupting medical imaging and predictive analytics. We talked about the challenges that come with data and the opportunities that these challenges present.

In this rapidly evolving field, its imperative that all healthcare stakeholders have a seat at the table and everyone's voice is heard. We also need to ensure that we don't lose the focus on the patient, with ethics and regulations guiding the path forward to get to a healthcare system empowered by AI and deep learning technology that is not only innovative but also reliable and robust.

REFERENCES

1. Press Release, (2023) Gartner survey finds CRO's cite AI as the top disruptive technology impacting industries. www.gartner.com/en/newsroom/press-releases/2023-05-17-gartner-survey-finds-ceos-cite-ai-as-the-top-disruptive-technology-impacting-industries
2. What is AI?, (2023) McKinsey and Company. www.mckinsey.com/featured-insights/mckinsey-explainers/what-is-ai
3. Wang, P., (2007) What do you mean by 'AI'? Temple University. https://linas.org/mirrors/nars.wang.googlepages.com/2007.06.27/wang.AI_Definitions.pdf
4. McCarthy, J., (2007) What is Artificial Intelligence? Stanford University. https://www-formal.stanford.edu/jmc/whatisai.pdf
5. Chowdhury, M., (2021) 7 business industries affected by AI disruption, Analytics Insight. www.analyticsinsight.net/7-business-industries-affected-by-ai-disruption/
6. Smith Goodson, P., (2023) IBM demonstrates groundbreaking Artificial Intelligence research using foundational models and generative AI, Forbes. www.forbes.com/sites/moorinsights/2023/02/13/ibm-demonstrates-groundbreaking-artificial-intelligence-research-using-foundational-models-and-generative-ai/?sh=be6ef62750de
7. Tyler, D., and Mandeep, M., (2023) AI use in healthcare a growing opportunity, Grant Thornton. www.grantthornton.com/insights/articles/health-care/2023/ai-use-in-healthcare-a-growing-opportunity
8. Rebitzer, J. B., and Rebitzer R. S., (2023) AI adoption in US health care won't be easy, Harvard Business Review. https://hbr.org/2023/09/ai-adoption-in-u-s-health-care-wont-be-easy
9. Health AI for good rather than evil? The need for a new regulatory framework for AI based medical devices. https://ideas.dickinsonlaw.psu.edu/cgi/viewcontent.cgi?article=1286&context=fac-works
10. Samoili, S., López, C. M., Gómez, E., De Prato, G., Martínez-Plumed, F., and Delipetrev, B., (2020) AI watch. Defining Artificial Intelligence. Towards an operational definition and taxonomy of Artificial Intelligence, EUR 30117 EN, Publications Office of the European Union, Luxembourg, doi: 10.2760/382730, JRC118163. https://eprints.ugd.edu.mk/28047/1/3.%20jrc118163_ai_watch._defining_artificial_intelligence_1.pdf
11. Schank, R., (1987) What is AI anyway? AI Magazine. https://ojs.aaai.org/aimagazine/index.php/aimagazine/article/view/623
12. Bruce Giles, (2023) Predictive or generative AI: which will change healthcare the most? Becker's Hospital Review. www.beckershospitalreview.com/innovation/predictive-or-generative-ai-which-will-change-healthcare-the-most.html

13. Rajpurkar, P., Chen, E., Banerjee, O., and Topol, E. J., (2022) AI in health and medicine. Nature Medicine 28, 31–38. https://doi.org/10.1038/s41591-021-01614-0
14. Bine, S. A., (2018) Artificial Intelligence, machine learning, deep learning and cognitive computing: what do these terms mean and how will they impact health care? The Journal of Arthroplasty 33(8), 2358–2361. www.sciencedirect.com/science/article/abs/pii/S0883540318302158
15. de Hond, A. A. H., Leeuwenberg, A. M., Hooft, L., et al. (2022) Guidelines and quality criteria for artificial intelligence-based prediction models in healthcare: a scoping review. npj Digital Medicine 5(2). https://doi.org/10.1038/s41746-021-00549; www.nature.com/articles/s41746-021-00549-7
16. www.ibm.com/blog/ai-vs-machine-learning-vs-deep-learning-vs-neural-networks/
17. www.ncbi.nlm.nih.gov/pmc/articles/PMC8285156/
18. https://klab.tch.harvard.edu/academia/classes/BAI/pdfs/intro-deep-learning.pdf
19. https://svn.bmj.com/content/svnbmj/2/4/230.full.pdf
20. https://healthitanalytics.com/news/using-sdoh-data-to-enhance-artificial-intelligence-outcomes#:~:text=By%20connecting%20individuals%20to%20proper%20community%20resources%2C%20providers, while%20improving%20risk%20identification%20and%20eliminating%20health%20disparities
21. 10 promising AI applications in healthcare. https://hbr.org/2018/05/10-promising-ai-applications-in-health-care
22. Lavecchia, A., (2019) Deep learning in drug discovery: opportunities, challenges and future prospects. Drug Discovery Today 24(10), 2017–2032.
23. Zhang, L., Tan, J., Han, D., and Zhu, H. (2017) From machine learning to deep learning: progress in machine intelligence for rational drug discovery. Drug Discovery Today 22(11), 1680–1685.
24. How predictive analytics and generative AI can transform hospital operations. www.beckershospitalreview.com/strategy/how-predictive-analytics-and-generative-ai-can-transform-hospital-operations.html
25. Inside Google's plans to fix healthcare with Generative AI (2023) www.forbes.com/sites/katiejennings/2023/08/29/google-healthcare-generative-ai/?sh=1c912b37eab9
26. Features and usability assessment of a patient centered mobile application (HeartMapp) for self-management of heart failure. www.sciencedirect.com/science/article/abs/pii/S0897189716300520
27. Wearable health devices—vital sign monitoring systems and technologies. www.mdpi.com/1424-8220/18/8/2414
28. What is deep learning and how will it change healthcare. https://healthitanalytics.com/features/what-is-deep-learning-and-how-will-it-change-healthcare
29. www.ncbi.nlm.nih.gov/pmc/articles/PMC9669545/
30. 10 real-world examples of AI in healthcare. www.philips.com/a-w/about/news/archive/features/2022/20221124-10-real-world-examples-of-ai-in-healthcare.html
31. Phil, B., (2018) How AI-assisted surgery is improving surgical outcomes, Robotics Business Review. www.roboticsbusinessreview.com/health-medical/ai-assisted-surgery-improves-patient-outcomes/
32. Emerging surgical robotic technology: a progression toward microbots. https://ales.amegroups.org/article/view/5499/html
33. www.ncbi.nlm.nih.gov/pmc/articles/PMC7768095/
34. Deep learning for healthcare: review, opportunities and challenges. www.ncbi.nlm.nih.gov/pmc/articles/PMC6455466/
35. www.frontiersin.org/journals/oncology/articles/10.3389/fonc.2022.773840/full
36. Speech recognition for medical conversations. https://arxiv.org/pdf/1711.07274.pdf
37. www.technologyreview.com/2022/03/09/1046976/ai-is-helping-treat-healthcare-as-if-its-a-supply-chain-problem/
38. Scalable and accurate deep learning with electronic health records. www.nature.com/articles/s41746-018-0029-1
39. AI based innovations at Mayo Clinic. https://sloanreview.mit.edu/article/ai-based-innovations-at-mayo-clinic/
40. https://news.stanford.edu/2017/01/25/artificial-intelligence-used-identify-skin-cancer/
41. Real world application, challenges and implication of artificial intelligence in healthcare: as essay. www.ncbi.nlm.nih.gov/pmc/articles/PMC9557803/#ref32
42. Former IBM CEO Rometty says AI focus should be on people and building trust, (2023) Goldman Sachs. www.goldmansachs.com/intelligence/pages/former-ibm-ceo-rometty-says-ai-focus-should-be-on-people-and-building-trust.html

Index

N

O

P

Q

R

S

T

U

V

W

For Product Safety Concerns and Information please contact our EU
representative GPSR@taylorandfrancis.com
Taylor & Francis Verlag GmbH, Kaufingerstraße 24, 80331 München, Germany

www.ingramcontent.com/pod-product-compliance
Lightning Source LLC
LaVergne TN
LVHW081315110826
845149LV00006B/1511